PSYCHOBIOLOGY OF SUICIDAL BEHAVIOR

ANNOUNCING OF THE NEW YORK ACADEMY OF SCIENCES
Volume 487

PSYCHOBIOLOGY OF SUICIDAL BEHAVIOR

Edited by J. John Mann and Michael Stanley

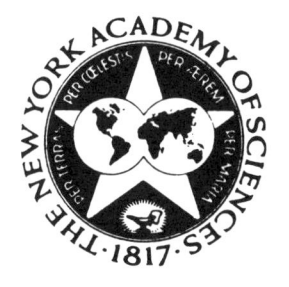

The New York Academy of Sciences
New York, New York
1986

Copyright © 1986 by The New York Academy of Sciences. All rights reserved. Under the provisions of the United States Copyright Act of 1976, individual readers of the Annals are permitted to make fair use of the material in them for teaching or research. Permission is granted to quote from the Annals provided that the customary acknowledgment is made of the source. Material in the Annals may be republished only by permission of The Academy. Address inquiries to the Executive Editor of The New York Academy of Sciences.

Copying fees. For each copy of an article made beyond the free copying permitted under Section 107 or 108 of the 1976 Copyright Act, a fee should be paid through the Copyright Clearance Center, 21 Congress Street, Salem, MA 01970. For articles more than 3 pages, the copying fee is $1.75.

Library of Congress Cataloging-in-Publication Data

Psychobiology of suicidal behavior.

(Annals of the New York Academy of Sciences, ISSN 0077-8923 ; v. 487)
Proceedings of a conference held Sept. 18-20, in New York, N.Y., and sponsored by the New York Academy of Sciences and the National Institute of Mental Health.
Includes bibliographies and index.
 1. Suicide—Physiological aspects—Congresses.
2. Psychobiology—Congresses. 3. Neuropsychiatry—Congresses. I. Mann, J. John (Joseph John) II. Stanley, Michael. III. New York Academy of Sciences. IV. National Institute of Mental Health (U.S.) V. Series. [DNLM: 1. Suicide—congresses. 2. Suicide—psychology—congresses. W1 AN626YL v.487/HV 6545 P974 1985]
 Q11.N5 vol. 487   500 s   87-1640
 [RC569]   [616.85'8445]
 ISBN 0-89766-369-1
 ISBN 0-89766-370-5 (pbk.)

PCP
Printed in the United States of America
ISBN 0-89766-369-1 (Cloth)
ISBN 0-89766-370-5 (Paper)
ISSN 0077-8923

ANNALS OF THE NEW YORK ACADEMY OF SCIENCES

Volume 487
December 31, 1986

PSYCHOBIOLOGY OF SUICIDAL BEHAVIOR[a]

Editors and Conference Organizers
J. JOHN MANN and MICHAEL STANLEY

CONTENTS

Preface. *By* J. JOHN MANN and MICHAEL STANLEY ix

Part I. Epidemiology, Ethical, Assessment, and Descriptive Studies of Suicide and Suicidal Behavior

Methodological Strategies in Suicide. *By* LEE N. ROBINS and PAMELA A. KULBOK 1

Suidical People: One Population or Two? *By* MARSHA M. LINEHAN 16

Statistical Approaches to Suicidal Risk Factor Analysis. *By* JACOB COHEN 34

Ethical Considerations in Biological Research on Suicide. *By* BARBARA STANLEY 42

Conceptualizing a Serotonin Trait: A Behavioral Dimension of Constraint. *By* RICHARD A. DEPUE and MICHELE R. SPOONT 47

Part II. Risk Factors and Psychosocial Correlates of Suicide

Early Family Influences on Suicidal Behavior. *By* KENNETH S. ADAM 63

Psychosocial Factors and Suicidal Behavior: Life Events, Early Loss, and Personality. *By* CHRISTINE K. CROSS and ROBERT M. A. HIRSCHFELD 77

Hopelessness as a Predictor of Eventual Suicide. *By* AARON T. BECK 90

[a]This volume is the result of a conference entitled Psychobiology of Suicidal Behavior held from September 18 to September 20, 1985 in New York, N.Y., sponsored by The New York Academy of Sciences and by the National Institute of Mental Health through Public Health Service Grant 1 R13 MH40612-01.

Genetics of Suicide. *By* ALEC ROY 97

Prospective Studies of Suicide and Mortality in Psychiatric Patients. *By* DONALD W. BLACK and GEORGE WINOKUR 106

Part III. Postmortem Neurochemical Studies of Suicide and Depression

Postmortem Monoamine Receptor and Enzyme Studies in Suicide. *By* J. JOHN MANN, P. ANNE MCBRIDE, and MICHAEL STANLEY 114

Serotonin and Serotonergic Receptors in Suicide. *By* MICHAEL STANLEY, J. JOHN MANN, and LEE S. COHEN 122

Postmortem Neurochemical Studies in Depression. *By* I. N. FERRIER, I. G. MCKEITH, A. J. CROSS, E. K. PERRY, J. M. CANDY, and R. H. PERRY....................................... 128

Muscarinic Receptor Density in Skin Fibroblasts and Autopsied Brain Tissue in Affective Disorder. *By* J. CHRISTIAN GILLIN, JOHN R. KELSOE, JR., CHARLES A. KAUFMAN, JOEL E. KLEINMAN, S. CRAIG RISCH, and DAVID S. JANOWSKY........ 143

The Serotonin Hypothesis of (Auto)Agression: Critical Appraisal of the Evidence. *By* H. M. VAN PRAAG, R. PLUTCHIK, and H. CONTE 150

Part IV. Suicide Attempts and Psychobiological Studies *In Vivo*

Serotonergic Function and Suicidal Behavior in Personality Disorders. *By* LIL TRÄSKMAN-BENDZ, MARIE ÅSBERG, and DAISY SCHALLING 168

Cerebrospinal Fluid Correlates of Suicide Attempts and Aggression. *By* GERALD L. BROWN and FREDERICK K. GOODWIN 175

Suicide and Aggression in Schizophrenia: Neurobiologic Correlates. *By* DAVID PICKAR, ALEC ROY, ALAN BREIER, ALLEN DORAN, OWEN WOLKOWITZ, JEAN COLISON, and HANS AGREN 189

Cerebrospinal Fluid Studies of Bipolar Patients with and without a History of Suicide Attempts. *By* WADE H. BERRETTINI, JOHN I. NURNBERGER, JR., WILLIAM NARROW, SUSAN SIMMONS-ALLING, and ELLIOT S. GERSHON 197

Indices of Serotonin and Glucose Metabolism in Violent Offenders, Arsonists, and Alcoholics. *By* ALEC ROY, MATTI VIRKKUNEN, SALLY GUTHRIE, and MARKKU LINNOILA 202

Aminergic Studies and Cerebrospinal Fluid Cations in Suicide. *By* CSABA M. BANKI, MIHÁLY ARATÓ, and CLINTON D. KILTS... 221

Studies of Amine Metabolites in Depressed Patients: Relationship to Suicidal Behavior. *By* STEVEN K. SECUNDA, CHRISTINE K. CROSS, STEPHEN KOSLOW, MARTIN M. KATZ, JAMES H. KOCSIS, and JAMES W. MAAS....................................... 231

Cerebrospinal Fluid Studies in Suicide: An Overview. *By* MARIE
ÅSBERG, PETER NORDSTRÖM, and LIL TRÄSKMAN-BENDZ..... 243

Part V. Neuroendocrine and Platelet Studies and Suicidal Behavior

Neuroendocrine Studies in Depression: Relationship to Suicidal
Behavior. *By* JAMES H. KOCSIS, SARA KENNEDY, RICHARD P.
BROWN, J. JOHN MANN, and BARBARA MASON 256

Hypothalamic-Pituitary-Adrenal Axis and Suicide. *By* MIHÁLY
ARATÓ, CSABA M. BANKI, CHARLES B. NEMEROFF, and
GARTH BISSETTE 263

Platelet Markers of Suicidality. *By* H. Y. MELTZER and R. C.
ARORA... 271

Part VI. Suicidal Behavior in Major Psychiatric Syndromes: Descriptive and Management Issues

Personality and Suicide. *By* ALLEN FRANCIS, MINNA FYER, and
JOHN CLARKIN... 281

Suicide in Schizophrenia. *By* CELESTE A. JOHNS, MICHAEL
STANLEY, and BARBARA STANLEY............................. 294

Suicide and Bipolar Disorders. *By* KAY REDFIELD JAMISON......... 301

Suicide and Alcoholism. *By* RICHARD J. FRANCES, JOHN
FRANKLIN, and DANIEL K. FLAVIN 316

Generalizable Treatment Strategies for Suicidal Behavior. *By* SUSAN
J. BLUMENTHAL and DAVID J. KUPFER........................ 327

Part VII. Current Formulations and Future Directions

Suicide Prevention: Current Efficacy and Future Promise. *By*
CYNTHIA R. PFEFFER... 341

Suicide, Aggression, and Depression: A Theoretical Framework for
Future Research. *By* FREDERICK K. GOODWIN 351

Index of Contributors.. 357

Major funding for this conference was provided by:
- THE NATIONAL INSTITUTE OF MENTAL HEALTH

Financial assistance was received from:
- BRISTOL-MYERS COMPANY
- HOECHST-ROUSSEL PHARMACEUTICALS INC.
- LEDERLE LABORATORIES
- ELI LILLY AND COMPANY
- NATIONAL INSTITUTE OF MENTAL HEALTH—NIH
- A. H. ROBINS COMPANY
- ROCHE LABORATORIES/DIVISION OF AMERICAN CYANAMID COMPANY
- SANDOZ RESEARCH INSTITUTE/SANDOZ, INC.
- SCHERING-PLOUGH CORPORATION
- SQUIBB CORPORATION
- THE UPJOHN COMPANY

The New York Academy of Sciences believes that it has a responsibility to provide an open forum for discussion of scientific questions. The positions taken by the participants in the reported conferences are their own and not necessarily those of The Academy. The Academy has no intent to influence legislation by providing such forums.

Preface

J. JOHN MANN[a] AND MICHAEL STANLEY[b]

[a] Laboratory of Psychopharmacology
Department of Psychiatry
Cornell University Medical College
1300 York Avenue
New York, New York 10021

[b] Departments of Psychiatry and Pharmacology
Columbia University and
New York State Psychiatric Institute
722 West 168th Street
New York, New York 10032

Approximately 25,000-30,000 Americans die by suicide each year. The rate of suicide among people under the age of 40 years has doubled in the last 25 years. Suicide was once assumed to be a component of largely depressive disorders. Today it is a recognized component of many nondepressive psychiatric syndromes. This has led to reformulation of the factors contributing to suicide. It is now regarded as the end point of some combination of genetic, psychobiological, psychosocial, and drug-related factors.

A multidisciplinary approach is required to understand the interplay of these factors. To meet this challenge, this volume brings together social scientists, epidemiologists, psychiatrists, psychologists, statisticians, and geneticists from the United States and overseas. An interactive model of suicide evolves from these contributions that will facilitate hypothesis generation, design of experiments, and communications between scientific disciplines. This volume is unique in highlighting neurobiological correlates of suicidal behavior and thereby has the dual goal of, firstly, complementing the information from psychosocial risk factors in the assessment of suicidality; and secondly, the data presented suggest immediately feasible psychopharmacological treatment programs that target the suicidal behavior directly. Improved detection of at-risk individuals will lead to contact with skilled professionals who can diagnose and treat the underlying psychiatric disorders that also contribute to suicide risk. Finally and most importantly, we hope that informed public opinion will divert resources sufficient to initiate and sustain the research and treatment advances that can grow out of these ideas.

Methodological Strategies in Suicide[a]

LEE N. ROBINS AND PAMELA A. KULBOK

Department of Psychiatry
Washington University School of Medicine
4940 Audubon Avenue
St. Louis, Missouri 63110

INTRODUCTION

This paper is concerned with methods employed in suicide research. Its purpose is to assess the contribution of various strategies in the search for understanding of suicide behavior and to recommend useful approaches for future research.

While methodological strategies used in suicide research include the basic nonexperimental research designs of retrospective case-control studies and prospective studies, because suicide is recorded as a cause of death on the death certificate required by law, there is also the opportunity for ecological analyses across total populations, an option available for no other event of psychiatric interest except perhaps mental retardation so severe as to exempt children from school attendance. From death certificates come aggregate data such as national and regional suicide rates. Analytical approaches in the study of aggregate data include the classic epidemiological designs such as ecologic comparison studies, time trend analyses, and natural experiments. With the advent of modern computer technology, it becomes possible also to link suicide records to other official records and to use the demographic characteristics of suicides found on death certificates to look in more detail at their special characteristics.

ECOLOGIC ANALYSIS

Patterns of Suicide Behavior

Ecologic studies compare suicide rates between nations or within a nation between regions or between sex and age groups. Trend analyses examine the patterns of suicide mortality in various populations over time.

---

[a]This work was supported in part by Research Grant MH 31302, Research Scientist Award MH 00334, and Research Training Grant in Psychiatric Epidemiology and Biostatics MH 17104 from the National Institute of Mental Health.

As an example of comparisons across groups, we have the World Health Organization's comparison of suicide rates for 1975-1980 in 24 European countries.[1] Rates were extremely variable, ranging from 45 per 100,000 in Hungary to less than 3 per 100,000 in Greece. If the United States had been included in the comparison, it would have ranked 15th, with a suicide rate of 12.

Countries vary greatly not only in their rates in a particular year, but also in the stability of their rates. The rate for the United States has been quite stable over the last 15 or 20 years, while rates in England and Wales, Scotland, and Greece have fallen and rates in all other European countries have risen.

The striking differences between suicide rates in different countries and in the same country over time are in marked contrast to, for example, prevalence rates of schizophrenia, which show great cross-national and cross-era stability. This variation encourages speculation that suicide must be very much influenced by local cultures and attitudes. However, except for the fact that the three European countries with the lowest rates are all predominantly Catholic, there is nothing known about differences among these cultures that would explain the ranking observed.

Before searching for cultural explanations, however, there are a number of cautions that researchers have stressed. Attractive as is the availability of rates across countries and across time for hypothesis building, there are reasons to question the comparability of these rates. Since suicide is extremely rare before age 15, it is to be expected that rates will be low in countries with high fertility rates. And since rates for white males increase with age, high health standards that protect against early deaths from natural causes are associated with more persons surviving into ages at which risk for suicide is high. Clearly then, rates should not be compared without age standardization when cultural explanations are sought.

It is also suspected that variations in ascertainment procedures account for a good deal of the variation in rates. Where more cases are referred to coroners and more autopsies performed, more suicides will be discovered. Thus a high suicide rate in a country with good public health and high standards for ascertaining cause of death does not necessarily mean that there is something in the culture conducive to suicide. It may be only that rates in other countries appear low due to poor ascertainment and early deaths from other causes.

Time trends need to be examined cautiously not only because ascertainment procedures can change locally, but because in all countries a change in the international system for listing causes of death in 1968 probably had some effect on suicide rates. A "cause-undetermined" category was added, removing the need for making a forced choice between accident and suicide in doubtful cases. This presumably decreased suicide rates somewhat, although it probably decreased accident rates more, since it is generally believed that in every country doubtful decisions usually go against suicide.

When despite these opportunities for artifactual influences a common trend across time is found, one tends to believe that it is correct. One such trend exists: rates of suicide in the 15- to 24-year age group have been rising. Between 1970 and 1980 in the United States there was a 50% increase in rates for males in the 15- to 24-year age group.[2] Lower (13% to 32%) but still alarming increases in male suicide rates in this age group were reported in European countries between 1973 and 1980.[3]

This observation of a rapidly increasing rate for young people needs to be seen in the context of changes in the total rate. In the United States this rise while the overall rate has been stable implies two important facts: first, rates for older men in the United States have been declining. This good news tends to be overlooked in the concern over rising suicide rates among the young. Second, these very large increases in rate occurred in a group that began with an almost negligible rate 40 years ago, so that while the percent increase is large, the numbers are still relatively small as compared with other age groups, and youths still contribute relatively little to the overall rate. FIGURE 1 shows these time trends dramatically for white males. Rates are presented by 10-year age brackets from 1950 to 1981.[4] For the final three years, annual rates are available; before that, rates by decade. In 1950, suicide rates were strongly and positively associated with age for white males, increasing steadily with age from only 6 per 100,000 for those 15-24 to 10 times that rate for those 75 or older. Since then, rates have fallen for all age groups above 44. Despite these changes, the ratio of rates of those 75 or older remains about double the rate of those 45-54.

There has been little or no change over this period for persons aged 35-44, while rates for the young have been increasing. As a result, the range has narrowed. In 1970, the rates were still perfectly correlated with age, but the ratio of rates for the oldest to youngest had dropped from 10 to 1 to 3.6 to 1. In the next dozen years, as

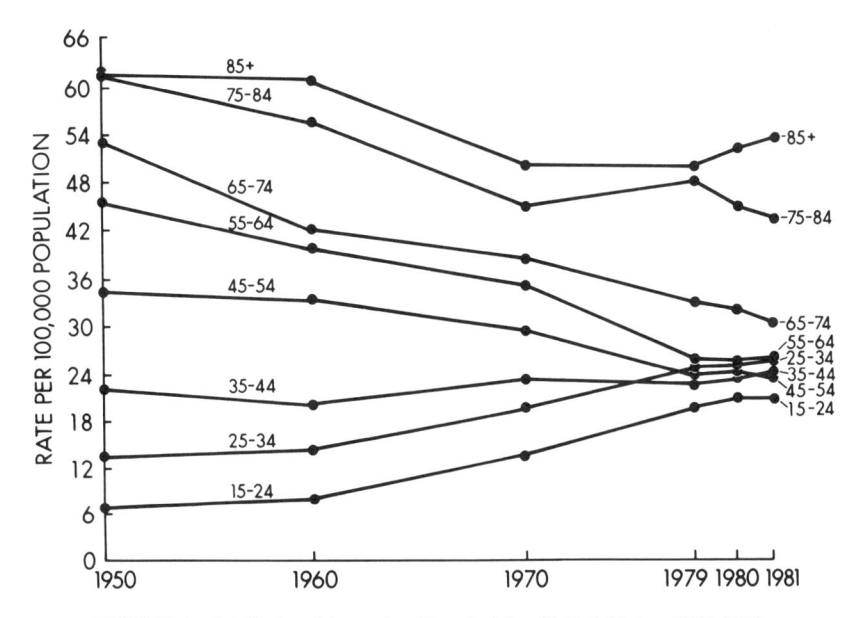

FIGURE 1. Suicide in white males 15 and older, United States, 1950-1981.

the rates of the elderly declined and the rates of the young rose, the 25- to 34-year-olds' rate became as high as the rate of 55- to 64-year-olds.

Women and black males showed much less variation by age in 1950 and have experienced less dramatic changes since then. FIGURE 2 shows results for black males. In 1950, while the youngest group had the lowest rate, there was no clear relationship with age overall. However, 25- to 34-year-old black male deaths have paralleled the sharply rising rates in white men in that age range so that by the 1980s, they had the highest rates among black males.

This pattern of rising rates among the young, stable rates in middle age, and falling rates among the elderly has also been found in England, showing that these changes are not accidental or local.[5]

These results by age, sex, and race show how much findings of a stable rate over time for the United States population can hide about the patterns for subpopulations. These fascinating, but so far uninterpretable, results are achieved by using death certificates as a source not only for the fact of suicide but of the age, race, and sex of the suicide. This allows calculating suicide rates for specific age-race-sex groups. Contrasting age/sex/race rates overcomes much of the scepticism about the validity of ecological comparisons across areas or nations or even across time within a single nation. While ascertainment practices may vary across nations or may have changed over time, it is not obvious that they would change differentially by age, race, and sex within a single country. Not that analyses contrasting rates by age-sex-race groups are proof against artifacts. If, for example, older white males shifted from guns and hanging to pills as their means of suicide, or quit writing suicide notes, the apparent decline in their rates might be due only to a lower proportion ascertained. Part of the rise in young black suicides might be only apparent, due to increased ascertainment because of the black migration to cities, where ascertainment is presumably more complete, but the fact that the increase occurs in both races shows that such artifacts are not the sole explanation.

The hypothesis that place of residence affects ascertainment could in principle be tested by analyzing suicide rates holding constant place of residence and place of death, both of which appear on death certificates along with age, sex, and race, to

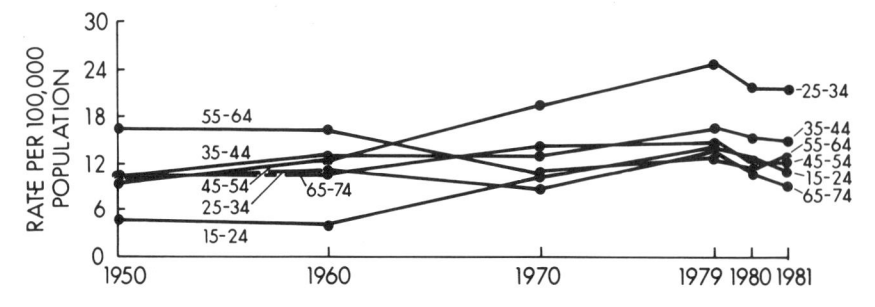

FIGURE 2. Suicide in black males 15-74, United States, 1950-1981.

learn whether the increase in rates among younger persons is found in both rural and urban settings. There are certainly grounds for suspecting that migration might affect rates, since enormous local variation in ascertainment procedures has been found. Nelson et al. studied the practices of certifying suicide by 191 coroners in 11 western states.[6] They found extensive variation in the educational backgrounds of coroners, in professional resources available to them, in the statutes under which they function, and in their procedures. For example, 30% of the coroners reported that autopsies are almost always performed if suicide is suspected; the remainder rarely performed autopsies under these circumstances. The authors cite the work of Litman, who found that the frequency with which death from self-inflicted gunshot was called suicide varied from 50% to 95%.

However, without proof that such artifacts are of a magnitude sufficient to account for the striking shifts in FIGURE 1, both the decline in suicides in elderly white males and the increase in young blacks and whites appear worthy of study.

The reporting of changes by age, race, and sex groups as well as total rates has been made practical by the computerization of death certificates. In the United States, the death certificate provides not only immediate causes of death and conditions contributing to death, but also age, sex, race, place of birth, marital status, veteran status, usual occupation, place of residence, and parents' names, in addition to features of the death itself such as where and when it occurred, who made the certification, and to which undertaker the body was turned over. All of these data can now be used to learn more about how persons who commit suicide differ from those with other causes of deaths and from the total population. So far, little advantage has been taken of these additional items.

Stability despite Variation in Ascertainment

The individual determination of suicide on each death certificate reflects the judgment and professional opinion of the physician, coroner, or medical examiner who certified the cause of death.[2] Criteria to guide professional medical examiners in decision making have never been established.[7] Errors in reporting suicides are generally supposed to be chiefly underreporting, particularly if the evidence is equivocal. In this circumstance, most coroners probably prefer to err in the direction of overestimating natural deaths or accidents rather than suicides, in order to avoid unnecessary upset for the family. Deliberately obscuring or withholding information necessary to make a suicide determination may also occur, particularly when the coroner is a local official, subject to political pressure or pressure from the family or friends of the suicide. Suicides are also missed if no body is found, since in this case a death certificate is not filed even if there is circumstantial evidence for suicide, such as a note. Even cases that come to autopsy may be missed if a preexisting illness is found that could conceivably have caused the death, or if large amounts of drugs or alcohol are found in the blood which might have caused the death by accidental overdose. Without an adequate history of the deceased's substance use and consequent tolerance, coroners may assume the observed levels were fatal when they were not.

Coroners clearly need uniform standards for deciding when a suicide has occurred, but as yet there are none. A national committee was recently established by the Centers for Disease Control to address the issues of standard criteria for the certification of suicides and minimal educational requirements for certifiers of the cause of death. Given the variation in ascertainment practices, it is of interest to see whether that variation is so severe that national comparisons become meaningless.

Barraclough alone,[8] with Sainsbury,[9] and Sainsbury and Jenkins[5] used two ingenious methods to see whether the large differences across nations noted above were artifacts of differential ascertainment. First, they compared the rank order of rates by nations with the rank order of suicide rates of immigrants from those countries to the United States. It was presumed that in the United States ascertainment would not be correlated with the nation of origin. Therefore, if the rank order was similar to that found in the countries of origin, the explanation for the variation must lie in the culture or in the biology of the national group, not in ascertainment procedures. The rank order correlation between rates in native countries and among immigrants from those countries was very high. Similar results were obtained by Lester for migrants to Australia.[10]

Barraclough's second method was to compare ranks for suicide rates with ranks for suicide plus undetermined causes across countries. Again the correlation between ranks for suicide alone and for suicide plus undetermined cause was very high, 0.89 in 1968 for 22 countries and 0.96 for 19 countries in 1970-1973. In addition, the spread in rates across countries was little reduced. Barraclough argued that if the difference in rates across countries was only due to the fact that some countries were using much more rigid criteria than others, there should be much less variation in rates of suicides plus undetermined causes than in suicide rates alone. On the basis of these findings, he concluded that national differences were real.

Similarly, Malla and Hoenig, asking whether the low rate of suicides in Newfoundland compared with the rest of Canada could be due to ascertainment problems, combined cases called suicides with unexplained and undetermined deaths.[11] The resulting suicide rate in Newfoundland (6.36 per 100,000) was still less than half the overall Canadian rate of 14. They too concluded that underreporting alone could not account for the lower rate.

Sainsbury compared rates over a decade in districts in England where coroners had changed with rates in districts where the same coroner had been active over the decade.[12] The change in coroners did not change the districts' ranks in suicide rates. Nor was the ranking changed by counting accidental poisonings and undetermined deaths as suicides.

Showing that adding deaths by unascertained cause to suicides does not change rankings by area is helpful in arguing for the meaningfulness of national or regional differences. However, it does not cope with the fact that an unknown proportion of suicides are reported as accidents, homicides, and natural deaths. It is difficult to see how these misclassified suicides can be recovered short of the onerous task of sampling *all* deaths for a specified period and attempting an independent ascertainment procedure according to well-specified criteria. Nonetheless, the failure of each experiment in accounting for regional differences by reducing the likelihood of ascertainment biases suggests that variation in rates across geographic areas is probably real, and therefore needs explanation.

Searching for Explanations

These studies which showed that regional differences in suicide rates were probably real shed little light on why such regional differences might exist. A more complex form of ecologic analysis is needed to test hypotheses about social, economic, religious, and political factors that may contribute to suicide rates. The classic work of Emil Durkheim is an excellent example of ecologic analysis that tests causal hypotheses.[13]

Durkheim explored differences in rates in rural and urban areas, in and out of the military, by age and marital status, by the dominant religion and ethnic affiliation, by occupation and climate. He concluded that suicide mortality varies with social integration, social structure, and social change.[14] While his work still stimulates research, it has also been cited as a prime example of the dangers of ecologic fallacy.[15] Having found that predominantly Protestant provinces in Western Europe had higher suicide rates than did predominantly Catholic provinces, he concluded that Protestants are more likely to commit suicide than are Catholics. While possibly correct, this inference cannot be made with certainty so long as there are both Catholics and Protestants in all provinces. In predominantly Protestant provinces it could have been the Catholics who were taking their own lives. The risk of ecological fallacy exists whenever the composition of each group in the analysis is not homogenous with respect to the study factor.

If Durkheim had had computerized death certificates, he might have been able to do a more definitive analysis. While religion does not appear on the death certificate, there is a strong correlation between choice of undertaker and religious preference. But even now there are serious limitations in using the items on death certificates for ecological analyses. The fact that a death certificate exists for a particular individual can be ascertained from the National Death Register. The register also shows in which jurisdiction the certificate is filed to make possible its retrieval. But the cause of death is not available until the certificate is retrieved. This means that the death register is a help in follow-up studies, where a sample has been selected prior to death so that individual identifiers can be checked in the register, but it is of no help in developing suicide rates. While the National Center for Health Statistics does have data tapes, the nongovernmental researcher must approach local departments of vital statistics. Not all states have entered all of the death certificate variables onto computers, and in any case, access to these data is restricted by various privacy concerns. In addition, there are problems with missing information and the information available may be misleading. For example, Monday has been found to be the day of the week with the largest proportion of suicides. But rather than meaning that it is depressing to have to return to work, this may actually only mean that Monday is the day for *discovering* suicides committed over the weekend.[16]

Suicide and Social Change

A number of studies have attempted to relate changes in suicide rates to concomitant historical changes. As an example, Henry and Short related changes in suicide rates to fluctuations in official crime statistics in a sample of cities.[17] They found an inverse relationship between suicide and homicide, which they interpreted on the basis of psychoanalytic theory which sees suicide and homicide as alternative ways of expressing aggression, i.e., it sees suicide as aggression turned inward. Therefore, on the assumption that the amount of aggression in the population is constant, suicide should increase as homicide decreases, and vice versa. Holinger and Kelmen extended the span of years covered and included the total United States.[18] They found a direct rather than an inverse relationship between suicide and homicide that held for all race-sex groups, a finding consistent with the earlier work of Brenner, which indicated that suicide and homicide increase in parallel when unemployment rises,[19] and with clinical studies that find high rates of suicidal behavior in violent patients.

A high rate of suicide associated with unemployment has been observed with considerable regularity,[20-22] both in ecological studies showing correlations among rates of unemployment and suicide across geographic areas and in studies noting that the rate of joblessness on death certificates of suicides is well above the concurrent population rate.

These results, however, might be explained in ways other than arguing that unemployment leads to suicide. Community unemployment rates are correlated with many other social variables that indicate what Durkheim called "social disorganization," which might be the more important predictor. The high frequency of unemployment on death certificates of suicides might only reflect the impaired performance associated with the psychiatric disorder that was the true cause of the suicide. More convincing evidence for a causal relationship would be the finding that a national increase in unemployment is followed by an increase in suicide, which then is reversed when the employment picture changes. This must be studied on the national level because changes in local rates might simply show that the local area is changing character due to migration in or out.

There was an increase in suicides during the Great Depression, but it has been difficult to show a consistent relationship with less dramatic fluctuations in employment, in part perhaps because there is no agreement about what the proper lag time is between changes in employment levels and changes in suicide rates. An interesting technique was developed by Wasserman, who used increase in the average length of unemployment rather than in the number unemployed as the indicator of a depressed economy and found a significant increase in suicide nine months after the beginning of an economic depression.[21]

While crime rates and levels of unemployment fluctuate over time, some changes are unique and datable. Examples are the occurrence of wars, changes in medical practice with regard to prescription of lethal sedatives (e.g., the shift from barbiturates to benzodiazepines),[23] or the enactment of laws that markedly change access to common means of suicide, such as restrictions on the sale of guns or the removal of carbon monoxide from cooking gas.[24,25] If it can be assumed that nothing has changed except these historical events, changes in suicide rates following such events can be attributed to these "natural experiments." When a sustained drop in rates follows restriction of a single important means of committing suicide, as occurred in England, Vienna, and Brisbane, Australia, when cooking gas was detoxified, it demonstrates that intervention is worthwhile, because barring suicide by one means does not simply lead to the substitution of some other method.

Unlike a true experiment in which the experimenter controls the exposure to the experimental condition, arguments for the effect of a natural experiment are always suspect, and ways must be found to support the probability that any statistical relationship discovered is not spurious. Wars, for example, are associated with low rates of suicide,[1] but this may only reflect departure for the battlefield of medical examiners and the ease with which suicides in war zones can be misreported as combat deaths.

Brown offered two observations in support of the effect of detoxifying cooking gas that addressed the possibility of a spurious relationship with the drop in rates.[26] First, there was the essential temporal correspondence in which the detoxification of cooking gas preceded the decline in the British suicide rate. Second, the total decline in suicides was numerically equivalent to the decline in suicide mortality from carbon monoxide over the relevant period. This demonstrated that the two events were probably related, i.e., the finding was not due to a coincidence between passage of the law at a time when rates of suicide happened to be declining independently.

When there is no fixed date at which a historical event took place, the causal argument is more difficult to make. In the United States, the number of handguns in private possession has been rising sharply, but there is no date on which they can be said to have become common. Boyd argued that an increased availability of guns had caused a rise in suicide by following the same line of argument used in the cooking gas example.[27] First he showed that the increasing rate of suicide by firearms from 1953 to 1978, from 4.9 per 100,000 to 7.1 per 100,000, paralleled the increase in the overall suicide rate during this 25-year period. Next, he showed that nonfirearm suicides did not increase during this period. Finally, he showed that accidental deaths by firearms did not increase during that period, so that one could conclude that the effect was specific to suicides, not just a general increase in gun deaths. Lester and Murrell tested the same hypothesis by comparing suicide rates in states that differed in the strictness of their gun control laws.[24] States with stricter laws had lower suicide rates for males during 1969 to 1971. The fact that only males were affected was consistent with (although not definitive proof for) the argument that the availability of guns was the reason for the differences, because men are twice as likely as women to use firearms as their method. Markush and Bartolucci examined regional United States suicide rates in the mid-1970s and found a statistically significant correlation between gun and pistol prevalence and suicide rates.[28] Farmer and Rohde examined methods of suicide and self-injury in 11 countries from 1969 to 1973.[29] They compared total rates with rates excluding use of firearms and hangings. Excluding these methods reduced the variation across countries, suggesting that higher rates might be attributable to greater availability of firearms.

Each of these demonstrations, while suggestive, is also consistent with the theory that violent people buy guns, vote against laws restricting their ownership, *and* commit suicide.

Closer to a true experiment has been the establishment of suicide prevention centers since the 1960s, since these were intended to lower suicide rates. Even had rates declined following their establishment, showing that the centers were responsible for the decline would have been difficult. But, in fact, there has been no decline in rates since the prevention movement began.[30] The probable reason for their lack of success seems to be that they have attracted primarily young white women, the demographic group that has high rates of attempts but low rates of successful suicides.

Linking Records

Another ecological approach depends on linking suicide records with records from other rosters. Where there are cancer registers, for example, which can be assumed to offer reasonably complete coverage, the effect on suicide risk of knowing that one has a potentially fatal disorder can be studied ecologically so long as the rosters are computerized. When names in a tumor registry were linked with vital statistics records, a twofold increase in the risk of suicide was found for the cancer patients.[31]

Linking the 16-year accumulation of records in the Monroe County psychiatric register to suicides[32] allowed ascertaining the proportion of suicides who had been patients within that 16-year period (45%) or in the 30 days before death (half of these). Record linkage provided two sets of controls for the treated suicides—untreated suicides and nonsuiciding patients. Comparing the treated suicides to these two groups shows how vital the choice of control subjects is, since they produce diametrically opposite findings. As compared to untreated suicides, treated ones tended to be young, female, black, and of low social class. Compared with nonsuiciding patients, patients who committed suicide tended to be old, white, male, and of higher social status. Thus psychiatric patients as a group have a very different demographic profile from suicides, and the suicides who are also patients fall between the two. Record linkage studies of suicide are rare in the United States because there are so few rosters other than those available through vital statistics that cover complete populations. The psychiatric register is virtually defunct these days because it is expensive to maintain, was not used as much as expected for research, and ran afoul of privacy laws. But even had registers thrived, record linkage has its own problems. If the updating of the two registers is not in synchrony, a case in one register may be missed in the other simply because the data entry has been delayed. There are always problems in matching names and identifiers due to misspellings or absence of a middle initial. These problems lead to missing cases and thus underestimating the proportion of suicides who are in the register. Nonetheless, the ability to link rosters greatly increases the potential for finding explanatory variables.

These ecologic designs have suggested a variety of causal factors in suicide, among them national attitudes, availability of means, economic stress, age and sex roles, psychiatric and physical illness. They have simultaneously raised questions as to whether apparent differences in rates are real or are artifacts of ascertainment and reporting. Other methods, linking individuals' histories to their suicidal behavior, are necessary to make the causal arguments more convincing.

RETROSPECTIVE STUDIES OF COMPLETED SUICIDE

Retrospective clinical studies are investigations in which the researcher collects data on events or circumstances of affected persons prior to the onset of an illness in hopes of identifying a single antecedent or a pattern of distinctive antecedents of its onset. The preferred design for retrospective clinical studies is generally the case-control design, in which those affected and control subjects similar to them in ways thought not to be causes of the disorder of interest are interviewed or investigated through records about circumstances present before those affected became sick. The chief design issues with case-control studies are getting representative samples of those affected, choosing the proper control subjects, and dating onset, so that the time frame of inquiry is appropriate. Retrospective studies of suicide have two advantages: representativeness of the cases is generally not an issue, because a consecutive series or random sample of all suicides known to vital statistics within a specified time period can be studied, and the date is certain. However, it is obviously impossible to interview affected persons, and it is so unclear who the relevant controls should be that most studies include none.

Lacking the opportunity to interview the proband, retrospective studies have utilized a variety of sources of information, principally relatives, physicians, employers, medical records, suicide notes, and coroners' reconstructions of events surrounding the suicide itself. When this technique has centered on reconstructing the events immediately surrounding the death, it has been called the "psychological autopsy."[33] But the search for causes has also entailed earlier histories, such as earlier suicide attempts, histories of psychiatric treatment, and losses or threats of losses that might explain the suicide's hopelessness.

The studies of Dorpat and Ripley,[34] Barraclough and others,[35] and Robins,[36] which all used retrospective reconstruction of events preceding the suicide, agree that almost all suicides were psychiatrically ill at the time of death. In all three studies, depression and alcoholism were the diagnoses predominantly associated with completed suicide, and all three echoed the results of ecological studies that emphasize the importance of being an elderly white male.[36] The uniformity of results shows that relatives of the suicide are well enough informed to allow making retrospective diagnoses. Also, confirmation by evidence that the suicide had often been in treatment prior to the event suggests that relatives probably do not greatly exaggerate the attendant psychiatric problems in an effort to understand reasons for the suicide.

None of these studies provided a control group for comparison. However, the rates of psychiatric disorder reported were so high that there is little doubt that suicides have higher than expected rates of disorder. What is lacking is a quantitative measure of the excess and the opportunity to distinguish those signs or symptoms of the illness that might help to identify which psychiatrically disordered persons are at highest risk. Studies that have employed control groups have offered a variety of choices. Farberow and Shneidman compared 32 male patients in a Veterans Administration mental hospital who committed suicide with patients who attempted suicide, threatened suicide, or were nonsuicidal.[37] The suicidal patients were distinguished from the nonsuicidal group by a diagnosis of depression or paranoid schizophrenia. A family history of mental hospitalization differentiated the completed suicides from the other groups. Social and environmental factors revealed no differences between groups. Breed selected controls matched by age, sex, and race with male suicides from the neighborhoods where the suicides had lived.[38] He found the suicides to have had more occupational problems, including downward mobility, lower income, and more unemployment.

In addition to adding information about high treatment frequency and the frequency and type of psychiatric disorders associated with suicide to the demographic information from ecological studies, these retrospective studies have permitted contrasting diagnostic groups with respect to their apparent motives for suicide[39] and the methods selected.[40] What is still lacking are the figures needed for preventive planning—knowing how high the risks of suicide are for each high-risk group such as elderly white males, and the unemployed with alcohol problems or depression who have suffered certain types of loss, and how long the risk persists after its first signs appear. Prospective studies have addressed some of these issues.

PROSPECTIVE STUDIES OF HIGH-RISK POPULATIONS

To be financially feasible, prospective studies require samples enriched by subjects known to be at high risk on the basis of clinical, sociodemographic characteristics, or critical life events. But even high-risk samples must be very large to yield a reasonable number of suicides in a reasonable time span. Cobb and Kasl, for example, followed a large sample of men working for a plant that was about to be closed, but found only two suicides.[41] It was impossible to identify factors related to suicide with such a small result. MacKinnon and Farberow addressed this problem when they noted that even with the most conservative estimates of predictive error in a psychiatric inpatient population, suicide would be too rare to warrant intervention.[42] A number of studies confirm their conclusion. A follow-up of suicide attempters over an eight-month period found only 2% who actually completed the suicide.[43] Motto attempted to predict suicide in depressed and suicidal psychiatric inpatients on the basis of social and situational factors derived by discriminant analysis and found statistically significant results, but results of limited practical utility for intervention.[44] Pokorny followed a sample of 4800 psychiatric inpatients to assess the number of completed suicides and parasuicides.[45] A total of 67 suicides were identified and 179 suicide attempts. The predictors derived produced too many false-positive cases to be useful. Dorpat and Ripley summarized 15 studies of the rate of committed suicide following attempted suicide.[46] The percentage who were found at follow-up to have committed suicide ranged from 0.03% to 22.0%, depending on the duration of the follow-up.

Even with large, high-risk samples, there are problems in using prospective studies to explain suicide. Murphy points out that although a prospective study allows personal interviews with the prospective suicide, and thus provides more and better quality information than that obtainable after death, it yields fewer data about circumstances immediately antecedent to the suicide act, since it is unlikely that the suicide will follow closely upon an interview.[47] In addition, the ethical requirement to attempt to prevent a suicide if there is a clear and imminent danger compromises the scientific objectivity of prospective studies.

Despite these difficulties, prospective studies have provided some correlates of suicide. Attempters have been found to be a group with a much elevated risk. Tuchman and Youngman compared the suicide risk in 1112 consecutive attempted suicides with the risk for the general population, and found a 139-fold increase (1.9% vs. 0.01%),[48] despite the fact that attempters tend to be female, young, and nonwhite while suicides tend to be older white males. Attempters are at considerably higher risk, for example, than persons with terminal illnesses such as cancer,[31] where the excess is only 2-fold.

Suicide as One of Many Outcomes

The studies discussed thus far were designed specifically to study suicide. An alternative design is to follow a high-risk population with respect to a variety of outcomes, of which suicide is one. The advantage of this design is that it allows comparing the frequency of suicide with that of other possible results and identifying intermediate outcomes that may facilitate or inhibit suicides in persons at risk. It also makes follow-up more attractive economically, since a single study can yield a number of important results even when suicide rates are low. However, the study will be most useful if there are several follow-up contacts so that intermediate outcomes can be identified, and if the cases are all followed to death, so that all the suicides that will ever occur will be discovered.

A study of children seen in a child guidance clinic who were followed into their mid-40s[49] and Terman and Oden's follow-up of children with very high IQs[50] through approximately their 40s and 50s are examples of studies that discovered many childhood predictors of adult outcomes but that fell short of achieving these goals for suicide. The child guidance clinic study found a slightly higher rate of suicide (2%) in those who received a consensus diagnosis of antisocial personality than in those with other adult disorders or in a control group of nonpatients.[49] However, the numbers were too small to conclude that antisocial personality is a risk factor for suicide. But even had differences been statistically significant, the fact that follow-up ended when the subjects were in their mid-40s meant that the results might only indicate that antisocial personality is associated with earlier suicide, not more suicides. The follow-up of children with high IQs was reanalyzed to seek childhood antecedents and intercurrent events differentiating five who shot themselves from a control group who died a natural death.[51] Despite the special sample and small number, the familiar variables of alcoholism and occupational instability were noted.

UNIFYING ECOLOGIC AND INDIVIDUAL STUDIES

The studies we have reviewed sought predictors of suicide either by comparing aggregate data across time or place or by comparing individual cases of suicides with nonsuicides. These studies have produced a host of correlates, both demographic (i.e., age, sex, and race, nationality) and specific personal experiences such as psychiatric disorder, terminal illness, losses, and threatened losses. What has not yet happened is some bridging of these two approaches so that personal experiences can be extrapolated to aggregate data to explain why rates are high in these demographically defined populations. Accomplishing this is difficult for the reasons outlined above—suicides are rare and they cannot be interviewed.

There have been two attempts to circumvent these problems by approaching the problem obliquely. The argument goes as follows. If suicide is more common in certain populations than in others, and if suicidal individuals have characteristics that distinguish them from nonsuicidal persons, then those distinguishing characteristics should be particularly common in the populations that provide the highest suicide rates. This approach has been applied by Hendin in an attempt to explain the fact that suicide rates are high in Denmark and low in Norway[52] and by Robins et al. in attempting to explain the high rate in older white American males as compared with other groups.[53] Both studies began with interviews comparing patients at high and low risk for suicide, and then carried out interviews in the general populations that produce high and low suicide rates to see whether the characteristics that distinguished suicidal from nonsuicidal patients also distinguished general populations at high risk from general populations at low risk. In the study seeking to explain the high suicide rate in older white men, six findings from clinical studies were confirmed as relatively common both in suicidal patients and in the general population of older white men. Both high-risk groups had a higher incidence of depression and alcohol abuse, were more secular and less religious, more often had family members or friends who had committed suicide, were more often without a spouse, and expected a less rewarding old age.

This indirect approach is only one necessary step in producing a unified body of theory that can accommodate findings at both the macro and micro levels. It allows weeding out hypotheses that are not promising on the aggregate level, but fails to prove the correctness of the hypotheses that are sustained. A next step should be a prospective study of members of high-risk populations with and without the postulated risk characteristics. In the United States, such a sample would be white men over 65 who are allocated to high- and low-risk groups on the basis of their history of alcohol problems and depression, their family histories of suicide, their religiousness, their marital status, and their attitudes toward aging. They should be men without a known physical illness that is likely to carry them off through death by natural causes within the projected follow-up period before their risk of suicide can be ascertained. If our hypotheses are correct, the suicide rate in the high-risk population will be so high that it will be possible to validate the potency of these predictors even for an event as rare in the general population as suicide within a reasonable study period—perhaps 10 years—and in a sample of only moderate size. The most exciting finding that such a study could yield would be that older white men *without* the personal risk factors of psychiatric illness, family history of suicide, separation from spouse, secular views, and pessimism about aging had suicide rates no higher than those found in low-risk demographic categories (women, blacks, and young white men). With such results, we would be encouraged to believe that if older white men could be protected from these risk factors, their rates might decline to the levels experienced by the rest of the population. The next step would be experimental epidemiology: an effort to change the experience of older white men in a few communities to see whether the rate can in fact be reduced. If this step were to succeed, we would be ready for a national trial, and some expectation that the promise of what epidemiological and clinical studies of suicide can offer will be fulfilled—a successful program of prevention.

REFERENCES

1. World Health Organization Regional Office for Europe. 1982. Changing Patterns in Suicide Behaviour, Report on WHO Working Group. EURO Reports and Studies 74. Copenhagen, Denmark.
2. Centers for Disease Control 1985. Suicide Surveillance, 1970-1980. Department of Health and Human Services, United States Public Health Service. Atlanta, Ga.
3. DIEKSTRA, R. F. W. 1985. Suicide and suicide attempts in the European Economic Community: an analysis of trends, with special emphasis upon trends among the young. Suicide Life-threatening Behav. 15(1): 27-42.
4. National Center for Health Statistics. 1984. Health, United States. DHHS Publication No. (PHS) 85-1232. Public Health Service. U.S. Government Printing Office. Washington, D.C.
5. SAINSBURY, P. & J. S. JENKINS. 1982. The accuracy of officially reported suicide statistics for purposes of epidemiological research. J. Community Health 36: 43-48.
6. NELSON, F. L., N. L. FARBEROW & D. R. MACKINNON. 1978. The certification of suicide in eleven western states: an inquiry into the validity of reported suicide rates. Suicide Life-threatening Behav. 8(2): 75-88.
7. MURPHY, G. E., G. E. GANTNER, R. D. WETZEL, S. KATZ & M. R. ERNST. 1984. On the improvement of suicide determination. J. Forensic Sci. 19(2): 276-283.
8. BARRACLOUGH, B. M. 1973. Differences between national suicide rates. Br. J. Psychiatry 122: 95-96.
9. SAINSBURY, P. & B. M. BARRACLOUGH. 1968. Differences between suicide rates. Nature 220: 1252.
10. LESTER, D. 1972. Letter. Med. J. Aust. i: 941.
11. MALLA, A. & J. HOENIG. 1983. Differences in suicide rates: an examination of underreporting. Can. J. Psychiatry 28: 291-293.
12. SAINSBURY, P. 1983. Validity and reliability of trends in suicide statistics. World Health Statist. Q. 36: 339-345.
13. DURKHEIM, E. 1951. Suicide. Free Press. New York, N.Y.
14. SELKIN, J. 1983. The legacy of Emile Durkheim. Suicide Life-threatening Behav. 13(1): 3-13.
15. KLEINBAUM, D. G., L. L. KUPPER & H. MORGENSTERN. 1982. Epidemiologic Research: Principles and Quanitative Methods. Lifetime Learning Publications. Belmont, Calif.
16. MACMAHON, K. 1983. Short-term temporal cycles in the frequency of suicide, United States, 1972-1978. Am. J. Epidemiol. 117(6): 744-750.
17. HENRY, A. F. & J. F. SHORT. 1954. Suicide and Homicide. The Free Press of Glencoe. London, England.
18. HOLINGER, P. C. & E. KLEMEN. 1982. Violent deaths in the United States, 1900-1975. Relationships between suicide, homicide, and accidental deaths. Soc. Sci. Med. 16: 1929-1938.
19. BRENNER, M. H. 1979. Mortality and the national economy: a review, and the experiences of England and Wales, 1936-1976. Lancet (Sept.): 568-573.
20. PLATT, S. 1984. Unemployment and suicidal behavior: a review of the literature. Soc. Sci. Med. 19(2): 93-115.
21. WASSERMAN, I. M. 1984. The influence of economic business cycles on United States suicide rates. Suicide Life-threatening Behav. 14(3): 143-156.
22. PLATT, S. & N. KREITMAN. 1985. Parasuicide and unemployment among men in Edinburgh 1968-1982. Psychol. Med. 15: 113-123.
23. OLIVER, R. G. & B. S. HETZEL. 1973. An analysis of recent trends in suicide rates in Australia. Int. J. Epidemiol. 2(1): 91-101.
24. LESTER, D. & M. E. MURRELL. 1980. The influence of gun control laws on suicidal behavior. Am. J. Psychiatry 137: 121-122.
25. KREITMAN, N. 1976. The coal gas story: United Kingdom suicide rates, 1960-1971. Br. J. Prev. Soc. Med. 30: 86-93.

26. BROWN, J. H. 1979. Suicide in Britain: more attempts, fewer deaths, lessons for public policy. Arch. Gen. Psychiatry 36(Sept.): 1119-1124.
27. BOYD, J. H. 1983. The increasing rate of suicide by firearms. N. Engl. J. Med. 308(15): 872-874.
28. MARKUSH, R. E. & A. E. BARTOLUCCI. 1984. Firearms and Suicide in the United States. Am J. Public Health 74(2): 123-127.
29. FARMER, R. & J. ROHDE. 1980. Effect of availability and acceptability of lethal instruments on suicide mortality: an analysis of some international data. Acta Psychiatr. Scand. 62: 436-446.
30. MILLER, H. L., D. W. COOMBS, J. D. LEEPER & S. N. BARTON. 1984. An analysis of the effects of suicide prevention facilities on suicide rates in the United States. Am. J. Public Health 74(4): 340-343.
31. MARSHALL, J. P., W. BURNETT & J. BRASURE. 1983. On precipitating factors: cancer as a cause of suicide. Suicide Life-threatening Behav. 13(1): 15-27.
32. KRAFT, D. P. & H. M. BABIGIAN. 1976. Suicide by persons with and without psychiatric contacts. Arch. Gen. Psychiatry 33: 209-215.
33. SHNEIDMAN, E. S. 1981. The psychological autopsy. Suicide Life-threatening Behav. 11(4): 325-340.
34. DORPAT, T. L. & H. S. RIPLEY. 1960. A study of suicide in the Seattle area. Compr. Psychiatry 1(6): 349-359.
35. BARRACLOUGH, B., J. BUNCH, B. NELSON & P. SAINSBURY. 1974. A hundred cases of suicide: clinical aspects. Br. J. Psychiatry 125: 355-373.
36. ROBINS, E. 1981. The Final Months. Oxford University Press. New York, N.Y.
37. FARBEROW, N. L. & E. S. SHNEIDMAN. 1955. Attempted, threatened, and completed suicide. J. Abnorm. Soc. Psychol. 50: 230.
38. BREED, W. 1963. Occupational mobility and suicide among white males. Am. Sociol. Rev. 28(2): 179-188.
39. MURPHY, G. E. & E. ROBINS. 1967. Social factors in suicide. J. Am. Med. Assoc. 199(5): 303-308.
40. MURPHY, G. E. 1975. The physician's responsibility for suicide. I. An error of commission. Ann. Intern. Med. 82(3): 301-304.
41. COBB, S. & S. V. KASL. 1972. Some medical aspects of unemployment. Ind. Gerontol. 8: 8-15.
42. MACKINNON, D. R. & N. L. FARBEROW. 1976. An assessment of the utility of suicide prediction. Suicide Life-threatening Behav. 6(2): 86-91.
43. SCHMIDT, E. H., P. O'NEAL & E. ROBINS. 1954. Evaluation of suicide attempts as a guide to therapy: clinical and follow-up study of one-hundred-nine patients. J. Am. Med. Assoc. 155(6): 549-555.
44. MOTTO, J. A. 1979. The psychopathology of suicide: a clinical model approach. Am. J. Psychiatry 136: 516-520.
45. POKORNY, A. D. 1983. Prediction of suicide in psychiatric patients: report of a prospective study. Arch. Gen. Psychiatry 40(March): 249-257.
46. DORPAT, T. L. & H. S. RIPLEY. 1967. The relationship between attempted suicide and committed suicide. Compr. Psychiatry 8(2): 74-79.
47. MURPHY, G. E. 1984. The prediction of suicide: why is it so difficult? Am. J. Psychother. 38(3): 341-349.
48. TUCKMAN, J. & W. F. YOUNGMAN. 1968. Assessment of suicide risk in attempted suicides. In Suicide Behaviors. H. L. P. Resnik, Ed.: 190-197. Little, Brown & Co. Boston, Mass.
49. ROBINS, L. N. 1966. Deviant Children Grown Up. Williams and Wilkins Co. Baltimore, Md.
50. TERMAN, L. M. & M. H. ODEN. 1947. The Gifted Child Grows Up. 4. Genetic Studies of Genius. Stanford University Press. Stanford, Calif.
51. SHNEIDMAN, E. S. 1981. Suicide among the gifted. Suicide Life-threatening Behav. 11(4): 254-281.
52. HENDIN, H. 1964. Suicide and Scandinavia. Grune & Stratton, Inc. New York, N. Y.
53. ROBINS, L. N., P. W. WEST & G. E. MURPHY. 1977. The high rate of suicide in older white men: a study testing ten hypotheses. Soc. Psychiatry 12: 1-20.

Suicidal People[a]

One Population or Two?

MARSHA M. LINEHAN

*Department of Psychology, NI-25
University of Washington
Seattle, Washington 98195*

A continuing controversy in the field of suicidology has been how to characterize and label the subject under study. The generic term suicidal behavior variously includes completed suicide, nonfatal deliberate self-harm (e.g., suicide attempts, suicide gestures, parasuicide, self-injury, self-poisoning, self-harm) with or without suicidal intent, suicide communications, including suicide threats, and suicide ideation. It is not unusual to find studies where subjects are mixed together from each of these categories with little attention to differences that might exist between the groups. Less common but still too frequent is the practice of studying one group, e.g., individuals who deliberately harm themselves but do not die, and drawing conclusions about another group, e.g., suicide. This terminological and methodological confusion reflects a similar confusion about the nature of the population under study.

In an influential 1958 monograph, Stengel, Cook, and Kreeger made a controversial argument that individuals who suicide and those who deliberately but nonfatally harm themselves (suicide attempters) represent two separate populations.[1] Their primary rationale was that the two groups could be distinguished both epidemiologically and in terms of the observed and functional characteristics of the suicidal acts. More recently, Kreitman and his colleagues have made a similar argument, contending that parasuicides (a term they introduced) form a population distinct from suicides.[2] The basis of their argument is that many nonfatal parasuicidal acts do not appear motivated by an intent to die, and thus are improperly viewed as unsuccessful attempts to suicide. Furthermore, they contend that intent at the time of a suicidal act is difficult to measure and is often based on questionable clinical inferences. Intent to die, therefore, should not be part of the criteria for defining suicidal behavior.

This point of view is in marked contrast to the previous assumption that individuals who contemplate suicide, threaten suicide, attempt suicide, or otherwise harm themselves, and those who in fact kill themselves, are drawn from a single population. Suicidal behavior is seen as on a continuum of intensity with suicide ideation at one end and completed suicide at the other. Lester and Beck[3,4] and Lester *et al.*[5] have argued that individuals who deliberately harm themselves are members of a single suicide population. Weiss has taken a similar position, labeling those who are characterized by high medical risk and high intent to die as "aborted successful suicides."[6]

---

[a] This paper was supported in part by National Institute of Mental Health Grant NIHM No. 5 ROI MH34486-03 to Dr. Linehan.

The term applies to cases where the individual would have been dead had it not been for medical intervention. Weiss is obviously assuming that "aborted successful suicides" are individuals from the suicide population misclassified by the accident of remaining alive as nonsuicides. More recently, Farmer has argued against a two-population theory suggesting that whether an act of self-harm results in death (suicide) or not is due, in part, to the accidental availability of a lethal method.[7]

The two points of view are represented in FIGURES 1 and 2. As can be seen in FIGURE 1, in the single-population view the common bond between the three groups is the contemplation of suicide. Differences between the three groups are minimized rather than enhanced. As seen in FIGURE 2, the multipopulation approach suggests that a substantial portion of the self-harm group are drawn from a population who are not primarily contemplating suicide when they injure themselves.

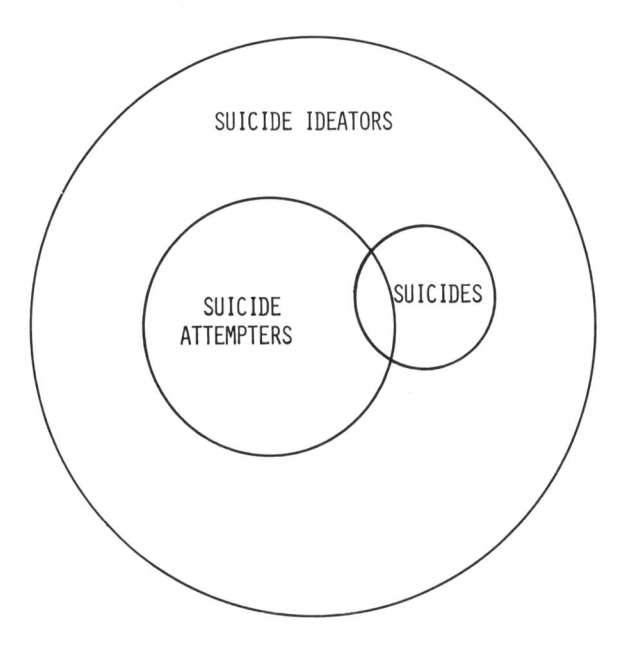

FIGURE 1. Single population.

A resolution of this controversy is important for several reasons. First, the overlap among suicidal categories has important implications for which individuals are included and excluded from research samples. To date, the ambiguity in definitions of suicidal behavior has led to a virtual quagmire where comparisons among studies are extremely difficult due to variations in entrance requirements and shifting boundaries for the behavioral categories. Although this is less problematic in the case of suicide, where inclusion/exclusion decisions are usually a matter of legal definition, it is a substantial problem in the case of nonfatal suicidal behavior. Second, whether one can generalize results obtained from one category, e.g., nonfatal self-harm, to describe members of other categories is dependent on whether the members of each category come from the same population. Third, and crucially important from a treatment standpoint, there are important attitudinal implications inherent in how we define and characterize the subjects under study. The single-population theory defines all subjects with reference to the extreme minority who actually die. The importance of the majority who do not die is contingent on their relationship to the minority who do. It is the risk of suicide that makes suicide ideation and intentional self-harm important. To the extent that individuals who contemplate suicide and intentionally harm themselves

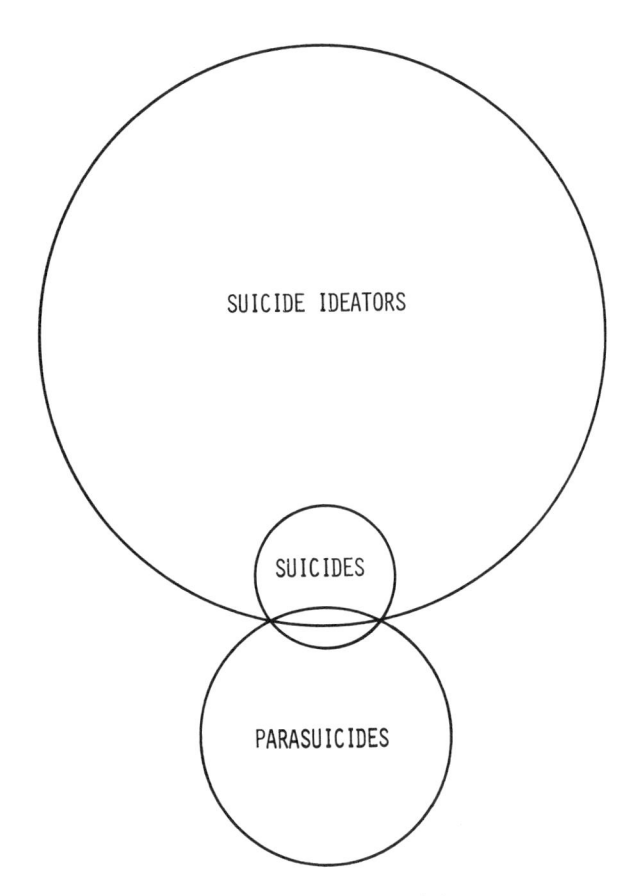

FIGURE 2. Separate populations.

nonfatally differ from suicides, then not only may the behavior be viewed as non-important but attitudes toward the individuals can be hostile rather than sympathetic. In contrast a multipopulation perspective views each type of behavior—ideation, self-harm, and suicide—as important in its own right, independent of the relationship of one population to the other. The purpose of this paper is to examine systematically the relative merits of a single-population vs. a multipopulation view of suicidal behavior. Since many investigations of deliberate nonfatal self-harm include individuals of varying levels of suicide intent, in the remainder of this paper I will use the broader term parasuicide to refer both to suicide attempts and deliberate self-harm (or attempts to inflict self-harm).

THE CASE FOR THE MULTIPLE-POPULATION THEORY

The characteristics of individuals who suicide and parasuicide have been reviewed extensively. Space prevents me from a detailed comparison of that literature here. The results of thousands of studies, however, shed little light on the controversy. In a previous paper I presented a social-behavioral model as a basis for comparing individuals engaging in each category of suicidal behavior.[8] Overall, findings indicate that suicides are similar in many ways to those who parasuicide and different from them in other ways. Differences that have been consistently found across numerous studies include the demographic variables of sex, age, and race and the behavioral characteristics of personality disorder and irritability or hostility. The latter two characteristics may represent a similar dimension since hostility and interpersonal difficulties are an important dimension of the personality disorder diagnoses. Important as these distinctions may be, it is nonetheless the case that similarities between parasuicides and suicides are extensive. In two recent, large-scale studies comparing suicides with parasuicides, approximately one-third of the variables in each study discriminated the two groups while two-thirds did not.[9,10]

Another line of argument has to do with the similarity of parasuicides and suicides to suicide ideators. If parasuicides and suicides are separate populations, ideators should be more similar to suicides than to parasuicides. Fewer studies have been conducted on suicide ideation per se, and even fewer investigations compare ideators with other suicidal populations. Interestingly, survey studies both of the general population[11,12] and of psychiatric patients[13,14] have not shown the age and sex differences between ideators vs. nonideators characteristically found in studies of parasuicide and suicide. The significant differences that have been found, however, suggest that individuals with suicide ideation serious enough to come to professional attention may differ little from parasuicides or suicides. In one study conducted by Mark and Haller, ideators differed from parasuicides on only 10 of 1250 variables.[15] In my own research program, we have found that ideators and parasuicides differ in both interpersonal problem solving styles and presenting problems[16,17] but do not significantly differ on a range of other variables including reasons for living,[18] hopelessness, depression, hostility, assertion, and life stress. When differences are found between ideators and parasuicides, the ideators are generally more disturbed than the parasuicides across a number of variables. As noted above, these studies generally focus on individuals who have come to professional attention because of their suicide ideation. Thus, the individuals had to communicate the ideation. It is unclear whether the population under study might more appropriately be labeled suicide threateners. Several studies, however, have found that suicides to a greater extent than parasuicides threaten or communicate suicide intent before their action. Thus, the overlap between suicide ideation and suicide may be greater than that between ideation and parasuicide.

THE CASE FOR THE SINGLE-POPULATION THEORY: OVERLAPPING POPULATIONS

The between-group differences described above are relatively noncontroversial. A single-population theory, therefore, cannot be based on a premise that *all* parasuicides are drawn from the same population as suicides. It can be derived, however, on a contention that *some* parasuicides are. Within-group variability among parasuicides, as this group is typically defined, is much greater than among suicides. This greater heterogeneity is due to the classification under a single rubric (whether labeled parasuicide or suicide attempt) of quite disparate types of self-injurious behaviors. Thus, parasuicide vs. suicide differences are a result of the improper inclusion of many people into one parasuicide group. In other words, the parasuicide group itself consists of multiple populations lumped together (see FIGURE 3). This misclassification of many individuals into the parasuicide group, together with the correct classification of others, can account for the ambiguity of results across studies as well as the findings of consistent similarities and differences between the groups. Thus, while not all parasuicides come from the single population of suicides, a substantial subgroup does.

To demonstrate the validity of this point of view the following is required. First, one must show that in studies demonstrating differences between parasuicides and suicides the variability in the parasuicide sample is greater than in the corresponding suicide sample. Second, a reasonable way must be found to divide the parasuicide sample into more than one group who differ from each other in important ways. Third, the subgroup of parasuicides hypothesized to come from the suicide population must be shown to be more similar to suicides than are the other subgroups.

Within-Group Variability among Parasuicides and Suicides

To my knowledge, no analyses have been conducted comparing the heterogeneity among parasuicides to that among suicides. The most obvious difference is the variability in method lethality. All methods among suicides are at least capable of causing death. Among parasuicides, however, variability is much greater, ranging from light scratches on the wrist or a few medication tablets more than prescribed to behavior so lethal that avoidance of death is due to either accident or extensive medical intervention. Inclusion criteria are variable for both categories of behavior. A case can be made, however, for greater variability within parasuicide.

Inclusion Criteria

Douglas[19] lists six fundamentally independent but related dimensions used to define suicide.[19] In actuality, the definition is largely out of the control of the scientific community since classification is a legal rather than a scientific decision. Thus, the scientific study of individuals who suicide is limited by the particular decision rules used in one's community. There have been few attempts to compare what different individual officials mean by the term suicide or what inclusion and exclusion criteria they actually use.

The problems in defining suicide may be legion, but problems classifying nonfatal self-harm are a methodological nightmare. All investigators require at a minimum that the individual have some knowledge or belief that the activity engaged in poses a risk to life or health. Most investigators require the execution of an overt act that

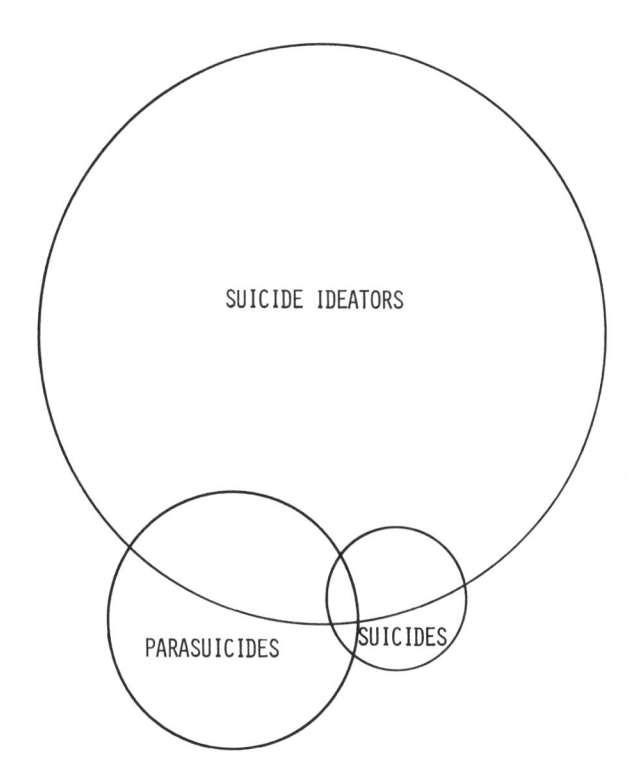

FIGURE 3. Overlapping populations.

is either believed to be or is potentially harmful. The primary definitional problems center around the role of deliberation and intent. Controversies have typically been framed in terms of the role of intent to die in defining parasuicide. In actuality, however, at least two other motivations are relevant: the intent to engage in the activity in question and the intent to incur harm. Investigators differ on how much intent they require to label the behavior suicidal. At one extreme, Dyer and Kreitman define parasuicide as "an act in which a person deliberately took a substance in excess of any prescribed or generally recognised therapeutic dosage . . . [including] . . . poisoning incidental to regular or experimental drug abuse."[20] Intent to perform the act is all that is required. At the other extreme, Silver et al. require a statement that the behavior was deliberately engaged in to terminate life.[21] At the midpoint, Fox and Weissman require at least *some* self-destructive intent.[22] As can be seen in FIGURE 4, the categories are progressively less inclusive. The problems in drawing comparative conclusions among studies with such diverse entrance restrictions are obvious. Kreitman and associates include all instances of drug poisoning with nontherapeutic drugs, including illegal recreational drugs but excluding alcohol. However, Petersen and Chambers, in a study of emergency room admissions for acute drug reactions, classified 47% as accidental;[23] 26% of the total involved toxic reactions to illegal street drugs, a category defined by Kreitman as parasuicide, even in the absence of any intent to incur self-harm.

Within-Group Classification Schemes for Parasuicides

If one contends that some suicides are misclassified as parasuicides due to the accident of living, then some way must be found to identify those individuals. A large number of studies have divided the sample according to the intensity of the suicidal behavior, defined by the suicidal intent accompanying the self-harm, the medical consequences or deadliness of the behavior, or a combination of the two. Common across studies is the tendency to categorize behaviors at the higher suicide intent or deadlier end of the continuum as more "serious" than behaviors at the other end. This is an unfortunate choice of terminology. Any time an individual is unhappy enough that deliberate, overt, acute self-harmful behavior results, the situation is serious indeed. Additionally, labeling self-destructive behavior as nonserious simply because the medical consequences are not as serious and/or intent to die is not high implies that the true importance of the behavior lies in its similarity to suicide.

There appears to be little or no consensus on how suicide intent should be measured. Some investigators rely on verbal responses to direct questions about suicide.[24-26] Many rely on Beck's Suicide Intent Scale (SIS) which includes a number of questions relating not only to the individual's self-reported intent, but also to the circumstances surrounding the act, the individual's expectations about outcome, desire to live or die, reasons for living, and so on. Some investigators rely on psychiatric opinion of suicide intent based on unspecified criteria. For example, Fox and Weissman state that "lack of intent was not assumed simply on the basis of patient's denial, absence of serious risk to life, or added manipulative elements [p. 32]."[22] Finally, many investigators use the medical consequences as an indirect measure of the individual's intent to die. The notion here is that the closer the person comes to actually dying, the more he or she actually intended to die. There is moderate empirical evidence for this proposition. In 12 studies where medical risk and intent to die were measured separately, a relationship between high risk and high intent was found in six. Four found no significant relationship and two did not report the relationship (see TABLE 1). If we assume that the failure to report the relationship indicates a greater probability of no relationship, then approximately half of the studies found a relationship and half did not. In all studies where a relationship was found, the direction was similar and positive, suggesting that a relationship does exist. The nonsignificant findings across many studies, however, suggest that the relationship is weak.

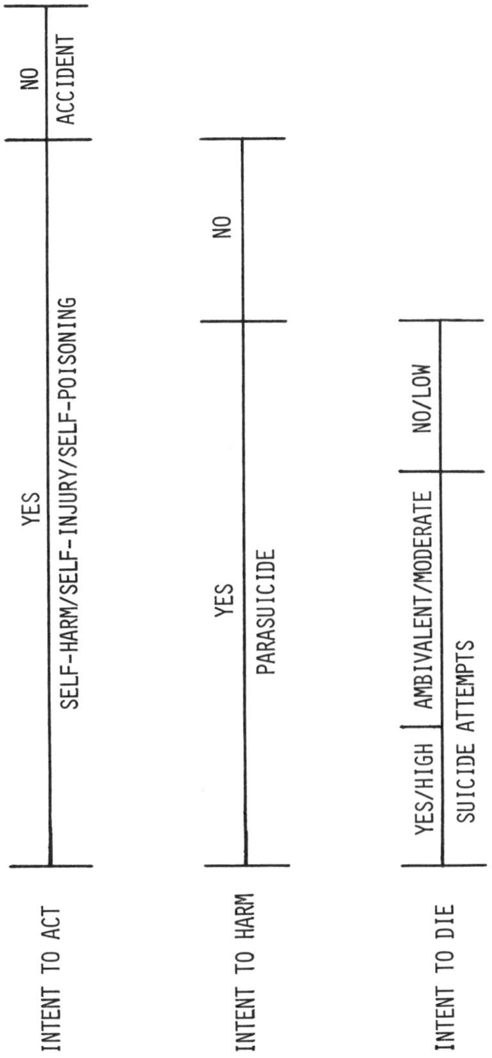

FIGURE 4. Nonfatal self-harm.

TABLE 1. Relationship between Lethality of Parasuicide and Individual Differences by Study[a]

Author	n	Rating	Level of Intensity (%) L	M	H	Age	Sex	Depression	Hopelessness	Diagnosis	Interpersonal Problems/Anger	Intent to Die	Time	FP	FS
Philadelphia General Hospital Group															
Beck et al.[27]	225GH	A	28	31	41	NR	NR	—	—	—	—	NS	—	—	—
Lester & Beck[3]	241GH	NR	←--NR--→			NR	NR	NS	NS	—	—	H>L	—	—	—
Lester et al.[5]												NS (ANOVA)			
Silver et al.[21]	45GH	A	73		27	NR	NR	NS	—	—	—	NR	—	—	—
Graylingwell Hospital (Sussex) Group															
Pallis & Barraclough[28]	46NR	C	continuous			NR	NR	—	—	—	—	—	—[b]	—	H>L
Pallis & Birtchnell[29]	84PR	C	42		42	NR	NR	NS	—	NS: diagnosis L>H: MMPI deviancy	NS: interpersonal problems L>H: hostility	—	—	—	—
Pallis & Sainsbury[30]	151GH	C	46	38	16	NR	NR	NR	NR	NR: symptoms	NR	H>L	—	—	—
Edinburgh Regional Poisoning Center															
Buglass & Horton[31]	1052ER	B	64	31	5	NR	NR	—	—	NR	NR	—	1 yr	NS	—
Kessell & McCulloch[32]	511ER	C	←--NR--→			NR	NR	—	—	NR	—	—	1 yr	—	—
Rosen[33]															
Rosen[34]	886ER	C	84		16	NR	NR	NR	NR	—	L>H: marital disharmony	NS	—	—	NS

Study		A	B				C							
University of Adelaide Group														
Goldney[35] Goldney[36] Goldney & Pilowsky[37]	110[c] ER	A	30	49			21	NR	—	NS	H > L	NS: psychiatric history NS: Axis I NS: Axis II	NS: violence	H > L	—	—
Other																
Birtchnell & Alarcon[24]	91 ER	B	42	33			25	NR	NS	—	—	—	NS	—	—
Card[38]	1640 CI	A	10	33	20	28	9	NR	—	—	—	—	—	1[d] yr	NS
Card reanalyzed (Pallis & Barraclough)[28]		C	50				50	NR	—	—	—	—	—	1[d] yr	H > L
Diekstra et al.[39]	171 GP	B	71				29	+	—	—	—	—	—	—	—
		A	56				40								
Garfinkel et al.[40]	505[c] ER	C	63	25			12	NR	—	—	—	H > L: symptoms NS: diagnosis	—	—	—
Fraser & Lawson[41]	246[f] ER	B	59	28	7	7	2	NR	—	—	—	—	NR	—	—
Gorenc et al.[42]	211 PR	C	←---NR---→					NR	NS	—	—	NS	—	0.48–0.58	—	—
Morgan et al.[25]	368 ER	B	←---NR---→					M < F	—	—	—	—	—	NR	—	—
Pierce[43]	500 GH	C	←---NR---→					M > F	—	—	—	—	—	H > L	—	—
Weiss et al.[44]	35 GH	C	43	31			26	NR	—	—	—	—	—	H > L	—	—

[a] A = degree of medical treatment required; B = level of coma; C = risk of death; L = low lethality; M = moderate lethality, H = high lethality; CI = city; ER = emergency room; FP = future parasuicide; FS = future suicide; GP = general practice; GH = general hospital; NR = results not reported by variable measured; PR = psychiatric referral; — = variable not measured, not relevant to study; NS = not significant; MMPI = Minnesota Multiphasic Personality Inventory.
[b] Retroactive, time unspecified.
[c] 18–30 year old females.
[d] Measured retroactively.
[e] Children.
[f] Only drug overdoses.

Comparisons between High- and Low-Intensity Parasuicides

After an extensive review of the literature, I located 52 studies where parasuicides of varying intensity were compared. The variables of most interest here would be those variables where differences have been found between parasuicides, as a whole, and suicides. As noted previously, those variables include age, sex, race, hostility/irritability, and diagnosis as well as method variability. Three variables—subsequent suicide, depression, and hopelessness—consistently measured in studies on intensity have not been shown to reliably discriminate parasuicides from suicides. Their inclusion in so many studies rests on the theoretical premise that either depression or hopelessness is the core defining characteristic of the suicidal population.

Results of each of the 52 studies are summarized by method of determining intensity in TABLES 1 to 4.[b] These tables are in turn summarized in TABLE 5. Results across studies lend themselves to tentative conclusions offered with much caution. Intensity appears to correlate positively with age. Fourteen of the studies report this finding; only 4 who report the analysis find no significant differences. Six studies report that males engage in more intense suicidal behavior than do females; 1 found a reverse pattern. Nine studies, however, report no significant differences. If there is a relationship, it is weak at best. Unfortunately, age and sex vs. intensity were not examined, or at least results were not reported, in over 34 studies. With the exception of one series of studies where all subjects were female, these analyses could have been conducted and reported. If the analyses were indeed carried out but nonsignificant results not reported, then the strength of the conclusions from those studies finding significant differences is reduced. Over a number of studies, significant differences could arise by chance. We would expect chance differences in 10%. However, one would also expect the differences to be equally distributed in both directions (i.e., between old vs. young, male vs. female). Such is not the case.

Examination of the psychological variables suggests that the strongest conclusion possible is that hopelessness is positively related to intensity of suicidal behavior. The ratio of significant to nonsignificant results in this direction is 3:1, and no study found a relationship in the opposite direction. A relationship between depression and intensity was also found in more studies than not, when analyses were reported. However, more often than not this relationship is mediated by the relationship between hopelessness and intensity. If there is a relationship between intensity and diagnosis, it appears that high-intense parasuicides are more often diagnosed as psychotic than are low-intense parasuicides. Unfortunately, it is impossible to ferret out how much the circumstances of the parasuicide had to do with the designation of psychosis, or how much the psychotic process interfered with the individuals' ability to give an accurate picture of intent at the time of the parasuicide. Interestingly, in contrast to popular opinion, evidence to date does not strongly confirm the notion that personality disorder is associated with low-intense parasuicides. Any conclusions here appear premature.

---

[b] When the authors provided the requisite data but not the statistical analyses, I performed the data analyses. Differences not achieving a significance level of at least $p < 0.05$ are reported as no significant difference found. This is in marked contrast to some reviews of the literature. It seems common in this field for original authors to note that a nonsignificant difference in a desired direction was found and then for the next person summarizing the study to ignore the fact that the findings were not significantly different from what could have arisen by chance. In my opinion, this practice is misleading and suggests a misunderstanding of scientific methodology. It seems to me that rather than less, we need more rigor in this field.

TABLE 2. Relationship between SIS and Individual Differences by Study[a]

Author	n	Age	Sex	Depression WO/H	Depression W/H	Hopelessness WO/D	Hopelessness W/D	Diagnosis	Interpersonal Problems/Anger	Intent to Die	Year	FP	NS
Philadelphia Hospital Group													
Beck et al.[45]	384GH	NS	—	0.30	NS	0.38	0.24	NR	—	0.48	—	—	—
Lester & Beck[4]	TABLE 1	—	—	—[b]	—	0.33	NR	—	NS: anger	H > L	—	—	—
Minkoff et al.[46]	68GH	—	—	0.26	NS	0.47	0.41	NS	—	NR	—	—	—
Silver et al.[21]	TABLE 1	NS	—	0.62	—	—	—	NS	—	NR	—	—	—
Graylingwell Hospital (Sussex) Group													
Pallis et al.[47]	1264ER	—	—	—	—	—	—	—	—	NR	1 yr	—	NS
											2 yr	—	H > L
Pallis & Jenkins[48]	151ER	—	—	—	—	—	—	—	NS: extraversion, sociability	H > L	—	—	—
Pallis & Sainsbury[30]	TABLE 1	—	—	NS	—	H > L	—	—	NS: social withdrawal, anger	—	—	—	—
Other													
Clum et al.[49]	47VA	—	—	—	—	—	—	NR	—	NR	—	—	—
Dyer & Krietman[20]	120ER	+	NS	0.43	NS	0.50[c]	0.32	—	—	NR	1	NS	—
Goldney[35]	TABLE 1	—	NS	NR	—	NR	—	—	—	NR	—	—	—
Hawton et al.[50]	50[d] GH	—	—	—	—	—	—	H > L: chronicity	NR	NR	—	—	—
Papa[51]	60GH	NS	NS	—	—	0.59	—	—	NS: interpersonal preferences	NR	—	—	—
Pokorny et al.[52]	55VA	—	—	0.52[e]	—	NS	—	—	—	NR	—	—	—
				0.39									
				0.02									
Kazdin[53]	11[f]ER	—	—	NS	—	0.35	0.31	—	—	NR	—	—	—

[a] WO/H = Without controlling for hopelessness; W/H = controlling for effects of hopelessness; See TABLE 1 for other abbreviations.
[b] Correlations were presented between SIS and subscales of the Beck Depression Scale. Results were comparable to those for full scale.
[c] Results held only for males over 34 years when sample stratified on age and sex.
[d] Adolescents.
[e] Correlation decreases from 0.52 to −0.02 as time between parasuicide and testing increases.
[f] Children.

TABLE 3. Relationship between Wanting to Die and Individual Differences by Study[a]

Author	n	Intensity (%) L	M	H	Age	Sex	Depression	Hopelessness	Diagnosis	Interpersonal Problems/Anger
Birtchnell & Alarcon[24]	TABLE 1	37	17	16	+	—	H>L	—	—	—
Comstock[54]	274ER	40	50	10	—	—	H>L	—	NR	—
Gorenc et al.[42]	TABLE 1	←--NR--→			—	—	H>L	—	—	—
Hawton et al.[55]	TABLE 2	91	9		+	—	—	—	H>L: chronicity	—
Lester et al.[5]	246ER	17	17	60	+	NS	H>L	H>L	NS: axis I NS: personality	NS: irritability
Kovacs et al.[26]	200ER	13	31	56	—	—	H>L	H>L	—	—
Morgan et al.[25]	TABLE 1	62	38		—	M>F	NR	—	NR	NR

[a] L = low, M = moderate, H = high; see TABLE 1 for other abbreviations.

TABLE 4. Relationship between Lethality plus Intent of Parasuicide and Individual Differences by Study[a]

Author	n	Level of Intensity (%) L	M	H	Age	Sex	Depression	Hopelessness	Diagnosis	Interpersonal Problems/Anger	Year	FP	FS
Dorpat & Boswell[56]	121GH	20	60	40	+	M>F	—	—	L>H: personality H>L: psychosis	—	—	—	—
Deykin et al.[57]	323ER[b]	52[c]	22	26	—	NS	—	—	—	—	4	NS[d]	—
Greer & Lee[58]	208GH	90		10	+		—	—	H>L: psychosis	—	2.5	—	NS[e]
Graham & Hitchens[59]	1736GH	11	24	27[f]	+	M>F	—	NR	NR	NR	—	—	—
McHugh & Goodell[60]	106GH	Continuous			+	—	H>L	—	H>L: depression L>H: personality	—	—	—	—
Motto[61]	193PR	16	38	26 20	NS	M<F	—	—	—	—	5-8	—	NS
Pierce[43]	TABLE 1				+	NS	—	—	H>L: chronicity	NS: antisocial	S	—	NS
Pierce[62]													
Pokorny[63]	252PR				—	—	—	—	—	NS: violence	4-6	—	NS
Rosen[33]	TABLE 1				+	NS	H>L	—	H>L: schizophrenia organic	L>H: marital problems	1	—	NS
Rosen[34] Rubenstein[64]	44ER	11 10 12	7	4	—	M>F	—	—	H>L: psychosis	L>H: marital problems, unrequited love	5	—	H>L
Schmidt et al.[65]	120ER	68		32	+	—	—	—	H>L: manic depression H>L: dementia	—	8 mo.	—	H>L
Weiss et al.[44]	TABLE 1	23 20	29	29	+	NS	H>L[g]	—	H>L: psychotic	L>H: family trouble	—	—	—
Weiss & Scott[66]	23GH				—	—	—	—	—	—	10	—	H>L

[a] See TABLE 1 for abbreviations.
[b] 13–17 year olds.
[c] Life-threatening behavior, includes risk-taking behavior.
[d] Intent of index parasuicide positively correlated with subsequent parasuicide.
[e] Serious parasuicides compared to unselected parasuicides.
[f] 36% were labeled accidents.
[g] Relationship lost when age controlled.

TABLE 5. Number of Studies Showing a Relationship between Degree of Intensity and Individual Difference[a]

Measures of Individual Difference	Measure of Intensity				
	Lethality (L)	SIS	Intent (I)	L+I	Total
Age					
+	2	2	2	8	14
NS	0	3	0	1	4
NR	19	17	5	3	34
Sex					
M < F	—	—	—	1	1
M > F	2	—	1	3	6
NS	1	3	1	4	9
NR	17	9	5	4	35
IR	1	—	—	—	1
Depression					
H > L	—	4-5	5	3	12-13
NS	6	2-3	0	0	8-9
NR	2	1	1	—	3
IR	13	4	1	9	27
Hopeless					
H > L	1	5-6	2	—	8-9
NS	1	1-2	0	—	2-3
NR	2	1	—	1	4
IR	17	4	5	11	37
Diagnosis					
H > L: psychosis	—	—	—	5	5
H > L: affective	—	—	—	2	2
H > L: personality	—	—	—	1	1
L > H: personality	—	—	—	1	1
NS	4	2	2	—	8
NR	3	2	2	—	7
IR	14	7	3	3	27
Interpersonal Problems/Anger					
L > H	2	—	—	3	5
NS	2	4	1	2	9
NR	5	—	2	1	8
IR	12	9	4	8	33
Future Parasuicide					
NS	1	1	—	1	3
IR	20	11	7	11	49
Future Suicide					
H > L	2	2 (2-5 yr)	—	3	7
NS	2	1 (1 yr)	—	5	8
IR	18	10	7	4	38

[a] IR = irrelevant, not measured in study.

Of great interest has been the relationship between intensity of an index parasuicide and the occurrence of future parasuicide and suicide. If high-intense parasuicides are in actuality members of the suicide population, then one might expect them to have a higher incidence of future suicide than do low-intense parasuicides. Conversely, one would expect low-intensity parasuicides to have a higher incidence of subsequent parasuicide than do high-intensity parasuicides. With respect to the latter hypothesis, supportive evidence is completely nonexistent. The 3 studies that conducted a follow-up for parasuicide report no significant differences between high- and low-intensity parasuicides on subsequent behavior. With respect to future suicide, the results are more ambiguous and somewhat controversial. Of the 15 follow-up studies found, 7 reported a higher suicide incidence for high-intensity parasuicides. Eight found no significant difference. In contrast to other variables, everyone who did a follow-up reported their results. It seems that the safest conclusion would be that the intensity of parasuicide is weakly related to the tendency to suicide at a later date.

CONCLUSION

The data presented here support the conclusion that parasuicides, broadly defined, are heterogeneous and represent more than one population of individuals who can be discriminated in terms of the intensity of the parasuicidal act. Furthermore, these differences are congruent with the hypothesis that the high-intensity parasuicide group, where intent to die and medical risk are significant, consists of individuals drawn from either the suicide population or one substantially overlapping it. These conclusions are extremely tentative. The policy across much of the suicidal literature of providing ambiguous definitions for the behavior in question, mixing groups of varying intensity together in one analysis, failing to report important analyses, especially those for sex, age, and race, together with the terminological obfuscation that characterizes much of the field, makes firm conclusions extremely difficult to come by. Until we reach some consensus on category definitions to describe our subject matter, agree on usual labels, report all relevant analyses, and include measurements that would test the generality of previous findings, progress will be slow. Further, because large numbers of subjects exhibiting suicidal behavior are hard to come by, we must do better at including relevant comparison groups in each and every study.

REFERENCES

1. STENGEL, E., N. COOK & R. I. KREEGER. 1958. Attempted Suicide. Maudsley Monograph No. 4. Chapman & Hall. London, England.
2. KREITMAN, N., Ed. 1977. Parasuicide. John Wiley & Sons. London, England.
3. LESTER, D. & A. T. BECK. 1975. J. Clin. Psychol. **31:** 11-12.
4. LESTER, D. & A. T. BECK. 1980-81. Omega **11**(3): 271-277.
5. LESTER, D., A. T. BECK & L. TREXLER. 1975. J. Abnorm. Psychol. **84**(5): 563-566.
6. WEISS, J. M. A.. 1966. The suicidal patient. *In* American Handbook of Psychiatry. S. Arieti, Ed. **3:** 115-130. Basic Books. New York, N.Y.
7. FARMER, R. D. T. 1980. The relationship between suicide and parasuicide. *In* The Suicide Syndrome. R. Farmer & S. Hirsch, Eds.: 19-35. Croom Helm. London, England.

8. LINEHAN, M. A. 1981. A social-behavioral analysis of suicide and parasuicide implications for clinical assessment and treatment. *In* Depression: Behavioral and Directive Intervention Strategies. H. G. Glazer & J. F. Clarkin, Eds.: 229-294. Garland Press. New York, N.Y.
9. PALLIS, D. J., B. M. BARRACLOUGH, A. B. LEVEY, J. S. JENKINS & P. SAINSBURY. 1982. Br. J. Psychiatry **141**: 37-44.
10. POKORNEY, A. D. 1983. Arch. Gen. Psychiatry **40**: 249-257.
11. PAYKEL, E. S., J. K. MYERS, J. J. LINDENTHAL & J. TANNER. 1974. Br. J. Psychiatry **124**: 460-469.
12. SCHWAB, J. J., G. J. WARHEIT & C. E. HOLZER III. 1972. Dis. Nerv. Syst. (Nov.): 745-748.
13. FOWLER, R. C., M. T. TSUANG & Z. KRONFOL. 1979. J. Affect. Disorders. **1**: 219-225.
14. MEYERS, E. D. 1982. Br. J. Psychiatry **140**: 132-137.
15. MARKS, P. & D. L. HALLER. 1977. J. Clin. Psychol. **33**(2): 390-400.
16. LINDHAN, M. A., J. A. CHILES, K. J. EGAN, R. H. DEVINE & J. A. LAFFAW. J. Consult. Clin. Psychol. (In press.)
17. LINEHAN, M. A., P. CAMPER, J. A. STILES, K. STROSAHL & E. SHEARIN. J. Cog. Ther. Res. (In press.)
18. LINEHAN, M. L., J. L. GOODSTEIN, S. L. NIELSEN & J. A. CHILES. 1983. J. Consult. Clin. Psychol. **51**(2): 276-286.
19. DOUGLAS, J. D. 1967. The Social Meaning of Suicide. Princeton University Press. Princeton, N.J.
20. DYER, J. A. T. & N. KRIETMAN. 1984. Br. J. Psychiatry. **144**: 127-133.
21. SILVER, M. A., M. BOHNERT, A. T. BECK & D. MARCUS. 1971. Arch. Gen. Psychiatry **25**(Dec.): 573-576.
22. FOX, K. & M. WEISSMAN. 1975. Soc. Psychiatry **10**: 31-38.
23. PETERSONN, C. M. & C. D. CHAMBERS. 1975. Int. J. Addictions **10**(6): 963-975.
24. BIRTCHNELL, J. & J. ALARCON. 1971. Br. J. Psychiatry **118**: 289-96.
25. MORGAN, H. G., C. J. BURNS-COX, H. POCOCK & S. POTTLE. 1975. Br. J. Psychiatry **127**: 564-574.
26. KOVACS, M., A. T. BECK & A. WEISSMAN. 1975. Am. J. Psychother. **29**: 363-368.
27. BECK, A. T., R. BECK & M. KOVACS. 1975. Am. J. Psychiatry **123**(3): 285-287.
28. PALLIS, D. J. & B. M. BARRACLOUGH. 1977. Omega **8**(2): 141-149.
29. PALLIS, D. J. & J. BIRTCHNEL. 1977. Br. J. Psychiatry **130**: 253-259.
30. PALLIS, D. J. & P. SAINSBURY. 1976. Psychol. Med.: 6487-6492.
31. BUGLASS, D. & J. HORTON. 1974. Br. J. Psychiatry **125**: 168-174.
32. KESSELL, N. & W. MCCULLOCH. 1966. Proc. R. Soc. Med. **59**: 89-95.
33. ROSEN, D. H. 1970. Am. J. Psychiatry **127**(6): 764-770.
34. ROSEN, D. H. 1976. J. Am. Med. Assoc. **235**(19): 2105-2109.
35. GOLDNEY, R. D. 1981. Br. J. Psychiatry **139**: 382-390.
36. GOLDNEY, R. D. 1981. Br. J. Psychiatry **138**: 1141-1146.
37. GOLDNEY, R. D. & I. PILKOWSKY. 1980. Austr. New Zealand J. Psychiatry **14**: 203-211.
38. CARD, J. J. 1974. Omega **5**(1): 37-45.
39. DIEKSTRA, R. F. W., A. C. DE GRAAF & M. VAN EGMOND. 1983. On the epidemiology of attempted suicide: a sample-survey study among general practicioners. *In* Depression et Suicide: 69-81. Pergamon Press. Paris, France.
40. GARFINKEL, B. D., A. FROESE & J. HOOD. 1982. Am. J. Psychiatry **139**(10): 1257-1261.
41. FRASER, D. M. & A. A. H. LAWSON. 1975. Health Bull. **33**: 97-101.
42. GORENC, K. D., F. KLEFF & R. WELZ. 1983. Intentionality and seriousness of suicide attempts in relation to depression. *In* Depression et Suicide: 566-570. Pergamon Press. Paris, France.
43. PIERCE, D. W. 1977. Br. J. Psychiatry **130**: 377-385.
44. WEISS, J. M. A., N. NUNEZ & K. W. SCHAIE. 1961. Quantification of certain trends in attempted suicide. *In* 3rd World Congress of Psychiatry **2**: 1236-1240. University of Toronto Press & McGill University Press. Montreal, Canada.
45. BECK, A. T., M. KOVACS & A. WEISSMAN. 1975. J. Am. Med. Assoc. **234**(11): 1146-1149.
46. MINKOFF, K., E. BERGMAN, A. BECK & R. BECK. 1973. Am. J. Psychiatry **130**(4): 455-459.
47. PALLIS, D. J., J. S. GIBBONS & D. W. PIERCE. 1984. Br. J. Psychiatry **144**: 139-148.

48. PALLIS, D. J. & J. S. JENKINS. 1977. Psychol. Rep. **41:** 19-22.
49. CLUM, G., L. LUSCOMB & A. T. PATSIOKAS. J. Clin. Psychol. (In press.)
50. HAWTON, K., M. OSBORN, J. O'GRADY & D. COLE. 1982. Br. J. Psychiatry **130:** 124-131.
51. PAPA, L. L. 1980. Nursing Res. **29**(6): 362-369.
52. POKORNEY, A. D., H. B. KAPLAN & S. Y. TSAI. 1975. Am. J. Psychiatry **132**(9): 954-956.
53. KAZDIN, J. E., N. H. FRENCH, A. S. UNIS, K. ESVELDT-DAWSON & R. B. SHERICK. 1983. J. Consult. Clin. Psychol. **51**(4): 504-510.
54. COMSTOCK, B. 1973. Low intentionality suicide attempts. *In* Proceedings of the Seventh International Congress on Suicide Prevention: 385-395. Swetts and Zeitlinger B.V. Amsterdam, Holland.
55. HAWTON, K., J. O'GRADY, M. OSBORN & D. COLE 1982. Br. J. Psychiatry **140:** 118-123.
56. DORPAT, T. L. & J. W. BOSWELL. 1963. Compr. Psychiatry **4**(2): 117-125.
57. DEYKIN, E. Y., R. PERLOW & J. MCNAMARRA. 1985. Am. J. Public Health **75**(1): 90-92.
58. GREER, S. & H. A. LEE. 1967. Acta Psychiatr. Scand. **43:** 361-371.
59. GRAHAM, J. D. P. & R. A. N. HITCHENS. 1967. Br. J. Prev. Soc. Med. **21:** 108-114.
60. MCHUGH, P. R. & H. GOODELL. 1971. Arch. Gen. Psychiatry **25:** 456-464.
61. MOTTO, J. A. 1965. Arch. Gen. Psychiatry **13:** 516-520.
62. PIERCE, D. W. 1981. Br. J. Psychiatry **139:** 391-396.
63. POKORNEY, A. D. 1966. Am. J. Psychiatry **112:** 1109-1116.
64. RUBENSTEIN, R., B. MOSES & T. LIDZ. 1958. AMA Arch. Neurol. Psychiatry **79:** 103-112.
65. SCHMIDT, E. H., P. O'NEAL & E. ROBINS. 1954. J. Am. Med. Assoc. **155**(6): 549-57.
66. WEISS, J. M. A. & K. F. SCOTT. 1974. Compr. Psychiatry **15**(2): 165-171.

Statistical Approaches to Suicidal Risk Factor Analysis

JACOB COHEN

Department of Psychology
New York University
6 Washington Place, Room 550
New York, New York 10003

The prediction of suicide using psychosocial risk factors has proven to be an unusually difficult one for two main reasons: the very low base rate (prevalence) of suicide and the difficulties attendant upon case finding.[1]

Even the most suicide prone populations (past attempters, depressives, schizophrenics) have prevalence rates no greater than 1% or 2% per year.[2] A high-risk group may have odds of committing suicide 30 or 40 times that of a control group (odds ratio), or a suicide rate 10 to 20 times higher (relative risk), so we are assured that there is some real validity underlying the prediction. Yet the base rate problem renders even this degree of discrimination of little practical predictive value. To appreciate the severity of this problem, consider a hypothetical superpredictor, one with 90% sensitivity and 90% specificity, which results in an odds ratio of 81. Now assume that it is used in a population with a 1% suicide rate. It turns out that the false-positive rate of our superpredictor comes to 92% (or, equivalently, its predictive value is 8%). This means that if we could mobilize the resources to screen 10,000 cases with our superpredictor, we would identify 1080 predicted suicides of whom 990 would be false positives. Expressed as a correlation coefficient (phi), our superpredictor's validity is 0.256; expressed as the percent of correctly predicted outcomes corrected for chance (i.e., kappa), it is 0.137. And this modest degree of association is statistically significant in a sample with as few as 60 cases!

Incomplete case finding for suicides and suicide attempts because of the lack of central registries and concealment further complicates research in suicidality.[1,3] With error in the outcome to be predicted, the validity of the predictor is necessarily underestimated. Matters here are made even worse by the likely interaction of predictors with inadequacy in case finding. For example, a stockbroker's suicidal attempt is more likely to be concealed than that of an unemployed dishwasher.

Neither of these problems has a statistical solution. Means for improving case finding must be implemented to purify the predictive criterion,[3] while substantial improvement in predictor validity will likely require research in other data domains, e.g., the biological.

Although the major problems in suicide research are not statistical, a sampling of the literature quickly reveals frequent errors in the choice and interpretation of statistical procedures whose consequences are not trivial. These include capitalization on chance in the selection of predictors, failure to cross-validate, failure to distinguish the statistical significance of a prediction from its magnitude, and ignoring the causal structure of the predictors.

CAPITALIZATION ON CHANCE

A frequent suicide research paradigm is borrowed from traditional item-analytic test construction methodology. The investigator begins with a sizable list of putative predictive elements (n in number) and applies them to cases of known suicidality and appropriate controls. The two groups are then compared, and the k items that yield a statistically significant difference at the 5% level (or almost do) are harvested as demonstrably valid. These are then applied to the original data as a checklist, with the number of indicators used as a suicidality score. The two groups are contrasted, and a cut-off score is found that yields an optimum combination of sensitivity and specificity; the latter are then offered as characteristic of that cut-off score.

Note first that it is statistically naive to accept on its face the validity of the k items. Some number m of the n original items are not truly valid, so an expected 0.05 m items are among the k items harvested. These rotten apples are indistinguishable from the truly valid items, but do not spoil the barrel unless m is large relative to n, which is not usually likely to be the case. Yet however many such items there are, they do constitute deadwood in the score.

A more serious problem with this procedure is that the application of the k items to the data that were the basis of their selection capitalizes on the chance factors that contributed to their selection. Not only is there the 0.05 m deadwood, but on the average the validities of the selective items found in the sample are overestimates of their true (population) values and their values in other samples. This error is further compounded by the fact that the optimal cut-off score also capitalizes on chance, and is therefore likely to overestimate the sensitivity and specificity it will yield in future samples.

The solution for this problem has long been known in psychometrics: cross-validation. One can determine the performance of the score and its cut-off, both determined from the sample in hand, on a new sample drawn from the same population. The new validity results, although subject to sampling error, are not subject to the positive bias of the original procedure.

Note that this difficulty is not solved by using more complex item selection procedures. Least-squares procedures such as multiple regression or discriminant function analysis provide weights to use in the combination of items into a score, but they are subject to the same positive bias due to capitalization on chance. Although these procedures come with means for estimating the amount of "shrinkage" that can be expected to occur on cross-validation, they make frequently untenable distribution assumptions leaving as the only reliable procedure an actual cross-validation on new data.

STATISTICAL SIGNIFICANCE AND DEGREE OF VALIDITY

Although the distinction between statistical and "practical" significance is ingrained in the consciousness of social scientists during the course of their graduate training, the scientific literature they produce frequently betrays lapses in their appreciation of this distinction. The suicide risk factor literature is apparently particularly subject to such lapses. It is well known to researchers that in a large enough sample, even the smallest degree of relationship will prove to be statistically significant. Because of the low base rate in suicide research, relatively large sample sizes are usually employed in order to obtain enough cases for study. Yet many articles in the literature conscientiously offer significance test results (often with several zeros in their p values), but supply misleading or inadequate information about the degree of validity obtained.

The percent agreement between prediction and outcome is misleading if it is not corrected for chance.[4] For the superpredictor described above, the observed proportion of agreement between prediction and outcome is 0.90 which, corrected for chance (i.e., kappa), is 0.137. Correcting proportion of agreement for chance always reduces its value, but the large discrepancy here reflects the insidious operation of the low base rate.

Sensitivity and specificity and their resultant odds ratio are useful indicators of the degree of validity, but they are designed to be independent of the base rate, so may be misleading as to their practical utility in prediction. Correlation coefficients, kappas, and relative risks are all dependent on the base rate. Now, if the data are gathered in such a way as to misrepresent the base rate, all these validity measures can be quite misleading. Consider a paradigm in which items are selected using a data base in which there are as many control cases as suicides. With our superpredictor's 90% sensitivity, 90% specificity, and an odds ratio of 81 in this sample, the correlation coefficient (phi) is now 0.799, and the chance-corrected proportion of agreement (kappa) is 0.800! (Compare these with the original values of 0.256 and 0.137, respectively, for a 1% base rate.) These spectacular values are the misleading result of having implicitly falsified the base rate as 50% by using equal numbers of cases in the two groups. It is not necessary to raise the sample base rate to as much as 50% to obtain impressive but misleading results. Had this research had a control group three times as large as the suicide group, hence a sample base rate of 25%, with the same sensitivity and specificity, phi would be found to equal 0.755 and kappa 0.750. Even for a sample base rate of 10%, phi is 0.624 and kappa 0.590.

What if we employ more reasonable validity specifications than those of our superpredictor? Let us posit more attainable values for a set of psychosocial risk factors of 50% sensitivity and 90% specificity,[2] which produce an odds ratio of 9. Using the very high suicide rate of 2% per year (higher than that of the highest risk group—psychiatric patients admitted for a suicide attempt),[2] one finds that phi equals 0.180 and kappa 0.126. But given samples of equal size, these specifications produce values for phi of 0.436 and kappa 0.400; for a sample size ratio of 1:3, phi equals 0.433 and kappa 0.428. Even for a sample size ratio of 1:9, the resulting phi of 0.345 and kappa of 0.339 are much higher than the 0.180, 0.126 values that the 2% rate would produce.

Again it should be noted that the use of more complex measures of association (e.g., multiple correlation) or variables with more information (scales rather than dichotomies) will not overcome the bias produced by unrepresentative base rates.

The combination of statistical significance assured by large sample sizes and insufficiently reported or biased measures of validity is deadly.

IGNORING THE CAUSAL STRUCTURE OF PREDICTORS

An investigator finds in a given research on suicidality that age, sex, marital status, social class, and employment status (among others) significantly relate to the outcome and reports them as risk factors for the population studied. When he then combines them into a predictive score he will have, in the latter, a "valid" measure, but is not likely to further our understanding of the phenomenon under study. Is marital status as such a contributory cause to the outcome or is it merely a surrogate for age? Similarly, is unemployment causal or is it merely an indication of the operation of social class?

The epidemiologist takes it for granted that rates generally need to be age and possibly sex adjusted to be usefully understood. The reason for this is that age and sex are fundamental, i.e., causally prior, variables whose operation must be taken into account in studying other putative causes. Similarly, the psychologist knows age must be partialled from the relationship between weight and sexual interest in elementary school boys to avoid the mistaken conclusion that fat boys are lovers.

Quite generally, then, to invoke an old saw, correlation does not mean causation. The fact that A and B are correlated with S does not necessarily mean that they both contribute to the causality of S. They may, but there are several other possibilities. For example, A may cause both B and S with B having no causal effect whatever on S. This latter circumstance nevertheless results in B being correlated with S, since they share the variation induced by A's causality. In the absence of information about the relationship between A and B, however, it is impossible to determine that B is not causally related to S, i.e., that their observed relationship is "spurious." When the epidemiologist "adjusts" S for A(ge), she literally revises S in such a way as to render it unrelated to A, and therefore unrelated to B and any other variable whose relationship to S is a spurious consequence of its dependence on A. In a correlation analytic framework, the same goal is accomplished by partialling A from S. With multiple predictor variables, it is possible to partial more than one variable, or, more generally, to employ multiple regression/correlation (MRC) analysis to distinguish true from spurious causal effects.

Another possibility when A and B are correlated with S is that neither of them causes S. This will occur when some other variable C which is outside the purview of the analyst and not included in the analysis causes A, B, and S. As before, this state of affairs results in A and B being (spuriously) correlated with S. (In causal analysis, this problem is identified as "unmeasured common causes.")

Before describing the proper application of MRC, I offer a critique of the misapplication in suicide research of this technique.

MRC may be employed in two quite different ways. It has traditionally been used for the purpose of forecasting the value of some future "dependent" variable from values of two or more currently available "independent" variables, i.e., literally for prediction. Recently, it has come into use as a general data-analytic system employed primarily for the understanding of the workings of phenomena.[5] Forecasting is a technological function while understanding a scientific one. To be sure, these functions are not unrelated, and each may contribute to the other, but they are nevertheless distinct.

Simultaneous Multiple Regression Analysis

The investigator with a batch of k potential predictor variables and an outcome S (committed or attempted suicide) may reject the procedure of harvesting those variables that are significantly correlated with S for use as a checklist set of risk factors as described above in favor of employing MRC. There are several pitfalls in his path.

He may do an ordinary MRC, regressing the k predictors simultaneously on S, and obtain regression coefficients for the predictors and a multiple correlation coefficient (R). The regression coefficients are optimal weights that, when applied to the values of the predictors and summed, produce a predicted S score that yields the largest possible correlation with the actual S; R is that correlation.

Now he is likely to find that several, possibly many, of the weights are not significant, particularly so if k is large relative to n (say, 0.1 or 0.2). This may be for several reasons. One is that some predictors are redundant—although they may be correlated with S, they are simply duplicating outcome-relevant information that other predictors are supplying. (The weights are *partial* regression coefficients reflecting "net" information.) Redundancy also has the effect of increasing the instability of all the results and thus reducing their computed statistical significance. Another reason for nonsignificant weights may be the psychometric unreliability of the predictors (often the case for ratings, clinical diagnoses, and short scales). Yet another reason may be that the sample size is too small to provide statistical power that is adequate to the task, given k and the level and pattern of correlation involved.[6]

The investigator may now purge the regression equation of the predictors whose weights are nonsignificant and offer the remainder as a prediction tool. Alternatively, he may recompute the regression equation for the surviving variables and provide new weights and a new R. In either case, he has capitalized on chance to some degree (as already noted). The final weights will not perform as well on a new sample as they did on the data from which they were generated.

Stepwise Multiple Regression Analysis

A popular form of MRC is called "stepwise" regression analysis. It proceeds by selecting from the k predictors the one with the largest correlation with S. It then pairs each of the $k-1$ remaining predictors in turn with the first and finds the one that produces the largest R. It continues by searching through the remaining $k-3$ for the one that most increases R, etc. The process is usually designed to end when none of the remaining variables "significantly" increases R. They are discarded, and the regression equation for the h selected predictors is offered as optimal.

Assume that our investigator uses this most seductive procedure, which seems to attain the maximum R with a minimum of relevant predictors. With the typically large k, the program has performed k significance tests in the first step, $k-1$ in the second, $k-2$ in the third, etc., and finally $k-h$ in the final step. This works out to a total of $kh-h(h-1)/2$ significance tests. Readers are invited to substitute their ideas of plausible values for k and h, but with the typically large values of k used in suicide research, the number of statistical tests is likely to be enormous. (For example, with a set of 40 predictor items from which 5 are selected by stepwise regression, the number of tests is 190.) Now, each of these tests proceeds in blissful ignorance of the typically large number of other such tests being simultaneously performed on the other competing predictors. The consequence is a serious capitalization on chance which renders invalid both the significance tests performed on the predictors and on the R at each step.

Furthermore, when there are two or more variables that differ trivially in the amount by which they would increase R, the program dutifully selects the best for the sample in hand, but of course not necessarily the one that would be selected in the population or in other samples. This problem is further compounded when the competing variables are redundant, i.e., materially correlated with each other, for then the nonselected variables are likely to be never selected, leaving the mistaken impression that they are not relevant to prediction. The bottom line is that neither the predictors selected for the final equation nor their order of selection, nor the magnitude of R (which is likely to be grossly overstated) can be relied upon as descriptive of the true state of affairs. Substantive interpretation of stepwise results is therefore particularly hazardous.

Whatever utility resides in either simultaneous or stepwise MRC as described above is its use in empirical prediction. When employed judiciously they may yield optimal recipes for forecasting. But neither is a tool for generating optimal scientific understanding on the phenomena represented by the data.

It should be noted that the strictures on simultaneous and stepwise MRC as described above hold also when the outcome is a categorical variable and discriminant function analysis is employed, since the methods are essentially equivalent.

One of the problems in the above research scenario is the use of a multiplicity of predictor *items*. However employed, MRC pays a price in power and stability as the number of predictors increases. Items are inherently unreliable in the psychometric sense so they relate weakly to S, and groups of items that reflect the same construct are the source of the redundancy that plagues MRC.

The solution to this problem is to identify these item groups and combine them into scales or indices. This process may be accomplished empirically (by factor or cluster analysis) or a priori, in any case independent of their correlations with S. This has the salutary effects of reducing the number of predictors, increasing their reliability, and reducing the redundancy among them. It also facilitates the interpretation of the results.

Hierarchical Multiple Regression

A form of MRC that takes into account the causal structure of the predictor variables and is therefore a scientific rather than a technological predictive tool is setwise hierarchical MRC.[5]

A "set" is a group of one or more variables that defines a research factor, for example, socioeconomic status, psychiatric history, education, and sex. It is possible in hierarchical MRC to represent categorical variables (e.g., diagnosis, marital status) or nonlinearly related variables (e.g., age, annual income) as sets as well.

In setwise hierarchial MRC, one orders the putative causal research factors in a hierarchy of hypothetical causal priority: the order of precedence is such that one is prepared to assume that no factor coming later in the series can causally effect one coming earlier. Thus, with S as the dependent or outcome variable, if the research factors, in order, are A, B, C, and D, then it is being assumed for example that neither C nor D can cause A or B and that D cannot cause C.

The squared multiple R (RSQ) in MRC may be interpreted as the proportion of the variance in the dependent variable (S) accounted for by the independent variables. The procedure is to perform a series of MRC analyses relating S first to A, then to

A and B, then to A, B, and C, etc. With each added research factor, one can determine the increment in the proportion of variance it accounts for by simply noting the increase in the RSQ from the previous level. Because of the presumed causal priority of the ordering, the increment due to the current research factor cannot be attributed to the previous factors, but must be a consequence of its unique casual effect on S. In a word, the procedure at each level *partials out* the causal effects of the preceding variables.

A simple example illustrates the logic. Assume that A is age, B is sex, C is marital status, and D is employment status. When C is added to A and B, the increment in the RSQ reflects the effect on S of marital status as such and not indirectly that of age or sex, since to the extent that age and sex have causal effects on S they are reflected in the RSQ for A and B; the increment due to C cannot be attributed to them. Similarly, the increment due to D can only reflect employment status as such and neither age, nor sex, nor marital status.

The size and statistical significance of these increments inform us of the causal relevance of each of the research factors provided that we have included all the materially relevant causes and in proper order. The omission of a factor that causes S and one of the factors included (e.g., the omission of a relevant biological factor) will mislead us about the included factor's causal effect. We would be similarly misled if we had placed C before A and B in the hierarchy.

The analytic yield from each of the MRCs in the series includes more than the RSQ attained at that level and its increment. Recall that each research factor is a set of one or more variables. The regression equation at each level includes the weights (partial regression coefficients) of the variables that make up that set, and their size and statistical significance are informative about these constituents.[5] For example, one of the constituents in the A research factor may carry information about the degree of curvilinearity in the relationship between age and S. As another example, one of the variables in the C set may effect a contrast between married/living with spouse and the other marital categories combined.[5] Note that all the variables in the equation are partialled from each of these.

MRC is a very powerful analytic tool with capabilities beyond those noted so far. The most important of these is the possibility of representing conditional relationships among research factors. Whatever may be the overall causal effects of age (A) and marital status (C), the possibility exists that the causal effects of marital status on S are conditional on age, i.e., that they vary across the age span. (In the analysis of variance such relationships are called "interactions.") Such conditional relationships can be modeled and represented as research factors in hierarchical MRC, and their causal effects assessed.[5]

In summary, setwise hierarchical MRC capitalizes on the analytic power of MRC in a context in which the causal relationships among the research factors are taken into account, thus facilitating an understanding of the phenomenon under study. It seems an ideal analytic tool for suicide research.

More complex causal theories that posit specific causal relationships among research factors require causal models analysis, a more advanced methodology with origins in plant genetics (path analysis) and econometrics (structural equation models) which has been under active development during the past two decades. This methodology seeks to provide the kind of mathematical and logical rigor to the analysis of observational data that has characterized the traditional experimental method. As suicide theory develops, the role of causal models is likely to increase. An exposition of this complex area is, however, beyond the scope of this paper. Accessible introductions are provided by Kenny,[7] Blalock,[8] and Cohen and Cohen.[5]

SUMMARY AND CONCLUSIONS

Suicide research is a particularly difficult area primarily because of the base rate problem and inadequate case finding. Traditional item-analytic and multiple regression or discriminant function data-analytic methods in suicide research are criticized on several technical grounds, including capitalization on chance, failure to cross-validate, and confusion of the degree of relationship with its statistical significance. These errors are further confounded when the research data base misrepresents the very low true base rate. However, the most serious defect in item-analytic and both conventional and stepwise multiple regression procedures is their failure to take into account the causal structure of suicide risk factors.

Setwise hierarchical multiple regression/correlation analysis is offered as an effective tool for suicide research. It capitalizes on the powerful general data-analytic features of regression analysis, but does so in a way that represents the causal structure of the putative risk factors. The more complex methods of causal models analysis are also recommended.

I do not believe, however, that progress in the understanding of suicide lies mainly in the improvement of the statistical procedures employed. Even with optimal procedures, the amount by which we can expect to increase the predictability of suicidality using psychosocial risk factors is not likely to be large. Recent research in the biochemistry of suicide offers some hope. If to the psychosocial factors now employed we can add relevant biological factors and their interactions with psychosocial factors, we may be able to develop the causal models necessary for the understanding, prediction, and prevention of suicide.

REFERENCES

1. WEISSMAN, M. M. 1974. The epidemiology of suicide attempts, 1960 to 1971. Arch. Gen. Psychiatry **30:** 737-746.
2. POKORNY, A. D. 1983. Prediction of suicide in psychiatric patients. Arch. Gen. Psychiatry **40:** 249-257.
3. WHITEHEAD, P. C., F. G. JOHNSON & R. FERRENCE. 1973. Measuring the incidence of self-injury: some methodological and design considerations. Am. J. Orthopsychiatry **43**(1): 142-148.
4. COHEN, J. 1960. A coefficient of agreement for nominal scales. Educ. Psychol. Measurement **20:** 37-46.
5. COHEN, J. & P. COHEN. 1983. Applied Multiple Regression/Correlation Analysis for the Behavioral Sciences. 2nd edit. Lawrence Erlbaum Associates. Hillsdale, N.J.
6. COHEN, J. 1977. Statistical Power Analysis for the Behavioral Sciences. Rev. edit. Academic Press. New York, N.Y.
7. KENNY, D. A. 1979. Correlation and Causality. Wiley-Interscience. New York, N.Y.
8. BLALOCK, H. M., JR., Ed. 1971. Causal Models in the Social Sciences. Aldine-Atherton. Chicago, Ill.

Ethical Considerations in Biological Research on Suicide

BARBARA STANLEY

*Department of Psychology
John Jay College of Criminal Justice
City University of New York
445 West 59th Street
New York, New York 10019*

and

*Department of Psychiatry
College of Physicians and Surgeons
Columbia University
722 West 168th Street
New York, New York 10032*

While suicide has been the subject of hundreds of investigations, very little has been written about the special ethical considerations in conducting this research. This lack of attention seems to stem not from a lack of ethical issues in suicide research but from a widely held belief by researchers in the field that suicide is the manifestation of a psychological disturbance and ought to be prevented whatever ethical compromises have to be made. Consequently, little time has been spent weighing the various ethical values in this research. Lettieri has argued that while labeling "at risk" individuals can have untoward consequences in many types of research, with suicide research the predictive label of "potentially suicidal" may be justified because the benefits of preventing possible suicide outweigh the risks of being labeled.[1] He contrasts this label with the label of "drug addict," which he believes has a far more negative impact without the positive benefits.

The limited discussion of ethical issues in suicide research stands in contrast to the extensive discussions during the past two decades of the ethics of suicide itself. In 1971, Thomas Szasz wrote a landmark article on the ethics of suicide in which he describes suicide as an individual's desire for greater autonomy and as an expression of self control.[2] He further emphasized that suicide should not be viewed as an expression of a disease but rather a desire. Although Szasz frequently proposes an "antidisease" model of psychiatric disturbances, he by no means stands alone in this view of suicide. Many others in recent years have written on "rational" suicide particularly, although not exclusively, as a reasonable and acceptable response to a terminal or debilitating illness.[3] The conclusion is then generally drawn that it is ethically proper to permit an individual to commit suicide in certain circumstances.[4] This may serve as a reminder that while most may start with a basic assumption that suicide is an expression of a disease process and that it ought to be prevented, there are others in the field who do not at all share this point of view and would question the validity of a biological approach to suicide.

Because of the limited discussion of ethical issues in suicide research more attention is needed in this area. This paper will address ethical questions raised once the decision has been made that research on the biochemistry of suicide is important. The purpose of this discussion is to help investigators to anticipate what the dilemmas will be and to take them into consideration in the planning stages of the research rather than halfway through the research project or after the project is complete.

There appear to be three points in the research process on suicide at which ethical concerns are prominent. The first concerns the decision to conduct a piece of research. Are there certain types of suicide research that, even if the results are likely to be of great benefit in furthering knowledge, present such serious ethical problems that they should not be done at all or done only with significant constraints? The second point at which ethical concerns are raised is during the actual course of the research. What ethical issues have a direct impact on the participants in the research? How do these issues intermingle with the integrity of the research design and the validity of the results? The third point of concern is the long-term consequences of positive findings, with respect to biological factors in suicide. In other words, what happens if the research is successful and a genetic marker that is associated with suicidal behavior can be identified with a high degree of certainty? Each of these areas warrants consideration by those choosing to do research in this area.

The first concern is the decision to conduct the research. With respect to the types of research to be done, one of the questions to be faced is the following. Are there certain research questions that are very important to answer but pose serious ethical dilemmas—so serious that some institutional review boards (IRBs) would not permit the potential risks to their patients? There are two types of studies that become increasingly likely to be conducted as positive findings on a biochemical link to suicide are amassed. The first type of study is a drug study designed to specifically target and diminish suicidal behavior. This would entail a wash-out period in which acutely suicidal patients would be maintained treatment free for usually a one- to two-week period. Is it justifiable to leave untreated the acutely suicidal patient for this period of time? If pharmacological treatments of suicidal behavior are to be found, some form of nontreatment—wash out—would have to be followed. While using other drug studies as models, for example, wash-out periods for antipsychotics using acutely ill schizophrenics, the imminent risk of death is not ordinarily present as it is with suicidal patients.

A second type of study which also poses an ethical concern is the use of biochemical probes to elicit suicidal behavior. This would be similar to the use of lactate infusions to elicit panic attacks[5] or amphetamines as a probe to study psychosis.[6] With suicidal behavior, it may be possible to elicit suicidal ideation using probes in patients who were not suicidal prior to the administration of the probe. In studying suicide, the case could be made that since the base rate is so low, elicitation of suicidality via probes may be more scientifically justified than other studies using probes. However, the ethical questions surrounding the induction of a suicidal state are serious. We are faced with balancing the importance and integrity of the research and ultimate potential benefit to patients against the issues involved in protecting the research participants.

Secondly, ethical concerns arise in the course of the research which have to do with protecting the subjects of the research. This area is principally the only one of the three areas of ethical concern identified here that your local IRB will typically consider in evaluating a proposal. Furthermore, protecting human subjects is frequently thought to be the only point of ethical concern and that once this area is adequately addressed there are no other ethical issues to evaluate. However, there are other issues that are important to consider during suicide research. Two such concerns are disclosure of information regarding the purpose of the research and the extent of confidentiality of the information subjects convey in the course of the research. One of the basic ethical principles in research is that the information conveyed in the course of a research project will be held in confidence. Most consent forms insure that all information will be kept confidential, and if conveyed to anyone it will be done without identifiers. The only exception usually seen is for drug research which places some limits on the confidentiality since the Food and Drug Administration (FDA) asserts a right to review patient records.[7] Usually this promise of confidentiality works well. However, there are times when ethical values have to be balanced against each other, making for difficult evaluations by the investigator. For example, in a research project examining the role of various biochemical correlates of suicidal behavior, this problem could easily be encountered. The project involved performing a lumbar puncture, blood work, and extensive psychiatric evaluations on subjects. Psychiatric patients who were suicide attempters were compared with those who had not attempted suicide. In addition, the currently suicidal patients were contrasted with those who were not currently suicidal. What would happen if during the course of the interviews for which confidentiality had been promised, a patient revealed that he/she was suicidal, a fact that he/she had not revealed to the treating staff. This may happen for a variety of reasons. First, the investigators spend quite a bit of time with the patients administering a diagnostic interview. Often this is more time than the clinical staff is able to spend with the patient, and so the patient may feel more comfortable with the investigator and thus reveal personal thoughts more freely. Secondly, it is generally made clear to the participants that the investigators would not be making clinical decisions regarding their care, whereas naturally the treatment staff would. In evaluating psychiatric inpatients, the clinical staff gives certain privileges to patients such as off-ward cards and weekend passes. Patients quickly learn that if they are suicidal, they do not gain these privileges. So while the patients may reveal genuine suicidal ideation to the investigators under the promise of confidentiality, they may not do so to treatment staff in order to gain their privileges. It is very difficult to decide what is the best route in these cases. While the patients are promised confidentiality, the investigators as employees of the institution and as members of the mental health profession have a duty to take care of the patient. There is a potential for legal problems if a patient reveals suicidal ideation, is given a pass, and then commits suicide.

The approach of encouraging the patient to discuss this information with the treating physician may often be utilized successfully. However, there is no guarantee that this will always work. In attempting to deal with this problem, the investigators may consider limiting the promise of confidentiality to confidentiality except in the case that information deemed important to clinical care is revealed in the course of assessments. In this instance, the treating staff would be notified. However, this route possesses the risk of compromising the validity of the data by possibly having patients deny genuine suicidal ideation. Thus there is a risk of classifying suicidal patients as nonsuicidal since a patient's verbal report is the source of this information. Furthermore, even if they were to decide to breach or limit confidentiality, it would be very difficult to determine which patients were truly suicidal. In addition to the usual problems of predicting suicidal behavior, investigators find that as research becomes known to the surrounding community, it tends to attract a small group of chronically suicidal individuals. These are people who are rarely nonsuicidal. If the investigators act upon the suicidal ideation of these individuals, i.e., commit these patients, deny off-ward privileges, these individuals would be hospitalized all the time and would never leave the ward.

A similar problem emerges with the issue of information disclosure. Integral to the research process is the obtaining of informed consent. As part of the informed consent procedure in the case described earlier, relevant information was disclosed to the potential research participants to assist them in deciding or refusing to participate in the project. Included in this information was the purpose of their research. This does not typically present problems with the psychiatric population. However, controls, normal individuals, are enrolled for payment. Disclosing the purpose of the project to them could lead to false denial of suicide ideation by individuals who either want to participate in the project for the payment attached to the research or who are curious about the research for personal reasons. Again the importance of valid data and the ethical principle of full disclosure must be balanced.

The third area of ethical concerns is the long-term consequences of positive findings in the biology of suicide. What should be done if a genetic marker or a strong biological predisposition is found to exist? What are the consequences of such a discovery? The following are some of the questions that arise from this. What should individuals who have been identified as having this marker be told? It is a difficult task to counsel someone and to let them know that he or she is at risk for suicide. Is there a chance that a self-fulfilling prophesy can emerge or that this information will serve as a significant psychosocial stressor and even precipitate a suicide attempt? A related question concerns what the family members should be told. As more studies are done examining families of suicides and suicide attempters, more knowledge will be gained about familial predispositions. These findings will have implications for vulnerable families and their decisions to have children.

Although they are not immediate concerns, at some point we must begin to think about what practical implications for daily life there will be for individuals identified as "at risk." For example, will individuals identified as at risk be able to obtain medical insurance? Will their families' claims to life insurance if the death occurs by accident be more suspect than other families' claims? Finally, regarding the question of clinical management, if we can successfully identify by biochemical means those at high risk for suicide, and yet have no effective biochemical treatment, what do we do? There is bound to be a lag between identification of the particular biological deficit and effective treatment of this deficit. How do we treat vulnerable individuals in this interim period?

In conclusion there are no easy solutions to these questions. It is important that investigators begin to think about the ethical implications of their research so that they can anticipate some of the problems they will face in the event that biological studies are successful. In this regard, investigators might consider that IRB review will not be very helpful because of the relatively narrow scope of their review and because investigators themselves with their intimate knowledge of the research findings and the affected patient population are in the best position to begin this discussion.

REFERENCES

1. LETTIERI, D. 1974. Suicidal death prediction scales. *In* The Prediction of Suicide. A. Beck, H. Resnik & D. Lettieri, Eds.: 119-140. Charles Press Publishers. Bowie, Md.
2. SZASZ, T. 1971. The ethics of suicide. Antioch Rev. **31:** 7-17.
3. MOTTO, J. 1981. Rational suicide and medical ethics. *In* Rights and Responsibilities in Modern Medicine. M. Basson, Ed.: 201-209. Alan R. Liss Inc. New York, N.Y.

4. MAYO, D. 1983. Contemporary philosophical literature on suicide. Suicide Life Threatening Behav. **13**(4): 313-345.
5. GORMAN, J. M., G. F. LEVY, M. R. LIEBOWITZ, P. MCGRATH, I. L. APPELBY, D. J. DILLON, S. O. DAVIES & D. F. KLEIN. 1983. Effect of acute β-adrenergic blockade on lactate-induced panic. Arch. Gen. Psychiatry **40**: 1079-1082.
6. ANGRIST, B. & S. GERSHON. 1970. The phenomenology of experimentally induced amphetamine psychosis—preliminary observations. Biol. Psychiatry **2**: 95-107.
7. Department of Health and Human Services. 1981. Food and Drug Administration rules and regulations. Fed. Reg. **46**(17): 8950, 8975-8980.

Conceptualizing a Serotonin Trait[a]

A Behavioral Dimension of Constraint

RICHARD A. DEPUE AND MICHELE R. SPOONT

Department of Psychology
University of Minnesota
75 East River Road
Minneapolis, Minnesota 55455

INTRODUCTION

Over the past decade there has been increasing evidence that reduced serotonergic (5HT) activity, as indexed by cerebrospinal fluid (CSF) 5-hydroxyindoleacetic acid (5HIAA) in living subjects or by postmortem imipramine or $5HT_2$ binding in brain,[1,2] is associated with a variety of human behavior patterns, including psychiatric and personality disturbance, suicide, and aggression. As the evidence increases, however, the manner in which these associations are to be conceptualized becomes less clear. This ambiguity may be due, in part, to the diverse set of behavioral correlates of 5HT functioning. Thus, whereas low CSF 5HIAA levels may hold a special relation to a subgroup of unipolar depressives,[3] similarly low levels have also been observed in patients with obsessive-compulsive,[4,5] schizoaffective,[6] alcohol-related,[7] anxiety,[6] schizophrenic,[8] and a variety of (but perhaps especially borderline)[9] personality disorders,[6,9] as well as in control subjects located at the low end of the metabolite distribution.[10] These findings have led to the suggestion that low 5HT functioning "may not be associated with psychiatric illness per se, but rather with an increased vulnerability to a range of psychiatric disturbances and to suicidal behavior [p. 635]."[6] But exactly what the nature of this vulnerability trait may be remains unclear.

Other 5HT correlates do not entirely clarify the situation. First of all, the two strongest correlates, suicide[6,8,11–13] and aggression,[9,14] are behaviorally quite different and often occur within divergent affective states (e.g., depression and anger, respectively). Moreover, suicide and aggression are heterogeneous behavioral domains, and it is unclear which aspects of these complex patterns relate to the 5HT trait. For instance, low CSF 5HIAA is not associated with suicidal behavior in general, but mainly with violent suicide attempts.[13] The term "violent" sheds little light on the nature of the 5HT trait because there are no clear criteria as to which behavioral characteristics violence refers, and because in some cases, such as gas poisoning, it is not clear why the method is more "violent" than drug overdosing (a nonviolent method).

---

[a] This work was supported in part by Research Grant MH 37195 from the National Institute of Mental Health.

In the case of Brown's elegant work on aggression and 5HT functioning,[9] ambiguity as to the nature of the behavioral correlates of low CSF 5HIAA arises again. For instance, whereas aggressive life history (−0.78) and Minnesota Multiphasic Personality Inventory (MMPI) Psychopathic Deviant (Pd) scale[15] items (−0.77) correlate similarly with CSF 5HIAA and 0.57 with each other, the aggressive history index correlates (0.77) with the Buss-Durkee Aggression Inventory (BDAI)[16] but the Pd scale does not. Thus, while each measure contains a domain related to 5HT functioning, these domains may not be identical. Interestingly, the Pd scale does not relate to the behavioral aggression subscale of the BDAI but does relate (0.64) to the hostility subscale, indicating that irritable hostility may be accounting for the Pd-5HIAA correlation. Furthermore, it is not even clear that aggression is the 5HT-relevant trait in Brown's findings. The aggression-5HT association was most pronounced in subjects with suicide attempts and personality disorders characterized by behavioral impulsivity, and two other studies showed that impulsive murderers who also have a history of suicide attempts have very low metabolite levels.

Perhaps suicidal and aggressive behaviors are merely different end-point indicators of a more central trait, such as impulsivity, which becomes most evident under states of strong affect (e.g., depression or anger). Note that the Eysenck Personality Questionnaire (EPQ) Psychoticism scale (which contains a large component of impulsivity) is inversely related to CSF 5HIAA levels[13] and that, on Beck's suicide scale, the only difference between high and low CSF 5HIAA suicide attempters (besides "violence" of method) was that the latter had a shorter period of planning for the attempt.[13] In any case, viewing suicide and aggression as two different indicators of a central (behavioral and biochemical) trait is consistent with the fact that their cooccurrence is often observed and is associated with the most extreme quantitative values of the trait (i.e., lowest CSF 5HIAA values).[9,14,17]

Three lines of inquiry may help to clarify the nature of the behavioral dimension(s) related to 5HT functioning: (a) analysis of 5HT functioning within the larger framework of major behavioral systems; (b) analysis of animal research in which 5HT functioning is manipulated within well-defined stimulus contexts; and (c) assessment of human personality dimensions that are hypothesized to be, and not to be, related to 5HT functioning.

BEHAVIORAL FACILITATION AND INHIBITION SYSTEMS

In order to provide a framework for the research on the effects of 5HT manipulations on animal behavior, it is necessary to outline the neurobiology and stimulus control of two major systems that function interactively to either facilitate or inhibit many specific forms of behavioral patterns. The behavioral facilitation system (BFS), which is a basic behavioral feature of all animals across phylogenetic levels,[18] functions to mobilize an animal's behavior so that active engagement with the environment occurs under appropriate stimulus conditions.[19-22] As shown in FIGURE 1, the BFS is a generalized system that facilitates, via activation of its locomotor and incentive-reward motivation components, a variety of more specific behavioral patterns.[19-25] These specific patterns may be grouped into two broad categories: (1) those related to positive engagement with the environment, such as social, sexual, consummatory, and achievement-related patterns;[20] and (2) those related to response to environmental threat;[19] although there are several threat-response systems, those relevant to our discussion are irritative aggression[26,27] and escape-avoidance.[19] Each of the specific behavioral patterns has its own specific neurobiology and trait dimension and is activated by its specific external and internal controlling stimuli, but each is facilitated by the BFS. This suggests that the BFS is sensitive to stimulus characteristics common to the stimuli eliciting each of the various specific behavioral patterns, as defined below.

The BFS facilitates two types of behavior:[22] (1) *unconditioned,* i.e., behaviors in an animal's repertoire that occur without specific learning experience, such as eating, drinking, mating, aggression, and spontaneous exploratory locomotion in response to

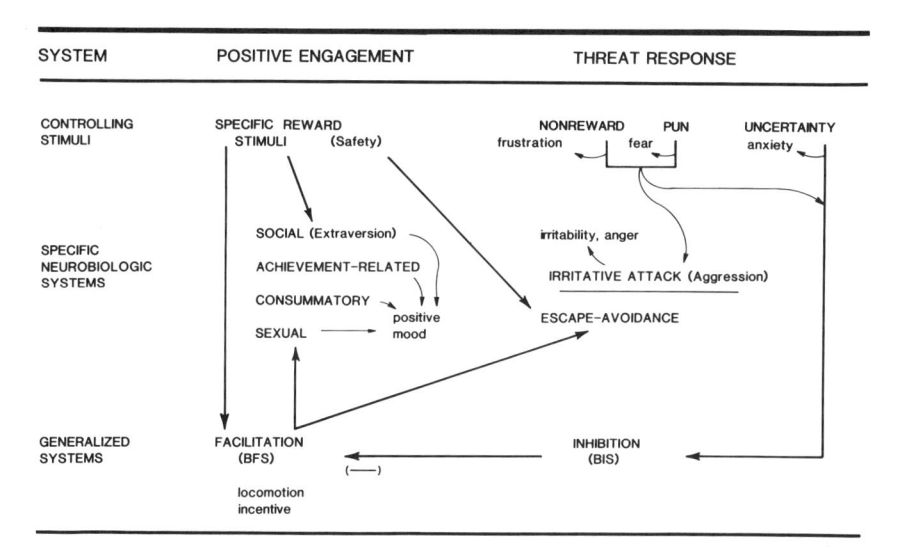

SYSTEM	POSITIVE ENGAGEMENT	THREAT RESPONSE
CONTROLLING STIMULI	SPECIFIC REWARD STIMULI (Safety)	NONREWARD PUN UNCERTAINTY frustration fear anxiety
SPECIFIC NEUROBIOLOGIC SYSTEMS	SOCIAL (Extraversion) ACHIEVEMENT-RELATED CONSUMMATORY SEXUAL → positive mood	irritability, anger IRRITATIVE ATTACK (Aggression) ESCAPE-AVOIDANCE
GENERALIZED SYSTEMS	FACILITATION (BFS) locomotion incentive	INHIBITION (BIS)

FIGURE 1. Structure and function of the behavioral facilitation (BFS) and behavioral inhibition (BIS) systems. The BFS is a generalized system, comprised of locomotion and incentive-reward motivation, which facilitates a number of specific environmental engagement patterns in response to signals of reward, including stimuli of safety and of goal-oriented irritative attack. The BIS is a generalized system which arrests behavior via inhibition of the BFS in response to signals of nonreward, punishment, and uncertainty. The specific engagement patterns are associated with their own neurobiology and specific stimuli, and with traits that provide variation in sensitivity to their controlling stimuli (such as extraversion and aggression). The positive engagement patterns are associated with positive mood, whereas stimuli controlling the BIS and irritative aggressive engagement are associated with a variety of moods as shown.

novel stimuli; and (2) *conditioned,* i.e., voluntary motivated behavior that occurs to signals denoting significant stimuli. In both of these types of behavior, the BFS is activated mainly by inherently rewarding stimuli (food, social, sexual, novelty) or conditioned signals of reward. However, the system is also activated by aversive stimulus contexts, or when signals of these contexts are present, when escape or avoidance responses are deemed possible—in this sense, the safe area is conceived as a positive reward, thus activating the BFS.[19] Moreover, the BFS is activated when specific, goal-oriented aggressive attack patterns require motivated motor support.[26,27] Thus, whereas the BFS is activated by a broad array of stimulus contexts, most of these contexts share a reward component. Furthermore, all contexts elicit incentive motivation, but the specific mood associated with BFS activity will vary as a function of stimulus context, as shown in FIGURE 1.[19,20]

The fact that the components of the BFS are locomotion and incentive-reward motivation is very important because, neurobiologically, these components are thought to be integrated in the mesolimbic dopaminergic (DA) pathway, shown on the left side of FIGURE 2.[21–23,25,28,29] As opposed to the nigrostriatal DA pathway, which is

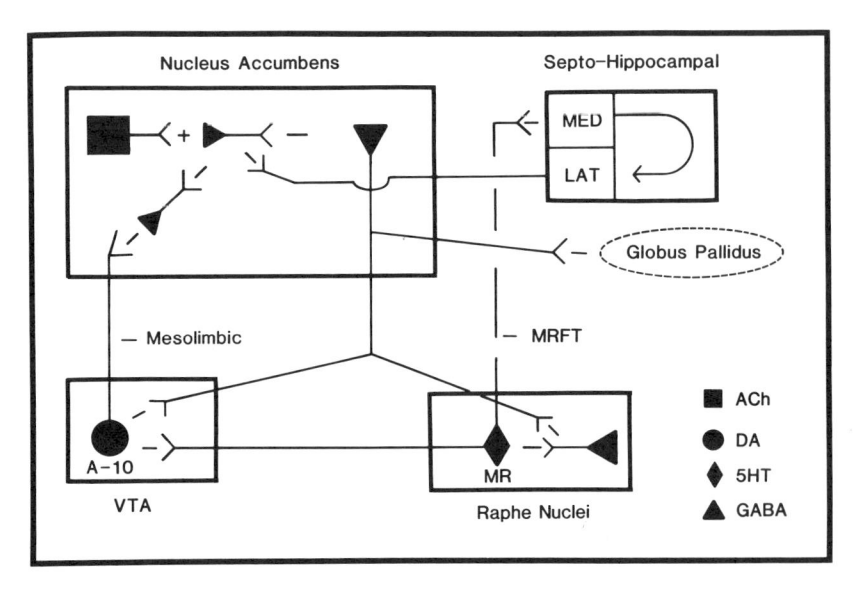

FIGURE 2. Neurobiology of the mesolimbic DA pathway [from the ventral tegmental area (VTA) A-10 cell group to the nucleus accumbens], and of the median raphe forebrain tract (MRFT), originating in the median raphe (MR), to the medial septal nuclei (MED), comprising the 5HT input to the septohippocampal system. The mesolimbic pathway is thought to subserve the BFS by DA's effects on a series of GABA neurons which, in the end, release the globus pallidus, and hence the extrapyramidal system, from GABAergic tonic inhibition (circuitry after Jones).[28] The septohippocampal system is thought to subserve the BIS. One source of output from the septohippocampal system is through the lateral (LAT) septal area, which projects to the nucleus accumbens. This projection is thought to provide the "downstream" 5HT influence in the nucleus accumbens (where response facilitation circuits are integrated), which inhibits response facilitation. ACh = acetylcholine.

more intimately involved in sensorimotor integration and response selection and co-ordination,[22,23,25] the mesolimbic system, in response to reward (rewarded behavior is often not acquired when the pathway is biochemically lesioned), modulates affective responses to the environment.[21–23,25,28,29] As shown in FIGURE 2 (where neural circuitry is after Jones),[28] this facilitation is thought to occur via DA's inhibiting effect in the nucleus accumbens (NAS) on a series of γ-aminobutyric acid (GABA) neurons which eventually tonically inhibit the globus pallidus. The end result of DA input is a disinhibition of the globus pallidus, and hence the extrapyramidal motor system, and increased incentive motivation.

Working interactively with the BFS is the behavioral inhibition system (BIS), as shown in FIGURE 1. The BIS is thought to act as a comparator, comparing actual environmental circumstances with concepts of expected outcome of behavior.[19] As such, the BIS functions continuously in a "just checking" mode. However, when significant mismatches between actual and expected outcomes of behavior occur, the BIS arrests ongoing behavior via inhibition of the BFS until other response strategies are formulated. The conditions constituting "mismatch" are nonreward, punishment, and uncertainty (as to future stimulus sequence and response strategy), and the BIS responds selectively to *signals* of these conditions.[19] Affective correlates of increased BIS activity may be conceptualized as frustration (accompanying signals of nonreward), fear (accompanying clear signals of punishment), and anxiety (accompanying stimulus contexts of uncertainty).

There is a substantial body of research which suggests that the neurobiologic foundation of the BIS is the septohippocampal system. The hippocampal formation is thought to perform the role of comparator, receiving a major portion of its information concerning the environment from the entorhinal area (EA) via the perforant path.[19] (The EA receives integrated information from the orbitofrontal and temporal cortices, collecting centers for information from the neocortical association areas.)[30] The medial area of the dorsal septal nuclei (medial septal nucleus and the nucleus of the diagonal band of Broca) is the second major source of input to the hippocampal formation, and it serves to modulate the mode in which the hippocampal comparator operates.[19] That is, the hippocampal formation typically displays a theta rhythm between 4 and 12 Hz (the range depending on species); the frequency of hippocampal theta is dependent on behavior, where high frequencies (> 8.5 Hz) are associated with instrumental movement, low frequencies (7.5-8 Hz) with attentive immobility, and very low frequencies (< 7.5 Hz) with fixed action patterns (e.g., drinking).[19] The medial septal area serves as a pacemaker of hippocampal theta, where theta frequency depends on the frequency of stimulation arriving at the medial septum from other brain areas.[19] In this sense, the medial septal area acts as an intensity-frequency transducer.

The important point for this discussion is that 5HT appears to decrease the threshold for septal driving of hippocampal theta at frequencies below and up to 7.7 Hz (whereas norepinephrine appears to lower the threshold for septal driving of theta at all frequencies).[31,32] This frequency (7.7 Hz) is most closely associated with attentive immobility in circumstances of nonreward and punishment. Moreover, this frequency is associated with potentiation of information coming into the hippocampus via the perforant path and with facilitated transmission of the information around hippocampal circuitry.[19] Thus, 5HT is believed to be intimately involved in transducing signals of nonreward, punishment, and uncertainty to (a) activation of the mismatch mode of the hippocampal comparator and (b) inhibition of behavior through efferent activity of the BIS to the nucleus accumbens (or BFS).[30,33]

As shown in the right side of FIGURE 2, 5HT efferents to the septohippocampal system arise almost entirely from median raphe (MR) cells (B-8), ascending via the MR forebrain tract of the ventral bundle of the medial forebrain bundle and perhaps innervating the medial area of the dorsal septal nuclei and the entire hippocampal cortical superstructure.[30,33] Thus, it is this pathway that is hypothesized to be one of those most intimately associated with the effects of nonreward, punishment, and uncertainty on behavior. [Dorsal raphe (DR) cells (B-7) project to the *lateral* area of the dorsal septal nuclei, perhaps influencing septohippocampal efferent activity which passes in part via this area, and then to the NAS.][33]

Neurobiologic interaction between the BFS and BIS exists at several levels (not all shown in FIGURE 2), including a hippocampal projection via the lateral septal area to the NAS, a collateral of the mesolimbic dopamine pathway to the lateral septum and EA, a DR projection to the lateral septal area and then to the NAS, a direct DR projection to the NAS (important because the MR can directly influence the DR), and an NAS projection to the raphe nuclei.[29,30,33] Moreover, the two systems operate interactively so as to modulate *behavior* depending on the environmental circumstances. This indicates that, as environmental context changes, the relative strength of the two systems will vary over time, and that the momentary balance between them will determine behavioral expression; that is, their balance will determine the occurrence (or nonoccurrence) and magnitude of environmental engagement behaviors, and the type and magnitude of the accompanying affective state.[19,20]

Relative strength or balance between the two systems is likely a function of at least two factors. First *state* factors, such as the type and strength of sensory input and internal drives, will have strong directional influence on one or the other system, momentarily shifting the balance toward the activated system. But of greater significance is the more enduring shift in the relative strength of the two systems that would result from *trait* factors that affect the activity, and sensitivity to the controlling signals, of one of the systems.[19,20] Considering the most relevant example for our discussion, if 5HT activity were traitwise low in an individual, the balance between the two systems would be shifted toward the BFS. Under these circumstances, three predictions about the interaction of the two systems can be delineated: (1) there will be increased responsiveness to *strong* controlling signals of the BFS (i.e., increased engagement); (2) there will be reduced responsiveness to strong controlling signals of the BIS (also increased engagement); and (3) both of these response biases will be particularly evident, relative to the "normal" case, in environmental contexts that contain strong controlling signals of both the BFS and BIS, the typical conflict situation (i.e., where the engagement response appears excessive in view of the strength of the existing BIS-relevant signals). These predictions can be assessed most effectively in animal research where 5HT manipulations are performed within controlled environmental contexts.

BEHAVIORAL RESPONSE TO SEROTONIN MANIPULATION

BFS Responsivity

BFS responsivity under conditions of 5HT manipulation has been assessed either in terms of its major component—locomotion—or in terms of engagement patterns influenced by the BFS (e.g., sexual behavior, aggression, social interaction). Although less work has been done on the effects of 5HT manipulations on sexual and social patterns, the work that is available indicates that decreased availability of 5HT is associated with significant increases in both of these behavioral patterns.[26,34-36] Most of the work relevant to this section has concerned locomotion and aggression, so these are reviewed in more detail.

Locomotion

There is a vast literature demonstrating that DA plays a major role in the induction of locomotor activity (LA).[21–25,28,29] Moreover, a recent extensive review concluded that "a formidable number of studies have demonstrated that DA and its agonists injected into the NAS induce a greater arousal of LA than equivalent injections in the striatum; there are virtually no studies in the literature to the contrary [p. 61]."[23] Although some role for the striatum in LA appears likely, its evaluation is confounded by the fact that larger doses of DA or its agonists injected into the striatum tend to produce stereotypy,[23] whereas lesions of the striatum or substantia nigra may interfere with the coordination of motor programs.[22,23,29]

There is also a large body of evidence (recently reviewed several times) indicating that increases in 5HT activity inhibit, whereas decreased activity potentiates, LA.[19,23,25,28,34,37,38] Although the data are inconsistent with some forms of 5HT manipulation when *spontaneous* LA is assessed,[b] consistency is much enhanced when the 5HT manipulation is complimented by the use of amphetamine (particularly in lower doses) or of apomorphine.[23,25,34] Put differently, effects of manipulation of BIS modulation of LA are more sensitively assessed when a strong excitatory signal to the BFS is provided. Thus, amphetamine-induced LA is typically attenuated when increased availability of 5HT is achieved by use of tryptophan or 5-hydroxytryptophan (5HTP) preamphetamine loads, or by ventricular, intraperitoneal, or subcutaneous injections of 5HT. These same effects have been found when the more selective DA agonist apomorphine is used to induce LA: 5HTP was not only found to inhibit apomorphine-induced LA, but also the duration of the apomorphine effect on LA was found to be inversely related to increases in brain 5HT.[39,40] On the other hand, amphetamine- or apomorphine-induced LA is potentiated when decreased availability of 5HT is achieved by use of electrolytic lesions of the raphe nuclei, tryptophan-free diets, *para*-chlorophenylalanine (PCPA), 5HT antagonists (e.g., cyproheptadine, methysergide), or dihydroxytryptamine compounds.

Not only does research suggest that DA activity in the NAS provides the most potent effect on LA, but also that 5HT injections directly in the NAS significantly attenuate or totally abolish DA-stimulated activity.[23,28,34] This evidence suggests that the 5HT input is not presynaptic to DA neurons but rather it must be "downstream" from the DA synapse (as shown in FIGURE 2).[28] Moreover, since both DA and 5HT inhibit NAS neurons, in order to have opposite effects on LA, there must be at least

---

[b]Other contradictory results of 5HT, leading both to inhibition of normal LA in rodents, and excitation of abnormal movement and of tremor (the so-called serotonin syndrome), may be the result of dissimilar neurophysiologic bases. The inhibitory 5HT effects on spontaneous LA may be mediated by *ascending* 5HT projections to the forebrain, while excitatory influences on other motor behaviors may be activated in *descending* or spinal tracts.[23,34] Additional problems associated with 5HT manipulation studies are (1) low doses of tryptophan seem less effective; (2) 5HTP in large doses can be taken up into DA neurons, displace endogenous DA, and perhaps increase LA as a result; (3) inconsistent effects of *para*-chloroamphetamine (PCA) may be due to either partially damaged 5HT neurons recovering over several days or, more likely, postsynaptic 5HT receptors increasing in sensitivity and other neurons not damaged by PCA compensating to maintain activity at normal levels; and (4) the degree to which the test environment is novel (vs. familiar), creating exploratory or fear responses, and thereby providing less BFS activation.[34] This latter problem appears to be less crucial when LA is induced by amphetamine or apomorphine.

one inhibitory interneuron between them on the locomotion pathway.[28] This is shown as a GABA interneuron in FIGURE 2.

That the 5HT inhibition effect in the NAS involves an MR projection (no 5HT interneurons have been identified in the NAS),[28,29] either via its effects on the septohippocampal system[19,31] and/or more directly on the NAS,[28,29] is suggested by the fact that lesions of the MR are fairly consistently associated with hyperactivity and increased LA to DA stimulants, whereas this is infrequently the case with DR lesions.[19,23,25,34,37] Furthermore, hyperactivity resulting from raphe lesions can be attenuated by direct 5HT administration into the NAS.[41]

An important finding is that MR, but not DR, electrolytic lesions produced selective decreases of 5HT in the hippocampus and limbic structures.[42,43] Concordantly, it has been found that hyperactivity seen after MR lesions or PCPA may also be mediated by 5HT depletion in the hippocampus selectively.[44] Moreover, lesions of the dorsal hippocampus cause an increase in LA, and raphe lesions or PCPA causes no further increase in LA in rats with dorsal hippocampal lesions.[34] Thus, it appears that *selective* 5HT reductions in the NAS and hippocampus are important, since general 5HT reductions in the forebrain of up to 85% via PCPA treatment have been found in some cases to have less of a potentiating effect on LA than do raphe lesions producing 5HT reductions of only 55%.[45]

Overall, then, it appears that 5HT plays an inhibitory interactive role with DA in the NAS in the modulation of LA. This inhibitory role appears to be exerted in large part by 5HT input arising from MR projections, projections that densely innervate the septohippocampal system,[33] the hypothesized foundation of the BIS. Thus, it is possible that the effect of reduced 5HT activity is to impair the functioning of the BIS, thereby reducing its inhibitory modulatory influence on the NAS response facilitation mechanism. The significance of these observations is that LA represents the strongest marker of the BFS[20] (and of incentive motivational state in general),[21,22,23,25] and its disinhibition by reduced 5HT activity provides a powerful conceptual model for the behavioral effects of a 5HT trait.

Aggression

Although in animals seven different forms of aggression have been identified, it has been difficult to identify all of these patterns in man.[26] At least four forms of aggression in man are more evident: defensive (or fear induced), sex related, competitive (intermale or agonistic), and irritative.[26] Although competitive aggression is one of the most important components of everyday human life in driving man to achievement in diverse areas of the arts and sciences, irritative aggression is most relevant to our discussion. Irritative aggression in man is evoked by stimuli of nonreward, punishment (including painful stimuli), and possibly heat, and, as shown in FIGURE 1, is accompanied by feelings of frustration-irritability, fear, or intense anger, depending on the stimulus context.[26,27] If the stimulus is sufficiently aversive, goal-oriented attack may occur.

In both animals and man, a large number of central nervous system (CNS) structures play activatory and inhibitory roles in the modulation of irritative aggression. For our discussion, two structures seem most relevant. Evidence indicates that, in animals, the basolateral and centromedial nuclei of the amygdala play inhibitory and facilitatory roles, respectively, in irritative aggression, whereas bilateral lesions of the amygdala dramatically reduce or eliminate irritative aggression altogether.[26] Similarly, electrical stimulation of the amygdala in man, at times most likely the centromedial area,[46] has elicited angry, verbally hostile, and overt assaultive behavior (although antiaggressive results have been found by stimulation of different loci in the amygdala), whereas unilateral or bilateral lesions of the amygdala have reduced or abolished outbursts of destructive violence by patients who had previously shown overt repetitive aggression, such as *assaults and suicidal attempts.*[26] Of interest, the mesolimbic DA pathway provides a projection to the amygdala,[30,31] and DA and its agonists have strong facilitatory effects on irritative aggression and slow the habituation of irritative attacks.[26,27,47,48] Norepinephrine modulates the DA facilitation, and so inhibition of norepinephrine activity, via use of 6-hydroxydopamine or clonidine by themselves or in combination with apomorphine challenge, results in exaggerated irritative aggression.[26,48]

The other relevant structure controlling irritative aggression is the septal region, which appears to provide an inhibitory (suppressive) influence.[26] For instance, in normal laboratory rats (and other species), bilateral lesions of the medial septal nuclei, depending on lesion size and location, induce hyperirritability which often is transformed into episodes of irritative aggression.[49] In man, stimulation of the septal region has been found to reduce violent behavior and to instantly alter rage to happiness.[50]

The role of 5HT in irritative aggression appears to be one of inhibitory modulation.[26,27] Thus, decreased availability of 5HT achieved by the use of PCPA, tryptophan-free diets, lesions of 5HT ascending projections or of the raphe nuclei themselves, methysergide, and 5,6-dihydroxytryptamine (DHT) have often been found to increase foot-shock- and tail-pinch-induced irritative aggression in rats and mice, whereas the initial increased release of 5HT induced by fenfluramine was found to have antiaggression effects in rats.[51]

Irritative aggression is also reliably increased in rodents that have been socially isolated, a procedure that has been shown to decrease tryptophan brain concentration in rats and mice and 5HT turnover in whole brain,[26,27] although the results vary particularly in mice by brain area as a function of strain.[52] Importantly, it has been observed that prolonged isolation in rats increases irritative aggression only if indices of 5HT functioning indicate decreased availability.[26,27] Moreover, the decrease in 5HT functioning may be relatively selective as to anatomical location: reduced tryptophan concentration and reduced tryptophan hydroxylase activity have been found in the septal area of rats subjected to prolonged isolation, whereas increases were detected in these two 5HT indicators in striatal nuclei.[27,52,53]

Serotonin's inhibitory action over irritative aggression may arise from two sources. First, the various results implicating the septal area in the suppression of irritative aggression suggest that the MR ascending projection may play an important role in this effect; if so, modulatory influence of irritative aggression by the BIS would be indicated. Second, the DR projects to the amygdala[33] and may provide a 5HT inhibitory influence directly on the aggression facilitation circuits in the amygdala. Although the effects of DR lesions on irritative aggression have apparently not been evaluated, DR lesions were sufficient to produce muricidal aggression in naturally nonkiller rats.[54]

There is a phenomenon that occurs with reduced 5HT availability that is described variously as hyperirritability, hyperexcitability, and hypersensitivity.[26,27,34] In general, it is an exaggerated emotional arousal and/or aggressive display (though not necessarily attack) to relatively mild stimuli, such as air puffs, novel stimuli, handling, and pain. One index of this hyperresponsiveness is degree of startle to air puffs. Interestingly, MR, but not DR, lesions produce an increased startle response,[34] and lesions to the medial septal nuclei (or PCPA) produce slower habituation of the response.[55-57] Thus, the septohippocampal system (BIS) may be involved in hyperexcitability to mild stimuli. Hyperexcitability induced by decreased 5HT availability is of theoretical interest, because it has been suggested that one effect of stress-induced corticosteroid secretion is to increase (lagged in time) 5HT turnover by as much as 150%, yielding a refractoriness of neural tissue to subsequent stressful stimuli for several hours.[33] Perhaps the efficacy of this stress-response mechanism is reduced in conditions of decreased 5HT functioning.

BIS Responsivity

Responsivity of the BIS under conditions of 5HT manipulation is assessed in terms of response rates to stimuli of nonreward (rate of extinction) and of the degree to which punishment suppresses behavior in passive and active avoidance tasks or in conflict situations. With only a few exceptions, results consistently indicate that 5HT synthesis inhibitors (PCPA) and 5HT receptor antagonists (including methysergide, D-2-bromolysergide acid diethylamide, and cianserin) counteract the suppressive effects of *punishment*, and this has also been true of 5,6- and 5,7-DHT, if only for a limited time period in one study.[19,58-60] These results have held over many different tasks, including passive avoidance and conflict, and the use of 5,7-DHT has been found to increase resistance to punished extinction of a one-way active avoidance response.[61,62] The antiserotonergic action of PCPA in these studies was confirmed by the demonstration that (a) it is reversed by a subsequent injection of 5HTP[19,58] and by the 5HT reuptake inhibitor Wy 25093,[60] and (b) the time courses of behavioral release and of 5HT depletion after PCPA injection coincide closely.[60,63,64] Moreover, the possibility that the release of behavior with reduced 5HT could be due to reduced sensitivity to pain is ruled out by experiment and by the fact that pain sensitivity is increased by reduced 5HT levels.[27] PCPA-induced increased resistance to extinction under conditions of *nonreward* has also been observed, even when PCPA is injected between acquisition and extinction, and this effect was reversed by 5HTP injection before each extinction session.[19,58,60] Conversely, 5HT agonists, such as 5HTP together with a monoamine oxidase inhibitor, a long-lasting 5HT receptor agonist (alphamethyltryptamine),[65,66] and 5HT injection into the cerebral ventricles (decreasing the antipunishment effects of oxazepam),[66] directly produce behavioral suppression.

Some evidence suggests that the effects of 5HT manipulations on punished and nonrewarded behavior are associated with the MR and the septohippocampal system. Electrical stimulation of the MR suppressed rewarded operant behavior and elicited signs of fear, and these effects were blocked by PCPA.[67] Conversely, electrolytic lesions of the MR impaired step-down passive avoidance[68] and produced deficits in punished extinction of one-way active avoidance, an effect not found for DR lesions.[69] Furthermore, methysergide, which reverses punishment-induced response suppression, has been shown to antagonize the effects of 5HT in the hippocampus[70,71] but not in a number of other brain areas.[72] Although 5HT injections into the DR produced response suppression,[73] this may be the result of (a) the DR's inhibitory interconnection with the MR[74] and/or (b) the DR's inhibitory interconnection with the substantia nigra, thereby reducing activity of the nigrostriatal pathway, since blockade of this interconnection releases punished behavior in a conflict task.[75]

Thus, there is strong support for the inhibitory role of 5HT in modulating responding to reward in contexts of nonreward and punishment. There is some evidence suggesting that this modulatory effect is, at least in part, carried out by the MR projection to the septohippocampal system, the possible anatomical location of the

BIS. Reduced availability of 5HT consistently produces excessive reward responding in spite of the presence of strong BIS-relevant stimuli.

IMPLICATIONS FOR A HUMAN BEHAVIORAL CONSTRAINT DIMENSION

The behavioral studies of 5HT manipulation indicate that 5HT subserves a neurobiologic system that modulates the activity of the BFS and, hence in turn, the amplitude of engagement responses. Due to the diversity of response patterns modulated by 5HT (LA, aggression, sexual, social interaction), two conclusions seem warranted. (1) The 5HT influence is not specific to any particular response system and, thereby, is best conceived as subserving a generalized behavioral constraint system which inhibits engagement patterns in reaction to signals of nonreward, punishment, or uncertainty. We have referred to this constraint system as the BIS, and, in view of the significant role of the MR ascending tract, the hippocampus, and the septal area in the behavioral effects of 5HT manipulation, the anatomical location of the BIS in the septohippocampal system gains strong support. (2) The BIS appears to exercise its influence on a more generalized behavioral facilitation system (BFS), as indicated by the potent effects of 5HT manipulation on LA and incentive motivational state which are not specific components of any one engagement pattern but which are common to all of them. In this way, the BIS achieves a potent, "upstream" modulatory influence over many specific engagement patterns. Thus, in interaction, the relative strength between the BFS and BIS would determine the *amplitude* of engagement observed at any point in time. FIGURE 3 illustrates this interrelation by plotting engagement amplitude across the range of BFS/BIS relative strengths as a *dashed* diagonal.

Relative strength is dynamical and will vary as a function of *state* changes in environmental context and internal drives of the organism. Theoretically, *trait* factors should affect the *mean* level and slope of the diagonal in FIGURE 3 across individuals, and at least two sets of trait factors can be defined. The most obvious of these are factors influencing the strength of the BFS and BIS. Evidence reviewed herein suggests that strength of the BIS, which may be viewed in terms of its sensitivity to signals of nonreward, punishment, and uncertainty, is influenced by 5HT functioning. Factors resulting in reduced availability of 5HT would be expected to increase the mean level and slope of the diagonal, as shown by the *solid* line in FIGURE 3. Certain state factors would mimic or potentiate this 5HT trait effect: alcohol (often associated with aggressive and suicidal behavior), or ingestion of barbiturates or benzodiazepines, has behavioral effects similar to those of reduced 5HT functioning,[19] is known to reduce the strength of BIS influence,[19] and hence should likewise increase the level and slope of the diagonal. Degree of increase in engagement resulting from these state and trait factors would theoretically depend on traitwise strength in the BFS (a DA activity trait?): the greater the reactivity of the BFS to signals of reward, the greater should be the increase in the engagement *slope* as a function of BIS weakening.

Because increased amplitude of engagement is associated with increased BFS but decreased BIS responsivity, behavioral manifestation of increased engagement should be most dramatic in environmental contexts that contain strong controlling signals of both systems. This is analogous to an experimental conflict situation under low-5HT conditions, where the BFS response appears excessive in view of the strength of the existing BIS-relevant signals. Both suicidal and aggressive behavior may be viewed as occurring within the context of a conflict situation. In the case of suicide, there is the rewarding value of escaping or avoiding life's difficulties, whereas the notion of taking one's life has obvious signals of punishment. But it is particularly in "violent" suicide, where the method itself has especially salient punishment cues—enough so that most individuals avoid these methods in favor of less aversive ones—that the "lure" of suicide appears so extreme. We hypothesize that the low-5HT individual is much less sensitive to these particularly strong signals of punishment and, thereby, may be said to "overrespond" to the rewarding aspects of suicide. Similarly, in a

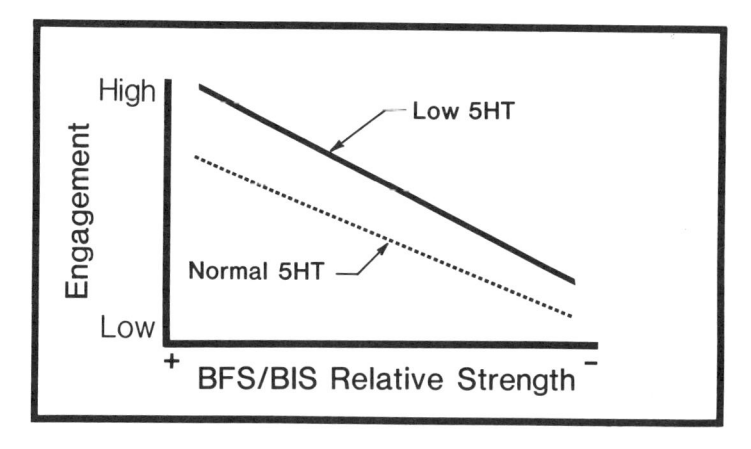

FIGURE 3. Interrelation between amplitude of behavioral engagement and relative strength of the BFS and BIS (where "+" denotes greater BFS strength and "−" denotes greater BIS strength). Relative strength varies as a function of state factors (such as environmental context and internal drives) and of trait factors which influence the strength of either the BFS or BIS (such as variations in the availability of the neurotransmitters subserving the systems). The *dashed* diagonal represents the level and slope of engagement under conditions of normal 5HT availability in the BIS: engagement increases with increasing strength of the BFS relative to the BIS. The *solid* diagonal represents a condition of low 5HT availability in the BIS, which results in reduced constraint of the BFS in general: the strength of the BFS relative to the BIS is greater under most stimulus contexts, and hence the level and slope of engagement are increased across the range of BFS/BIS relative strengths compared to the normal 5HT condition.

highly irritative aggressive or violent act, there are salient aversive cues, both internal (such as cognitions of harming or killing someone or of going to jail) and external (such as signs of fear in the victim), that would generally inhibit action or reduce its intensity, but which apparently do so much less effectively in the low-5HT individual.[c]

A second set of trait factors that could influence the amplitude of engagement is

---

[c]Although this behavioral profile may be described as one of impulsivity, this behavioral domain is very heterogeneous, and not all forms of impulsivity are likely to be related to reduced 5HT activity.[20] Studies that correlate the various forms of impulsivity with 5HT functioning are required to clarify this issue.

the neurobiologic sensitivity of the specific engagement patterns to their respective controlling stimuli. For instance, the extraversion dimension may be conceived as a dimension of sensitivity to rewarding social stimuli. Thus, a "low-5HT" individual who is also traitwise high on extraversion (or on an aggression dimension) would be expected to manifest not only increased engagement responsivity in general (due to decreased BIS constraint of the BFS) but also a strong sociability (or aggression) pattern in particular.

In addition to the aforementioned effects, one other characteristic may characterize "low-5HT" individuals. If the hyperemotional response to mild stressors found in animals with low 5HT also characterizes low-5HT humans, these individuals may often experience subjective feelings of negative affect, tension, alienation, and irritability. These feelings often cluster into a personality dimension of neuroticism or negative affect,[76] and suicidal patients have been found to be high on such measures.[13] Such a subjective state may *contribute* to the high levels of distress that often precede considerations of suicide, or to the impatience with frustrations (frustrative nonreward) that initiates irritative aggression.

What is lacking in this area of research is a sophisticated assessment of the behavioral trait correlates of the low-5HT individual (or of the 5HT dimension). Other correlates of the low-5HT *animal* are insomnia, increased susceptibility to convulsive seizures, increased sensitivity to pain, hyperdipsia, and increased alcohol preference.[27] Thus, taking these together with the other effects of low 5HT discussed above (i.e., the indicators of increased BFS responsivity and hyperemotionality), a rather broad behavioral profile is evident. Studies that assess the degree to which these behaviors covary among themselves and with other personality traits in humans have not been systematically undertaken but would be intriguing. In more extreme states of personality, such as borderline personality disorder (BPD) which is characterized by low CSF 5HIAA,[9] these behaviors do appear to covary. The *Diagnostic and Statistical Manual*, third edition, criteria for BPD include impulsivity; physically self-damaging acts (suicidal gestures, recurrent accidents, physical fights); and inappropriate, intense anger or lack of control of anger (frequent displays of anger).[77] Moreover, the overlap of other unstable personality disorders, such as narcissistic, antisocial, and histrionic, with BPD may indicate that low 5HT may be associated with a variety of extreme disturbances of personality.

We conceptualize the 5HT trait, then, as underlying a behavioral dimension of constraint and perhaps, via a DR effect on circuitry in the amygdala, a propensity to irritative aggression. Interestingly, constraint has reliably emerged as an independent dimension in recent inventory studies of personality structure and comprises an independent factor in two major personality inventories [the Eysenck Personality Questionnaire Psychoticism scale has a strong constraint component and Tellegen's Multidimensional Personality Questionnaire[76] (MPQ) defines quite clearly a constraint factor]. The fact that the concordance of CSF 5HIAA is significantly higher in monozygotic than dizygotic twins,[78] that Tellegen has found similar results for twins reared apart with his MPQ constraint factor,[79] and that suicidal behavior (if taken as an indicator of a low 5HT-constraint trait) exhibits familial transmission[80] suggests that the trait of constraint is subject to strong genetic variation. Apparently, the genetic influence on 5HT functioning does not have to be extreme quantitatively in that CSF 5HIAA values of "low"-5HT groups are generally about 20%-35% less than controls.[6,13] In terms of behavioral functioning, however, this magnitude may be large if animal work can be used as a reliable guideline for human behavior: it will be recalled that 5HT reductions of only approximately 50% had very significant effects on LA.

REFERENCES

1. STANLEY, M., J. VIRGILIO & S. GERSHON. 1982. Science 216: 1337-1339.
2. STANLEY, M. & J. MANN. 1983. Lancet 2: 214-216.
3. VAN PRAAG, H. 1984. Depression, suicide, and serotonin metabolism in the brain. *In* Neurobiology of Mood Disorders. R. Post & J. Ballenger, Eds.: 601-618. Williams & Wilkins. Baltimore, Md.
4. NIES, A., D. ROBINSON & K. LAMBORN. 1973. Arch. Gen. Psychiatry 28: 834-838.
5. BUCHSBAUM, M., R. COURSEY & D. MURPHY. 1976. Science 194: 339-341.
6. TRASKMAN, L., M. ASBERG, L. BERTILSSON & L. SJOSTRAND. 1981. Arch. Gen. Psychiatry 38: 631-636.
7. BALLENGER, J., F. GOODWIN & L. MAJOR. 1979. Arch. Gen. Psychiatry 36: 224-227.
8. VAN PRAAG, H. 1983. Lancet 2: 977-978.
9. BROWN, G., F. GOODWIN & W. BUNNEY. 1982. Human aggression and suicide: their relationship to neuropsychiatric diagnoses and serotonin metabolism. *In* Serotonin in Biological Psychiatry. B. Ho *et al.*, Eds.: 287-307 Raven Press. New York, N.Y.
10. SEDVALL, G., H. NYBACK, G. OXENSTIERNA, F. WIESEL & B. WODE-HELGODT. 1980. CINP Abstr. 607: 316-317.
11. ASBERG, M., P. THOREN & L. TRASKMAN. 1976. Science 191: 478-480.
12. ASBERG, M., L. TRASKMAN & P. THOREN. 1976. Arch. Gen. Psychiatry 33: 1193-1197.
13. ASBERG, M., D. SCHALLING, E. RYDIN & L. TRASKMAN-BENDZ. 1981. Suicide and depression. *In* Depression et Suicide. J. Soubrier & J. Vedrinne, Eds.: 367-404. Pergamon Press. New York, N.Y.
14. LINNOILA, M., M. VIRKKUNEN, M. SCHEININ, A. NUUTILA, R. RIMON & F. GOODWIN. 1983. Life Sci. 33: 2609-2614.
15. LANYON, R. 1961. A Handbook of MMPI Group Profiles. University of Minnesota Press. Minneapolis, Minn.
16. BUSS, A. 1961. The Psychology of Aggression. Wiley. New York, N.Y.
17. ACHTE, K., J. LONNQUIST & O. WALORANTA. 1981. Suicidal tendencies in violent individuals. *In* Depression et Suicide. J. Soubrier & J. Verdrinne, Eds.: 245-249. Pergamon Press. New York, N.Y.
18. SCHNEIRLA, T. 1959. An evolutionary and developmental theory of biphasic processes underlying approach and withdrawal. *In* Nebraska Symposium on Motivation. M. Jones, Ed.: 45-61. University of Nebraska Press. Lincoln, Neb.
19. GRAY, J. 1982. The Neuropsychology of Anxiety. Oxford University Press. New York, N.Y.
20. DEPUE, R., S. KRAUSS & M. SPOONT. A two dimensional threshold model of seasonal bipolar affective disorder. *In* Psychopathology: an Interactionist Perspective. D. Magnusson & A. Ohman, Eds. Academic Press. New York, N.Y. (In press.)
21. MILNER, P. 1977. Theories of reinforcement, drive, and motivation. *In* Handbook of Psychopharmacology. L. Iversen, S. Iversen, & S. Snyder, Eds. 7: 181-200. Plenum Press. New York, N.Y.
22. IVERSEN, S. 1978. Brain dopamine systems and behavior. *In* Handbook of Psychopharmacology. L. Iversen, S. Iversen & S. Snyder, Eds. 8: 333-384. Plenum Press. New York, N.Y.
23. FISHMAN, R., J. FEIGENBAUM, J. YANAI & H. KLAWANS. 1983. Progr. Neurobiol. 20: 55-88.
24. CROW, T. 1977. Neurotransmitter-related pathways: the structure and function of central monoamine neurones. *In* Biochemical Correlates of Brain Structure and Function. A. Davison, Ed.: 137-174. Academic Press. New York, N.Y.
25. KELLY, P. 1978. Drug-induced motor behavior. *In* Handbook of Psychopharmacology. L. Iversen, S. Iversen & S. Snyder, Eds. 8: 295-332. Plenum Press. New York, N.Y.
26. VALZELLI, L. 1981. Psychobiology of Aggression and Violence. Raven Press. New York, N.Y.
27. VALZELLI, L. 1982. Pharmacol. Res. Commun. 14: 1-13.
28. JONES, D., G. MOGENSON & M. WU. 1981. Neuropharmacology 20: 20-29.

29. MOGENSON, G., D. JONES & C. YIM. 1980. Progr. Neurobiol. **14:** 69-97.
30. NAUTA, W. & V. DOMESICK. 1981. Ramifications of the limbic system. *In* Psychiatry and the Biology of the Human Brain. S. Mathysse, Ed.: 165-188. Elsevier. New York, N.Y.
31. MCNAUGHTON, N., D. JAMES, J. STEWART, J. GRAY, I. VALERO & A. DREWNOWSKI. 1977. Neuroscience **2:** 1019-1027.
32. GRAY, J., D. JAMES & P. KELLY. 1975. Nature **258:** 424-425.
33. AZMITIA, E. 1978. The serotonin-producing neurons of the midbrain median and dorsal raphe nuclei. *In* Handbook of Psychopharmacology. L. Iversen, S. Iversen & S. Snyder, Eds. **9:** 233-314. Plenum Press. New York, N.Y.
34. GERSON, S. & R. BALDESSARINI. 1980. Life Sci. **27:** 1435-1451.
35. RALEIGH, M., G. BRAMMER & M. MCGUIRE. 1983. Male dominance, serotonergic systems, and the behavioral and physiological effects of drugs in vervet monkeys. *In* Ethopharmacology: Primate Models of Neuropsychiatric Disorders. A. Liss, Ed.: 185-197. Raven Press. New York, N.Y.
36. SANDLER, M. & L. GESSA. 1975. Sexual Behavior: Pharmacology and Biochemistry. Raven Press. New York, N.Y.
37. DRAY, A. 1981. J. Physiol. **77:** 393-403.
38. PLAZNIK, A., W. DANYSZ, W. KOSTOWSKI, A. BIDZINSKI & M. HAUPMANN. 1983. Pharmacol. Biochem. Behav. **19:** 27-32.
39. GRABOWSKA, M., L. ANKIEWICS, J. MAI & J. MICHALUK. 1973. Pol. J. Pharmacol. **25:** 29-39.
40. GRABOWSKA, M. & J. MICHALUK. 1974. Pharmacol. Biochem. Behav. **2:** 263-266.
41. COSTALL, B., R. NAYLOR & R. PINDER. 1976. Psychopharmacology **48:** 225-231.
42. GEYER, M., A. PUERTO, D. MENKES, D. SEGAL & A. MANDELL. 1976. Brain Res. **106:** 257-270.
43. DRAY, A., J. DAVIES, N. OAKLEY, P. TONGROACH & S. VELLUCCI. 1978. Brain Res. **151:** 431-442.
44. JACOBS, B., C. TRIMBACH, E. EUBANKS & M. TRULSON. 1975. Brain Res. **94:** 253-261.
45. KOHLER, C. & S. LORENS. 1978. Pharmacol. Biochem. Behav. **8:** 223-233.
46. KING, H. 1961. Psychological effects of excitation in the limbic system. *In* Electrical Stimulation of the Brain. D. Sheer, Ed.: 477-486. University of Texas Press. Austin, Tex.
47. WINSLOW, J. & K. MICZEK. 1983. Psychopharmacology **81:** 286-291.
48. HAHN, R. 1982. J. Pharm. Exp. Ther. **220:** 389-393.
49. WALLACE. T. & B. THORNE. 1978. Physiol. Psychol. **6:** 36-42.
50. HEATH, R. 1963. Am. J. Psychiatry **120:** 571-577.
51. MCKENZIE, G. 1980. Can. J. Physiol. Pharmacol. **59:** 830-836.
52. KEMPF, E., S. PUGLISI-ALLEGRA, S. CABIB, C. SCHLEFF & P. MANDEL. 1984. Prog. Neuro-Psychopharmacol. Biol. Psychiatry **8:** 365-371.
53. SEGAL, D., S. KNAPP, R. KUCZENSKI & A. MANDEL. 1973. Behav. Biol. **8:** 47-53.
54. WALDBILLIG, R. 1979. Brain Res. **160:** 341-346.
55. MILLER, S. & R. TREFT. 1979. Physiol. Behav. **23:** 645-648.
56. WILLIAMS, J., L. HAMILTON & P. CARLTON. 1974. J. Comp. Physiol. Psychol. **87:** 724-732.
57. DAVIS, M. & M. SHEARD. 1976. Eur. J. Pharmacol. **35:** 261-293.
58. STEIN, L. 1981. Behavioral pharmacology of benzodiazepines. *In* Anxiety: New Research and Changing Concepts. D. Klein & J. Rabkin, Eds.: 201-213. Raven Press. New York, N.Y.
59. SOUBRIE, P., M. THIEBOT, A. JOBERT & M. HAMON. 1981. J. Physiol. **77:** 449-453.
60. HODGES, H. & S. GREEN. 1984. Behav. Neural Biol. **40:** 127-154.
61. DAVIS, N. 1979. Doctor of Philosophy Thesis. University of Oxford. Oxford, England.
62. FUXE, K., S. OGREN, L. AGNATI, G. JONSSON & J. GUSTAFSSON. 1978. Ann. N.Y. Acad. Sci. **305:** 346-369.
63. GELLER, I. & K. BLUM. 1970. Eur. J. Pharmacol. **9:** 319-324.
64. WISE, C., G. BERGER & L. STEIN. 1973. Biol. Psychiatry **6:** 3-21.
65. GRAEFF, F. & R. SCHOENFELD. 1970. J. Pharmacol. Exp. Ther. **173:** 277-283.
66. STEIN, L., C. WISE & B. BERGER. 1973. Anti-anxiety action of benzodiazepines: decrease in activity of serotonin neurons in the punishment system. S. Garattini, E. Mussini & L. Randall, Eds.: 299-326. Raven Press. New York, N.Y.

67. GRAEFF, F. & N. SILVEIRA FILHO. 1978. Physiol. Behav. **21:** 477-484.
68. THORNTON, E. & A. GOUDIE. 1978. Psychopharmacology **60:** 73-79.
69. SREBO, B. & S. LORENS. 1975. Brain Res. **89:** 303-325.
70. SEGAL, M. 1975. Brain Res. **94:** 115-131.
71. SEGAL, M. 1976. Brain Res. **103:** 161-166.
72. HAIGLER, H. & G. AGHAJANIAN. 1974. J. Neural Transm. **35:** 257-273.
73. THIEBOT, M., A. JOBERT & P. SOUBRIE. 1980. Neurosci. Lett. **16:** 213-217.
74. SOUBRIE, P., A. JOBERT & M. THIEBOT. 1981. J. Physiol. **77:** 449-453.
75. THIEBOT, M., M. HAMON & P. SOUBRIE. 1983. Pharmacol. Biochem. Behav. **19:** 225-229.
76. TELLEGEN, A. 1986. Manual of the Multidimentional Personality Questionnaire. University of Minnesota, Minneapolis, Minn.
77. American Psychiatric Association. 1980. Diagnostic and Statistical Manual of Mental Disorders. Third Edition. Washington, D.C.
78. SEDVALL, G., B. FYRO, КB. GULLBERG, H. NYBACK, F. WIESEL & B. WODE-HELGODT. 1980. Br. J. Psychiatry **136:** 366-374.
79. TELLEGEN, A. Unpublished data.
80. ROY, A. 1983. Arch. Gen. Psychiatry **40:** 971-974.

Early Family Influences on Suicidal Behavior

KENNETH S. ADAM
Department of Psychiatry
McMaster University
1200 Main Street West
Hamilton, Ontario, Canada L8N 3ZS

INTRODUCTION

Suicidal behavior is manifest throughout most of the life cycle from early adolescence to old age with well-known epidemiological patterns for age and sex differentiating attempted suicide from suicide. It cuts across many diagnostic categories and is associated with a number of social, psychological, and biological variables. Yet its etiology remains controversial. Is suicidal behavior merely one of a number of depressive symptoms in the psychiatrically ill, or is it a more specific behavioral response with definable antecedents, an understandable course, and a range of more or less predictable outcomes? This paper will make a case for the latter alternative arguing that relatively specific events in the early social environment contribute to a vulnerability to suicidal behavior, while later events of related kind reactivate memories of those events and trigger overt suicidal behavior. Furthermore, we will propose, contrary to the prevailing view, that those who attempt suicide and those who succeed in killing themselves are not different but overlapping groups as the epidemiological data suggest, but the same individuals at different points of a developmental continuum. An overview of data supporting this case will be given, a theoretical model will be suggested, and an overall schema presented showing how this might account for some of the known data on suicidal behavior. While one must acknowledge that suicidal behavior is multidetermined and that biological and cultural factors influence its expression, this paper suggests that their role, at least in contemporary western society, is secondary to the social determinants.

EARLY SOCIAL ENVIRONMENT AS A PREDISPOSING FACTOR

That the early social environment of suicidal individuals is often markedly disorganized is well established in an extensive literature on suicide and attempted suicide.[50,56] Sociological studies have pointed to the strong association between indices of social disorganization and suicidal behavior, and psychoanalytic studies have reported on the self-destructive consequences to the individual of the psychological internalization of frustrating or disappointing early experiences.[20,38,39] Clinical studies looking at the early social environment have focused on the family. Of all the variables implicated in these studies the role of "broken homes" and "parental loss" has been most extensively studied. Since 1940 more than 30 studies have appeared reporting an incidence of broken homes in suicidal individuals ranging from a low of 17%[11] to a high of 76%[54] (see TABLE 1).

Where controls have been used for comparison, significant differences have been found with few exceptions.[2,6a,11,15,26,24,31,35,41] While the spread in these figures seems quite extreme at first glance, closer examination indicates that inconsistencies in the methodology of the studies account for much of the variation. Criteria for defining what constitutes a "broken home" vary considerably, with some studies restricting their examination to the death of parents in childhood, and some including divorce or permanent separation of parents or even briefer separations for other reasons. Similarly the age span over which these events are considered ranges from losses in the first 10 years of life to losses in early adulthood. Generally speaking, the broader the definition of loss used and the longer the period of early life under consideration, the higher the figures for loss in both suicidal subjects and controls. Walton, for example, who reported that 76.6% of his suicidal depressives had suffered "parental deprivation" before age 14, included the experience of parental strife in his criteria;[54] while Bunch et al., restricting their examination to losses from parental death alone, reported an incidence of 17% until age 16.[11] Nonetheless, if one corrects the data in these studies so that similar definitions of loss are considered over approximately the same period of time, there is a greater consistency in the data (see TABLE 2).

Data on the age of the subject at the time of loss are even more confusing. Many of the studies have simply examined globally for losses up to a certain age period (usually 15 or 16), while others have extended this time period and examined for smaller age periods separately. Where this has been done the findings are conflicting. Some studies report a higher incidence of loss in the early childhood years (0-5 or 0-10),[24,25,36,45] while others have reported a peak for loss in the adolescent years.[31,40,6a] One study found two peaks, one from 0-5 years and a second from 17-20,[4] and four other studies found no particular age period that stood out.[9a,17,35,41]

A number of factors confound interpretation of these findings. Firstly, loss from divorce or separation of parents is more likely to occur earlier in life than loss of a parent from death, so that studies that only consider parental death will report a peak at a later age than those that include all types of loss. Two studies, for example, which report peaks for loss in the 10-19 year age period only considered parental death,[31,6a] and in one study where two peaks for loss were found, the earlier peak at 0-5 years

TABLE 1. Parental Loss and Attempted Suicide (AS)—Various Studies

Reference	Age at Time of Loss	Percent Loss—AS	Percent Loss—Control Samples	Percent Loss—General Population
1953 Batchelor[9a]	16	58		
1962 Bruhn[10]	15	42	24	
1965 Dorpat[17]	18	63.8		
1966 Greer[24]	15	49	28 28	
1968 Koller[35]	15	30	17.5 16	
1970 Kearney[34a]	15	36	32 26	
1982 Adam[4]	16	31.6	16.7	
1958 Gregory[26a]				17.4-32.7
1982 Isherwood[31a]				15

TABLE 2. Incidence of Early Loss in Various Studies of Attempted Suicides Corrected for Similar Definition of Loss and Approximate Age at Time of Loss[a,b]

Author	Adam, Bouckoms, and Scarr, 1980[2]	Batchelor and Napier, 1953[9a]	Dorpat, Jackson, and Ripley, 1965[17]	Greer, 1966[24]
Losses to age	16	17	18	15
Attempted suicide (%)	31.6	33.0	40.0	41.6
Control 1	16.7% general practice patients			15.3% nonsuicidal psychiatric patients
Control 2	15.0% general population[c]			16.6% medical and surgical patients

[a] Losses from parental death or permanent separation.
[b] Reprinted from Adam, K. S. 1982. Loss, suicide and attachment. In The Place of Attachment in Human Behavior. C. M. Parkes & J. Stevenson-Hinde, Eds. Basic Books. New York, N.Y., with permission of the publisher. © 1982 by Tavistock Institute of Medical Psychology.
[c] From Isherwood, J. 1980. Doctoral Dissertation. University of Otago. Dunedin, New Zealand.

contained a predominance of losses from divorce/separation, and the later peak a predominance of losses from parental death.[4]

Secondly, while much effort has been devoted to determining the timing of loss, there is no good reason to assume that the point at which loss occurs is the most important factor determining its impact on the child. Rutter has pointed out that the effects of loss may differ depending on a range of factors including not only the age and developmental stage of the child but also the context in which the loss occurs, the presence or absence of alternative parental care, and the long-term consequences to the family of a deterioration in their social and economic situation.[47] Furthermore, while loss of parents from death, divorce, or separation is a dramatic event likely to have impact on the child, it is by no means the only circumstance leading to deficiencies in parental care. It is surprising therefore that so few studies have given attention to the context in which the experience of loss has taken place and its consequences on the family, and the circumstances other than loss that might detract from the consistency and reliability of parental care. A few exceptions must be noted.

Farberow found no significant difference in the incidence of loss among mental hospital patients who had attempted suicide but found more "family strife."[18] Bruhn found a high degree of gross social disorganization in the families of attempted suicides whether or not loss had occurred, noting that unemployment, residential mobility, and marital disharmony often acted in conjunction with parental deprivation.[10] Haider, in a study of 64 adolescents who had attempted suicide, noted that while there was a high incidence of broken homes, "the homes of the majority of those living with both parents was disorganized in many ways, such as an unsatisfactory relationship between parents, frequent quarrels, or a problem relative in the family."[27] Oliver and Kaminski, rating their subjects very simply, noted that only 35% of their attempted suicides came from "happy" homes.[41]

Few studies have looked at the consequences for the family following loss. Greer et al. found no differences between attempted suicides and controls in the numbers who remained with the surviving parent and those who were placed with other relatives or in orphanages,[25] and Koller and Castanos, using the same criteria, found the same information.[35] Neither rated the quality of the subsequent experience.

In two separate studies,[4,5] only one of which I will refer to here, we looked more closely at the early family life of suicidal patients examining not only for the presence of parental loss, but also for the whole question of the consistency and availability of caretaking figures throughout the whole developmental period of life right up to the age of 25. Considered in this inquiry were a broad spectrum of variables affecting the availability of parental figures including chronic illnesses, hospitalizations, parental alcoholism, and serious marital strife. In the first study, which compared 98 attempted suicides to 102 matched controls from a general practice, we examined for parent loss in the usual way looking at permanent losses from parental deaths or divorce and separation of parents up to the age of 25.

In keeping with other studies, we found significantly more parental loss in our attempted suicide subjects than in our general practice controls (48% vs. 23.5% $p < 0.001$). Then using simple and reliable global criteria we rated the early family environment of our subjects on the reliability, consistency, and availability of parental care throughout their developing years from early childhood until leaving home (the age of 25 was chosen as an outside limit.[a]

Ratings were made following review of the detailed protocols of each subject by two researchers who scored subjects independently. Where parental loss had occurred we rated the family stability prior to the loss, then for the period of 12 months or so immediately surrounding the loss, and finally for the long-term period after that. This gave us a measure of the context in which the loss had occurred, its immediate effects on family stability, and its long-term consequences. What we discovered was very revealing (see FIGURES 1 and 2).

Where loss had occurred in our suicidal subjects, the family was more likely to have been unstable beforehand, and to have experienced long-term disorganization of the family afterwards. In the control subjects with a history of loss we found family life was more likely to have been stable prior to the loss and, regardless of how the family had been immediately affected by the event, over the long term family stability returned to earlier levels. Moreover, when we examined those subjects whose homes were technically intact (i.e., with no loss), we found that most of the suicidal subjects had homes that were markedly disorganized and insecure even though no major loss had occurred TABLE 3.

Overall we found 91% of our attempted suicides had homes rated as either unstable or chaotic over the long term compared to only 40% of the controls. Furthermore, of the latter 40%, only 6% were in the more severe (chaotic) category compared to 38% of the attempted suicides. These findings were confirmed in another study in which we examined a group of university students with or without loss from the point

---

[a] Detailed information was collected on family background with particular emphasis on loss, separations, and other data relating to the presence or absence of adequate parental care. Family background data were recorded during the interview and rated as stable, unstable, or chaotic. Stable was defined as adequate parental care consistently available without material hardship. Unstable was defined as adequate parental care inconsistently available for physical or emotional reasons, with or without material hardship. Chaotic was defined as gross deprivation of adequate parental care associated with prolonged separation from parental figures and often with material and emotional deprivation for prolonged periods; it meant an environment of constant uncertainty.

of view of their suicidal ideation.[5] In both cases the data suggested that long-term family disorganization is strongly associated with the development of suicidal propensities and that it may well be the most important variable mediating the association with loss. Furthermore, the fact that loss in the suicidal subjects is superimposed on a family structure that is already disorganized suggested that the family's inability to respond constructively to such a crisis, as other families might, may be an important factor in effecting a pathological outcome.

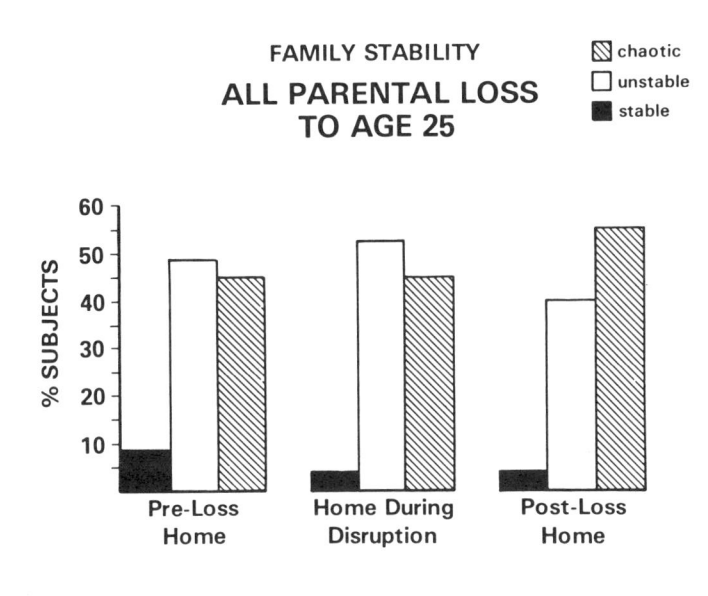

FAMILY STABILITY
ALL PARENTAL LOSS TO AGE 25

chaotic
unstable
stable

Attempted Suicides n = 47

FIGURE 1

STUDIES ON SUICIDAL CHILDREN AND ADOLESCENTS

While these findings are all based on retrospective studies in adults, they have general support in many studies of suicidal behavior in children and adolescents which report a high incidence of family disorganization with marital conflict, parental hospitalization, parental alcoholism, and mental illness repeatedly identified as variables along with the more obvious family disruptions caused by parental deaths, separations, and divorce. More subtle variables such as covert hostility, isolation, and rejection by parents have also been found.[27,37,48,49,14,23,44,53,16]

One recent study, which compared highly suicidal, depressed adolescents to matched nonsuicidal, depressed adolescents, found chronic illness of a parent during adolescence and latency distinguished between the two groups,[22] whereas a family history of suicidal behavior and lifetime psychiatric illness did not. The authors felt that diminished emotional involvement and decreased communication and affection

FAMILY STABILITY
ALL PARENTAL LOSS TO AGE 25

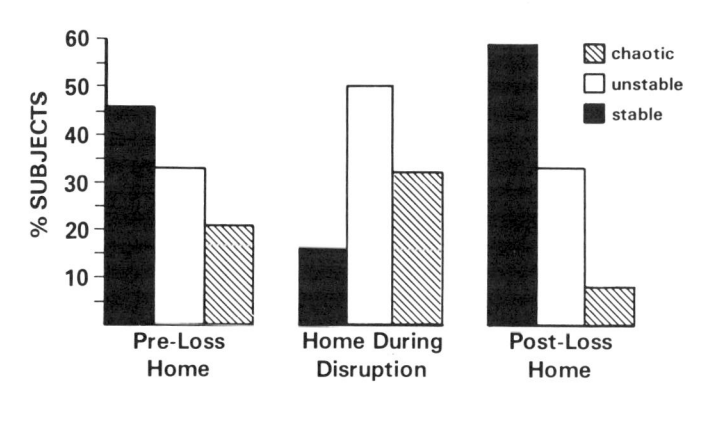

FIGURE 2. Controls n = 24

had been important factors in rendering a parent functionally nonavailable to the child. Another recent study by Hawton *et al.* found a relationship between the severity of family disorganization and the severity of behavioral disturbance and suicidal ideation in the child.[28] What all of these experiences have in common is the threat they pose to the continuity and availability of parental care and emotional support. Evidence that such disturbances can have a profound effect on emotional life and behavior comes from a number of sources which I will only briefly review making particular reference to those effects that appear relevant to self-destructive behavior.

ANIMAL STUDIES

Primate research has provided convincing evidence that deficits in the early social environment can have a profound and enduring influence on social behavior.[51] Rhesus monkeys raised under various conditions of isolation show important social deficits and abnormal behaviors which do not disappear spontaneously but which continue to plague them throughout their lives. Important among these are behavioral and physiological symptoms similar to those observed in depression in humans.[52] Disturbances in the control of aggression are a regular feature of monkeys raised in isolation, often taking the form of self-aggression and, when reunited with their peers, inappropriate aggression towards them. Jones and Barraclough have noted an extensive evidence linking self-injurious behavior in several nonhuman mammals to a number of biological and social variables, including stressful events, interference with sexual bonding, and isolation of confinement.[33] In an interesting study, Jones has pointed to striking similarities between the affective state and social situation preceding suicidal acts in humans and those in animal self-injury, suggesting that they may be homologous behaviors.[34] They feel that the feelings of depression and tension preceding suicidal acts in humans are similar to the agitation and depressionlike behavior observed in animals prior to self-injurious acts and note that conditions of bond disruption, isolation, and confinement are similar in both cases. While the similarities appear to be particularly strong for self-mutilators they hold for self-poisoners as well. Equally significant in terms of our own studies is the fact that these effects can be mediated and modified by varying the interactional conditions of rearing. Factors before, during, and following reunion alter the response of the infant monkey, and among high-risk infants individual responsiveness shows considerable variability.[13] Suomi notes, for example, that infants removed from their environment and raised separately show agitation but not depression, whereas those left in their social environment when their mother is removed show depression.[52] These observations may have a bearing on the differential responsiveness of children to varying conditions of parental deprivation in the early years.

STUDIES OF SEPARATION IN HUMAN CHILDREN

John Bowlby and his followers have demonstrated that human infants regularly show a marked behavioral response to even brief separations from principal caretaking figures in their early years.[7] The typical pattern of these responses is an initial phase of protest, characterized by agitation, tearfulness, and anger; a second phase of despair, during which the child appears quiet and socially withdrawn; and a phase of detachment after prolonged separation, where the child appears to lose interest in the attachment figure and rejects attempts made to approach him. It is hypothesized that the protest phase represents the child's efforts to retrieve his mother through a display of distress while his angry reproaches serve the function of maintaining her proximity to him through the anxiety and guilt engendered by his behavior. The phase of despair is seen as indicative of loss of hope, with the child's active attempts to retrieve the absent maternal figure replaced by preoccupation with thoughts of her and a withdrawal of interest in the external world. In the phase of detachment, the child is seen as giving up hope and having entered into a phase of emotional detachment where painful feelings directed towards the attachment figure are denied and interest with-

TABLE 3. Overall Stability of Home to Age 25[a]

Family Background Rating	Attempted Suicide	Controls	Total
Stable	9 (9.0%)	61 (59.8%)	70
Unstable	52 (53.0%)	35 (34.4%)	87
Chaotic	37 (38.0%)	6 (5.8%)	43
Total	98	102	200

[a] $p < 0.0001$.

drawn more completely from the world of humans. Detached children may alternatively display an insistent sociability but avoid attaching themselves to any one person. In each of these phases the child has been noted to be prone to tantrums and episodes of destructive behavior which Bowlby has described as being often "of a disquietingly destructive violent kind."[7] Upon being reunited with their mothers, children separated for several weeks appear unresponsive and undemanding and eventual recognition of the mother figure is usually accompanied by feelings of intense ambivalence and anger. For a long period thereafter these children demonstrate intense clinging behavior, and when left alone react with acute anxiety and rage. Bowlby has coined the term "attachment behavior" to refer to all such behaviors that result in a person attaining or retaining proximity to some other differentiated or preferred individual.[8] Recent studies have shown, as is the case with primates, that a variety of factors including the duration of the separation, the conditions under which it occurs, and the presence or absence of alternative caretakers can alter the child's responsiveness considerably.

While these effects of brief separations have been studied intensively, the effects of more prolonged, permanent, or repeated discontinuities in parental care have been less well documented. Raphael has reported on a study of families in the community during the first two months following the death of a parent.[44] Many of the children showed disturbances of attachment behavior, with girls showing more clinging and withdrawal, and boys more aggressive responses. Where surrogate figures were present and social supports available the families appeared to be doing well; where they were not, the outcome was poor. Arthur and Kemme, in a descriptive study of 83 children referred to a psychiatric clinic who had experienced the death of a parent, found a high incidence of emotional problems they felt were related to the loss.[6] Intense separation fears occurred in 19% of the children, and 15% of the sample had threatened or attempted suicide. Although dramatic events such as the death of a parent have attracted more attention, an accumulating body of data from clinical and psychoanalytic studies suggests that other forms of deficient parenting may also activate attachment behavior. Examples of these are discontinuities in parental care, unresponsive, rejecting or disparaging interactions, and threats of desertion or withdrawal of love.[9]

ATTACHMENT BEHAVIOR LATER IN LIFE

The relationship of earlier patterns of attachment behavior to attachment behavior later in life has only recently begun to attract attention. Weiss in his studies on the attachment of adolescents to their parents has shown that while attachment to parents continues in normal adolescents, it is eventually transferred from parental figures to another object.[55] His evidence seems to suggest that the quality of attachment remains the same, i.e., it is a "single perceptual system" with similar responses of separation distress and loneliness in the face of the absence of the attachment figure. Bowlby, has described a number of pathological patterns of attachment in later life which he feels are related to disturbed attachment earlier in life.[8] Among these are chronic yearnings for love and support, anxious attachment, compulsive self-reliance, and emotional detachment. These patterns of behavior reflect the lack of trust and insecurity that attachments hold for such individuals, which make it difficult for them to form stable relationships that maintain self-esteem and a sense of continuity in life. Henderson has described a number of behaviors in the interpersonal transactions of adult psychiatric patients as "care-eliciting behavior" which, though disruptive, appeared to function in bringing important others closer.[29,30] Examples he gives are parasuicide, neurotic depression, and abnormal illness behaviors.

"In abnormal care-eliciting, instead of crying, clinging, or using verbal appeals, the individual uses other signals. These signals cause distress to himself and to others, but their consequence is developmentally ancient: they bring others closer."[29]

SUICIDAL BEHAVIOR AND ATTACHMENT

The evidence that suicidal behavior and disturbances in attachment are closely related comes from several sources. Epidemiological studies of attempted suicide and suicide have regularly pointed to a higher incidence of single status and marital failure than in control populations, and many clinical studies have noted that these individuals experience major difficulties in their interpersonal relationships. In one of our studies, for example, only 10% of attempted suicides were rated as having a *stable* current relationship, compared to 75% of general practice controls, and 73% of the attempted suicides felt this relationship was likely to fail.[2] The acute suicidal crisis, more often than not, is precipitated by a crisis in a close interpersonal relationship in which the threat of rejection is imminent.[3,2,19,32] While the actual attempt often takes place impulsively, it is usually preceded by a period of increased stress and deteriorating relationships. Paykel *et al.* found attempted suicides to have experienced four times as many life events in the six months prior to this attempt than the general population and 50% more than depressive controls.[43] Prominent among these events were undesirable and uncontrolled events and serious arguments with a spouse. Similar findings have been reported in suicidal children. Cohen-Sandler *et al.* found that suicidal children not only had experienced more chaotic events throughout their life span than depressed nonsuicidal children and psychiatric controls did, but they experienced an increasing amount of these events as they matured.[14] Nearly all of the events described (parental marital separation, remarriages, hospitalizations, deaths of close grandparents, birth of siblings, and other psychological traumas like witnessing a murder) are likely to have threatened the availability of parental figures.

Clinical studies of individuals seen during the immediate period surrounding suicide attempts suggests a striking resemblance with the behavior of children following brief separations.[1] The actual suicide attempt is usually preceded by clear threats to a significant other person, and often takes place in a situation where discovery is certain. Significant others and caregivers are often subject to angry hostile behavior[57] intermingled with pleading and clinging alternating with aloofness and detachment. While the overt communication may appear to be "I want to die," the circumstances surrounding the events and the associated behavior usually clearly state "I don't want you to leave me." Such a suicidal crisis often takes place over a period of time during which the relationship in question has been deteriorating and may be accompanied by increasing depression and anxiety and increased alcohol or drug intake. The actual attempt usually takes place impulsively. The return of attachment figures ordinarily produces an abrupt abatement of the suicidal crisis with disruption of the relationship producing an escalation.

While many of the data described above come from the study of attempted suicide, similar factors have been identified in those who succeed in killing themselves. A high incidence of broken homes has been found in a number of studies,[17,50,46] with one exception,[11] and suicide is related to a number of indices of social disorganization with marital breakdown, isolation, and downward mobility prominent among these.[39,12] Ovenstone and Kreitman, in a study of 106 suicides, distinguished two syndromes of suicide in terms of their course and psychosocial characteristics.[42] One group characterized as "chronically disorganized" was composed of sociopaths, drug addicts, and alcoholics with long histories of psychological and social instability. They all had a history of previous suicide attempts, their sucidal acts were often precipitated by interpersonal conflicts, and took place in the vicinity of others following a communication of intent. A second group, with no history of previous attempts, was composed of relatively stable personalities with marginal adaptability and close dependency on one particular person. The final suicidal act in this group was more clearly precipitated by a recent bereavement or other personal loss such as major illness and was usually carried out alone using lethal methods. In both groups significant depression and heavy drinking were prominent prior to the suicidal act.

As much attention has been given in the literature to the role of major affective disorder in completed suicide, it is important to point to the role of social risk factors there. Roy, in a study of suicide in psychiatric patients, found 42.2% had a history of parental loss, 60% were unemployed, 55% were living alone, and 84.5% were unmarried.[45] Forty-four percent of this sample had a primary diagnosis of depressive disorder, 40% were schizophrenic, and 8.8% were dependent on alcohol. While it could be argued that these social variables are merely consequences of the primary diagnosis, several studies using nonsuicidal depressives as controls suggest this may not be the case. Walton found a much higher incidence of "parental deprivation" in suicidal depressives than in nonsuicidal depressives,[54] and Roy found a higher incidence of parental loss in patients with recurrent affective disorder who committed suicide than in controls with the same disorder who did not.[46] Moreover, significantly more in the suicidal group were living alone. Friedman *et al.*, in a recent study comparing highly suicidal depressed adolescents to matched nonsuicidal depressives, found chronic illness of a parent in latency to distinguish between the two groups, whereas a history of suicidal behavior and psychiatric illness in the parents did not.[22]

Viewed in these terms, I believe that much of what is called suicidal behavior can more usefully be conceptualized as attachment behavior, with its function not primarily a retreat from the world and its disappointments, but a desperate attempt to maintain relatedness to a vital attachment figure in the face of a threatening situation (FIGURE 3).

Using this model suicidal behavior can be seen in a developmental context with early insecurity about primary attachments linked to an impaired capacity to form and maintain the attachments that are essential to the maintenance of self-esteem and continuity throughout the life cycle. Early attachment failure may lead to the persistent patterns of attachment difficulties we associate with the disordered personality where excessive object hunger, anxious attachment, and emotional detachment place excessive demands on key relationships, leading to their breakdown. Such individuals are not only more prone to form insecure relationships but are unduly sensitive to threats to their continuation, reacting strongly with the activation of separation or abandonment anxiety of which suicidal ideation may be one component. Whatever other meanings suicidal behavior may have, it serves effectively in signaling distress to others in the social environment, admonishing them for neglect, punishing them for rejection, and coercing them to reestablish a needed bond. The successful formation of stable attachments, which may occur in spite of earlier difficulties, serves a protective function, whereas recurrent failure to achieve this end may lead to the social isolation and despair we associate with the successful suicide's final bitter statement to the world. Chronic alcoholism, major depressive disorder, and deterioration of the personality from other causes diminish the individual's capacity to respond to his situation and contribute to his downward social spiral. Viewed in attachment terms, the peaking of suicide attempts in the earlier years of life can be seen as a manifestation of more active attachment behavior in those prone to insecure attachments at a time when opportunities for relationships are more abundant. The less frequent event of completed suicide on the other hand may be related to the greater vulnerability to the effects of loss later in life when failing health and diminished productivity in other areas form a cumulative burden affecting self-esteem.

The well-known and puzzling association of attempted suicide with younger women

Attachment History	Psychological Response	Attachment Behavior	Associated Behavior
Insecure attachment	Separation anxiety	Protest Despair Detachment	
Failure of alternative attachments	Persistent anxiety Depression	Object hunger Anxious attachment Emotional detachment	Antisocial behavior Behavior disorder School Phobia Illness behavior
Impaired capacity to form attachments	Loneliness Low self-esteem Depression	Relationship difficulties Marital dysfunction	Personality disorder Alcohol and drug abuse
Threatened attachment	Abandonment anxiety Suicidal ideation	Suicidal threats Suicide attempts	Alcoholic binges Promiscuity Phobic states
Recurrent attachment failure	Chronic anxiety Severe depression Persistent suicidal ideation	Repeated suicide attempts	Major affective disorder Chronic alcoholism
Social isolation	Hopelessness Despair	SUICIDE	

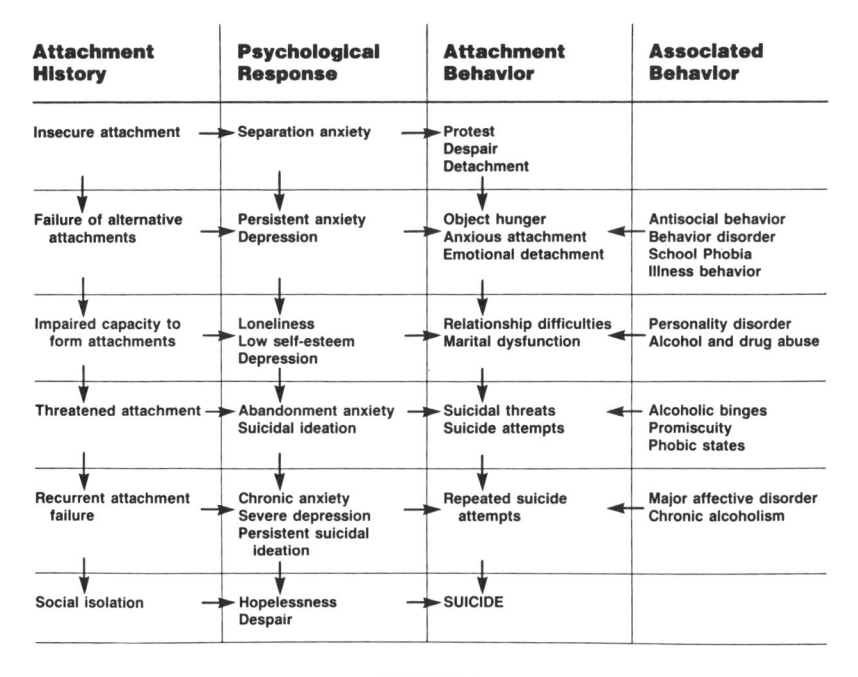

FIGURE 3

and completed suicide with older men may at least partially be explained in attachment terms. For whatever reason, women are more reliant than men on personal attachments for the maintenance of self-esteem, and this may result in more active attachment behavior and more enduring relationships over the long term. Men on the other hand are more likely to invest in work and other diversions to maintain self-esteem and may consequently be more vulnerable to the effects of bereavement, ill health, and retirement later on.

It has long been recognized that attempted suicide is more than just failed suicide but it has not generally been appreciated the extent to which suicide is really failed attachment.

REFERENCES

1. ADAM, K. S. & G. ADAM. 1978. Attachment theory and attempted suicide. Paper presented at the Fifteenth Annual Congress of Royal Australian and New Zealand College of Psychiatrists, Singapore.
2. ADAM, K. S., A. BOUCKOMS & G. SCARR. 1980. Attempted suicide in Christchurch: a controlled study. Aust. N. Z. J. Psychiatry 14(4): 305-314.
3. ADAM, K., G. BIANCHI, F. HAWKER, L. NAIRN, M. SANFORD & G. SCARR. 1978. Interpersonal factors in suicide attempts. A pilot study in Christchurch. Aust. N. Z. J. Psychiatry 12: 59-63.
4. ADAM, K. S., A. BOUCKOMS & D. STREINER. 1982. Parental loss and family stability in attempted suicide. Arch. Gen. Psychiatry 39: 1081-1085.
5. ADAM, K. S., J. LOHRENZ & D. HARPER. 1982. Early parental loss and suicide ideation in university students. Can. J. Psychiatry 27: 275-281.
6. ARTHUR, B. & M. KEMME. 1964. Bereavement in childhood. J. Child Psychol. Psychiatry 5: 37-49.
6a. BIRTCHNELL, J. 1970 The relationship between attempted suicide, depression, and parent death. Br. J. Psychiatry 116: 307-313.
7. BOWLBY, J. 1969. Attachment. *In* Attachment and Loss, 1. Basic Books. New York, N.Y.
8. BOWLBY, J. 1977. The making and breaking of affectional bonds. I. Aetiology and psychopathology in the light of attachment theory. Br. J. Psychiatry 130: 201-210.
9. BOWLBY, J. 1980. Loss, sadness, and depression. *In* Attachment and Loss, 3. Basic Books. New York, N.Y.
9a. BATCHELOR, L. & M. C. NAPIER. 1953. Broken homes and attempted suicide. Br. J. Delinquency 4: 99-108.
10. BRUHN, J. G. 1982. Broken homes among attempted suicides and psychiatric outpatients: a comparative study. J. Ment. Sci. 108: 772-779.
11. BUNCH, J., B. BARRACLOUGH, B. NELSON & P. SAINSBURY. 1971. Early parental bereavement and suicide. Soc. Psychiatry 6(4): 200-202.
12. BUNCH, J. 1972. Recent bereavement in relation to suicide. J. Psychosom. Res. 16: 361-366.
13. CAIRNS, R. B. 1977. Beyond social attachment: the dynamics of interactional development. *In* Attachment Behaviour: Advances in the Study of Communication and Affect. T. Alloway, P. Plinen & L. Krames, Eds.: 1-21. Plenum Press. New York, N.Y.
14. COHEN-SANDLER, R., A. L. BERMAN & R. A. KING, 1982. Life stress and symptomatology: determinants of suicidal behaviour in children. J. Am. Acad. Child Psychiatry 21: 178-186.
15. CROOK, T. & A. RASKIN. 1975. Association of childhood parental loss with attempted suicide and depression. J. Consult. Clin. Psychol. 43(2): 277.
16. CRUMLEY, F. E. 1981. Adolescent suicide attempts and borderline personality disorder: clinical features. South. Med. J. 74: 546-549.
17. DORPAT, T. L., J. K. JACKSON & H. S. RIPLEY. 1965. Broken homes and attempted suicide and completed suicide. Arch. Gen. Psychiatry 12: 213-216.
18. FARBEROW, N. 1950. Personality patterns of suicidal mental hospital patients. Genet. Psychol. Monogr. 42: 3-79.
19. FIELDSEND, R. & E. LOWENSTEIN. 1981. Quarrels, separations and infidelity in the two days preceding self-poisoning episodes. Br. J. Med. Psychol. 54: 349-352.
20. FREUD, S. 1957. Mourning and melancholia. *In* The Standard Edition of the Complete Psychological Works of Sigmund Freud. J. Strachey, Ed. 14: 232-258. Hogarth Press. London, England.
21. FRIEDMAN, R. C., M. S. ANONOFF, J. F. CLARKIN, *et al.* 1983. History of suicidal behaviour in depressed borderline inpatients. Am. J. Psychiatry 140: 1023-1026.
22. FRIEDMAN, R. C., R. CORN, S. HART, *et al.* 1984. Family history of illness in the seriously suicidal adolescent: a life-cycle approach. Am. J. Orthopsychiatry 54(3): 390-397.
23. GARFINKEL, B. D., A. FROESE & J. HOOD. 1982. Suicide attempts in children and adolescents. Am. J. Psychiatry 139(10): 1257-1261.
24. GREER, S. 1966. Parental loss and attempted suicide: a further report. Br. J. Psychiatry 112: 465-470.

25. GREER, S. C., J. C. GUNN & K. M. KOLLER. 1966. Aetiological factors in attempted suicide. Br. Med. J. 2: 1352-1355.
26. GOLDNEY, R. D. 1981. Parental loss and reported childhood stress in young women who attempt suicide. Acta Psychiatr. Scand. 64: 34-59.
26a. GREGORY, I. 1958. Studies of parental deprivation in psychiatric patients. Am. J. Psychiatry 115: 432-442.
27. HAIDER, I. 1968. Suicidal attempts in children and adolescents. Br. J. Psychiatry 114: 1133-1134.
28. HAWTON, K., M. OSBORN, J. O'GRADY, et al. 1982. Classification of adolescents who take overdoses. Br. J. Psychiatry 140: 124-131.
29. HENDERSON, A. S. 1974. Care-eliciting behaviour in man. J. Nerv. Ment. Dis. 159(3): 172-181.
30. HENDERSON, S. 1982. The significance of social relationships in the etiology of neurosis. In The Place of Attachment in Human Behaviour. C. M. Parkes & J. Stevenson-Hinde, Eds.: 205-231. Basic Books. New York, N.Y.
31. HILL, O. W. 1969. The association of childhood bereavement with suicidal attempt in depressive illness. Br. J. Psychiatry 115: 301-304.
31a. ISHERWOOD, J., K. S. ADAM & A. HORNBLOW. 1982. Life event stress, psychosocial factors, suicide attempt and auto-accident proclivity. J. Psychosom. Res. 26: 371-383.
32. JACOBSON, G. & S. PORTUGES. 1978. Relation of marital separation and divorce to suicide: a report. Suicide Life-Threat. Behav. 8(4): 217-224.
33. JONES, I. H. & B. M. BARRACLOUGH. 1978. Auto-mutilation in animals and its relevance to self-injury in man. Acta Psychiatr. Scand. 58: 40-47.
34. JONES, I. H., L. CONGIU, J. STEVENSON, et al. 1979. A biological approach to two forms of human self-injury. J. Nerv. Ment. Dis. 167(2): 74-78.
34a. KEARNEY, T. R. 1970. Aetiology of attempted suicide. In Proceedings of the Fifth International Conference on Suicide Prevention, London, England: 190-194. International Association for Suicide Prevention. Vienna, Austria.
35. KOLLER, K. M. & J. N. CASTANOS. 1968. The influence of childhood parental deprivation in attempted suicide. Med. J. Aust. 1: 396-399.
36. LEVI, L. D., C. H. FALES, M. STEIN, et al. 1966. Separation and attempted suicide. Arch. Gen. Psychiatry 15: 158-164.
37. LUKIANOWICZ, N. 1968. Attempted suicide in children. Acta Psychiatr. Scand. 44: 415-435.
38. MALTZBERGER, J. T. & D. H. BUIE. 1980. The devices of suicide. Int. Rev. Psychoanal. 7: 61-71.
39. MARIS, R. 1975. Sociology. In A Handbook for the Study of Suicide. S. Perlin, Ed.: 93-112. Oxford University Press. New York, N.Y.
40. MOSS, L. M. & D. M. HAMILTON. 1956. Psychotherapy of suicidal patients. Am. J. Psychiatry 112: 814-820.
41. OLIVER, R. G., Z. KAMINSKI, K. TUDOR, et al. 1971. The epidemiology of attempted suicide as seen in the casualty department, Alfred Hospital, Melbourne. Med. J. Aust. 1: 833-839.
42. OVENSTONE, I. M. K. & N. KREITMAN. 1974. Two syndromes of suicide. Br. J. Psychiatry 124: 336-345.
43. PAYKEL, E. S., B. PRUSOFF & J. K. MYERS. 1975. Suicide attempts and recent life events. Arch. Gen. Psychiatry 32: 327-333.
44. PFEFFER, C. R. 1985. Self-destructive behaviour in children and adolescents. Psychiatr. Clin. North Am. 8(2): 215-226.
45. RAPHAEL, B. 1982. The young child and death of a parent. In The Place of Attachment in Human Behavior. C. M. Parkes & J. Stevenson-Hinde, Eds.: 131-150. Basic Books. New York, N.Y.
46. ROY, A. 1982. Risk factors for suicide in psychiatric patients. Arch. Gen. Psychiatry 39: 1089-1095.
47. RUTTER, M. 1981. Maternal Deprivation Reassessed. 2nd edit. Penguin Books. Harmondsworth, England.
48. SHAFFER, D. 1974. Suicide in childhood and early adolescence. J. Child Psychol. Psychiatry 15: 275-291.

49. STANLEY, E. J. & J. T. BARTER. 1978. Adolescent suicidal behaviour. Am. J. Orthopsychiatry **132:** 180-185.
50. STENGEL, E. 1964. Suicide and Attempted Suicide. Penguin Books. Harmondsworth, England.
51. SUOMI, S. J. 1977. Development of attachment and other social behaviours in rhesus monkeys. *In* Attachment Behavior: Advances in the Study of Communication and Affect. T. Alloway, P. Plinen & L. Krames, Eds. **3:** 197-224. Plenum Press. New York, N.Y.
52. SUOMI, S. J. 1985. Ethology: animal models. *In* Comprehensive Textbook of Psychiatry. H. Kaplan & J. Sadock, Eds. 4th edit. **1:** 226-236. Williams & Wilkins. Baltimore, Md.
53. TISHLER, C. L. & P. C. MCKENNEY. 1982. Parental negative self and adolescent suicide attempts. J. Am. Acad. Child Psychiatry **21:** 404-408.
54. WALTON, H. J. 1958. Suicidal behaviour in depressive illness: a study of aetiological factors in suicide. J. Ment. Sci. **104:** 884-891.
55. WEISS, R. S. 1982. Attachment in adult life. *In* The Place of Attachment in Human Behaviour. C. M. Parkes & J. Stevenson-Hinde, Eds.: 171-184. Basic Books. New York, N.Y.
56. WEISMANN, M. 1974. The epidemiology of suicide attempts. Arch. Gen Psychiatry **30:** 737-746.
57. WEISMANN, M., K. FOX & G. L. KLERMAN. 1973. Hostility and depression associated with suicide attempts. Am. J. Psychiatry **130:** 450-455.

Psychosocial Factors and Suicidal Behavior

Life Events, Early Loss, and Personality

CHRISTINE K. CROSS

Group Operations, Incorporated
12750 Twinbrook Parkway
Rockville, Maryland 20852

ROBERT M. A. HIRSCHFELD

Center for Studies of Affective Disorders
Clinical Research Branch
Division of Extramural Research Programs
National Institute of Mental Health
Parklawn Building
5600 Fishers Lane
Rockville, Maryland 20857

INTRODUCTION

Investigations of the psychosocial factors associated with suicidal behavior are directed toward two goals: etiology and prediction. The etiologic question asks whether there are psychosocial factors, such as personality features, early life experiences, or stressful life events, that singly or in combination lead people to make attempts on and sometimes take their own lives. The prediction question parallels the etiologic one: Can certain psychosocial factors, singly or in combination, enable us to predict who will attempt or complete suicide, and, equally importantly, when?

This paper will review our current state of knowledge on the relationship between psychosocial factors and suicidal attempts and completions. Before proceeding with the review, the nature of this relationship will be placed in a conceptual framework and definitions of key variables will be presented.

The Relationship between Psychosocial Factors and Suicidal Behavior

Psychosocial factors may relate to suicidal behavior in any of three ways. First, they may relate indirectly, either predisposing a person to or mediating against suicidal behavior under certain conditions. Thus, early loss and certain personality characteristics, such as neuroticism and impulsivity, are generally viewed as predisposing factors, while social support and certain other personality characteristics such as restraint and objectivity may be viewed as mediating or protective factors. Second, psychosocial factors may act as precipitating or direct causal factors in suicidal behavior. Life events are, most notably, considered precipitating factors in suicidal behavior. And, third, psychosocial factors may be epiphenomenal. In other words, they may be related to a phenomenon—such as depression—which, in turn, is related to suicidal behavior, but with no real link between the psychosocial factor and suicidal behavior.

Definitions

The term attempted suicide refers to deliberate self-injurious acts committed by a person, with or without intent to die. Completed suicide refers to such acts that result in death. Suicide attempters and completers do share certain characteristics. For example both populations have high rates of psychiatric illness—in particular, depression—both groups have high divorce and unemployment rates, and a history of attempted suicide has been reported to characterize as many as 65% of completed suicides.[1-9] However, despite their overlap, the two populations are distinct. Suicide attempters are overwhelmingly young and female, while suicide completers tend to be older and overwhelmingly male. Moreover, only an estimated 10% to 20% suicide attempters subsequently commit suicide.

Recent life events refer to environmental occurrences that cause disruption to a person's customary life pattern with some degree of resulting distress or upset. Examples of life events include loss of a spouse due to death or divorce, change in residence, loss or change of employment, and the like. With regard to suicide, such events are viewed as precipitants when they occur in close proximity to the suicidal act.

Early loss refers to the loss of a parent or parents during childhood or adolescence due to death, divorce, or legal separation. A loss of this type may be considered a life event, but rather than recent, the event is remote and, as such, may be viewed as a predisposing rather than precipitating factor for suicidal behavior.

Personality refers to relatively enduring traits or characteristic modes of behavior exhibited by persons. As they relate to suicidal behavior, personality traits are viewed as predispositional. That is, certain personality characteristics such as neuroticism, dependency, or impulsivity may render a person vulnerable to suicidal acts under certain circumstances.

The primary source of data regarding psychosocial factors associated with suicidal behavior derives from retrospective investigations in which a group of suicide attempters or completers is identified, either among patients admitted to general hospital emergency rooms or among psychiatric patients, and compared on the variable(s) of interest to a group of nonattempter control subjects, selected either from the general population or from a psychiatric population. In addition, a few prospective studies of suicide have been conducted in the area of life events. The investigations follow a group of subjects selected from either the general population or from a psychiatric population and, after some specified period of time, identify those subjects who have suicided during the study period. The suicide group is then compared with the non-suicides on the variable(s) of interest.

An examination of existing literature provides some insights concerning psychosocial risk factors for suicidal behavior, despite certain limitations imposed by research design problems. In the sections that follow, a review and a synthesis of recent studies on the relationship of recent life events, early loss, and personality to attempted and completed suicide are presented. These studies are summarized in TABLES 1 and 2. The paper concludes with a summary of these findings and suggestions for future research.

ATTEMPTED SUICIDE

Life Events

Three relatively recent retrospective studies have examined the role of life events in suicide attempts. In their classic 1975 study, Paykel and his associates compared the frequency, type, and patterning of life events in 53 suicide attempters admitted to a general hospital emergency service to those in 53 age- and sex-matched nonsuicidal depressed patients and in 53 age- and sex-matched controls from the general population.[10] They found that the suicide attempters had four times as many life events (a mean of 3.3 per person) in the six months prior to the attempt as occurred in the general population controls (a mean of 0.8 per person) and one and one-half times as many as the depressed patients (a mean of 2.1 per person).

As compared to the normal controls, the suicide attempter group had more entrance (additions to social field), more exit (losses from social field), and more health, family, legal, and marriage-related events. In addition, the events experienced by the suicide attempters were more often undesirable, highly threatening, and uncontrollable than those experienced by the general population controls. Fewer differences in types of life events were found between suicide attempters and depressed controls, with only entrance and undesirable events occurring more frequently in attempters.

Event rates were relatively constant over the six-month period for normal controls. Depressed controls showed a moderated peak in event rates in the month before onset of the depressive episode. The suicide attempters had elevated rates throughout during the entire six-month period, with a marked peak occurring in the month before the attempt.

The results of this study may be limited in their generalizability, however, since the suicide attempter group was composed predominantly of young females (as were the depressed and normal control groups) whose attempts were relatively low in intent and lethality. Therefore, the results may not be representative of the more serious older male attempters who are at highest risk for completed suicide. Nonetheless, as the authors point out, these findings do suggest that suicide attempts are "often immediate reactions to stressful personal and interpersonal crises [p. 333]."[10]

Slater and Depue address the shortcomings of the Paykel *et al.* study in their investigation of life events and social supports in 14 suicidal and 14 nonsuicidal patients.[11] All subjects in this study met Research Diagnostic Criteria for primary major depressive disorder, and the attempts made by the suicidal group were moderately to severely lethal. The time period studied was the one year prior to hospitalization for either the suicide attempt or depression. Onset of depression and occurrence of life events were carefully dated and checked for reliability in both groups.

TABLE 1. Summary of Studies Relating Psychosocial Factors to Attempted Suicide[a]

Study	Sample	Methods	Major Findings
Life events			
Paykel et al.[10] 1975	53 SA admitted to general hospital 53 matched NSA depressed C 53 matched normal C	Semistructured LE inventory covering 6 mos. prior to attempt, onset of depressive episode, or interview.	SA had 4 times as many LE as normal C, 50% more than depressed C; event rates were increased for entire 6 mos. in SA, with a marked peak in the month before attempt.
Slater & Depue[11] 1981	14 SA with primary depression 14 NSA with primary depression	Semistructured LE inventory covering year prior to interview.	SA had no more LE prior to depression onset than depressed C but had significantly more in the postonset period; significantly fewer SA had social support in the form of a confidant.
Luscomb et al.[12] 1980	47 male SA admitted to VA hospital 51 male VA psychiatric patient C	Semistructured Life Stress inventory covering year prior to hospital admission.	Only older SA reported greater life stress and exit events compared to older C; no differences were found for younger groups.
Early loss			
Crook & Raskin[14] 1975	115 SA depressed patients 115 NSA depressed C 285 normal C		SA had experienced more early loss due to separation or divorce than depressed and normal C. No differences in parental loss due to death were found.
Morgan et al.[15] 1975	368 SA psychiatric patients		Approximately 50% of SA had been separated from one or both parents before age 15.
Goldney[16] 1981	110 female SA admitted to general hospital 25 female C		Higher percentage of SA had experienced earlier loss than C. Higher levels of childhood stress in SA also found. Incidence of loss did not differ between SA groups classified on the basis of lethality of attempt.
Adam et al.[17] 1982	98 SA admitted to general hospital 102 matched C		Significantly more SA had experienced parental loss due to separation or divorce, but not death, than C. Incidence of family instability almost twice as great in SA than C.

Adam et al.[18] 1982	75 subjects with history of parental loss 102 matched C without history of parental loss		Suicidal ideation and attempts more prevalent in parental loss group. Incidence of suicidal behavior was significantly high in those whose parental loss resulted in unstable or chaotic home environment.
Personality			
Pallis & Jenkins[20] 1977	124 SA classified as to seriousness of intent	Eysenck Personality Inventory	Male SA with low intent had higher impulsivity scores (Extraversion Subscale) than males with high intent.
Pallis & Birtchnell[19] 1977	42 serious SA psychiatric patients 42 nonserious SA psychiatric patients 126 matched NSA patient C	Minnesota Multiphasic Personality Inventory	No differences found between serious SA and C. Nonserious SA showed higher levels of dependency, hostility, and unconventionality than other two groups.
Goldney[21] 1982	110 female SA 25 female C	Adult Nowicki-Strickland Locus of Control Scale	SA had significantly higher externality scores than C. Within SA group, lethality of attempt was inversely related to externality scores.
Luscomb et al.[12] 1980	47 male SA admitted to VA hospital 51 male VA psychiatric C	Rotter Internal-External Locus of Control Scale	No between-group differences in Locus of Control.
Banki & Arato[22] 1983	19 female SA psychiatric 43 female NSA psychiatric patients 70 normal female C	Marke-Nyman Temperament Scale	SA scores higher on stability and lower on validity than NSA and normal C. Low validity scores were associated with violent attempts. No differences in solidity were found.

[a] SA = suicide attempters; NSA = non-suicide attempters; C = controls; LE = life events; VA = Veterans Administration.

TABLE 2. Summary of Studies Relating Psychosocial Factors to Completed Suicide[a]

Study	Sample	Methods	Major Findings
Life events			
Dorpat & Ripley[3] 1960	114 consecutive S	Information from official records and interviews with relatives.	Physical and psychiatric illness and recent loss of a loved one were found to contribute significantly to a large percentage of the suicides.
Hagnell & Rorsman[23] 1980	28 S from Lundby study 56 matched C 25 matched natural death C	Information gathered from official records and interviews with relatives for last year of life for S and ND, corresponding year for C (prospective).	Acute psychiatric illness most prominent LE preceding suicide. More S than C or ND had also experienced undesirable LE during year prior to death.
Borg & Stahl[24] 1982	34 psychiatric patient S 34 matched patient C	Semistructured interview information obtained at hospital intake; information from official records (prospective).	S more likely to be widowed or have lived alone than C. S tended to have "loss of a key person" judged as a significant precipitating factor in their psychiatric disorder more often than C.
Murphy et al.[25] 1979	50 unselected alcoholic S	Information from interview with relative.	26% of S suffered loss of a close interpersonal relationship within 6 weeks of suicide.
Early loss			
Dorpat et al.[13] 1965	88 S		50% of S came from broken homes and more than 20% had experienced early loss due to death.
Roy[26] 1984	13 manic-depressive S 13 matched manic-depressive C		More than half of S had experienced early loss due to death, divorce, or separation, while only 1 C had experienced such loss.
Personality			
No studies available employing formal psychometric methods.			

[a] S = suicides; C = controls; LE = life events; ND = natural death.

Slater and Depue report that although the percentage of subjects reporting at least one moderately to severely distressing life event in the preonset period did not differ between the two groups (all 14 attempters versus 11 of the 14 nonattempters), overwhelmingly more of the suicide attempters reported at least one such event during the postonset period than did nonattempters (10 versus 1, respectively).

Differences between the two groups emerged in social support as well. Significantly fewer of the suicide attempters than controls had the support of a confidant. In fact, less than half of the suicide attempters as compared to 12 of the 14 controls had such support. Moreover, of the suicide attempters without social support, 75% had experienced the loss of their confidant during the study period.

These findings indicate that onset of depressive episodes is associated with the occurrence of distressing life events. What distinguishes suicidal from nonsuicidal depressives is the continued occurrence of such events after the onset of depression in the suicidal group and the supportive presence of a confidant in the nonsuicidal group.

Results inconsistent with those described above were reported by Luscomb and his colleagues in their study of male suicide attempters in a veteran's hospital.[12] These authors found that, in general, suicide attempters did not differ from nonsuicidal psychiatric patients in level of stress experienced during the year preceding hospital admission, although older suicide attempters did report greater stress and more exit events than did older controls. Several serious methodological flaws may account for these discrepant findings, including the fact that the suicide attempter group was significantly younger and less psychotic than the psychiatric control group and the lack of restrictions placed on lethality or seriousness of the attempts.

Early Loss

A substantial literature exists on the relationship between early loss and suicidal behavior. Although the results of these studies are not entirely consistent, overall they do suggest that individuals who experience such losses constitute a high-risk group for suicidal behavior in adulthood. For example, Dorpat and his associates reported that approximately 69% of their 121 suicide attempters had come from broken homes.[13] Crook and Raskin found that parental loss due to divorce, desertion, or legal separation—but not death—was significantly more common in a group of 115 suicidal depressives as compared to groups of nonsuicidal depressives and normal controls;[14] and, Morgan and associates found that half of their 368 suicide attempters had been separated from one or both parents before age 15.[15]

While earlier studies tended to focus on the discrete loss event, more recent research has extended the emphasis to include the quality of the early environment of suicide attempters. Three recent studies of the early environment of suicide attempters indicate that family stability in childhood rather than early loss per se may be associated with suicidal behavior in adulthood. Goldney compared the incidence of early loss and ratings of childhood stress in a group of 110 female suicide attempters, aged 18 to 30, and a group of 25 similarly aged normal female controls.[16] A significantly higher percentage of suicide attempters (approximately one-third) than controls (none) had lost one or both parents due to death, divorce, or separation before the age of 15. In terms of type of loss, however, only loss due to divorce or separation, not death, differed significantly between the two groups (22% versus 0). Childhood stress ratings were also significantly higher in the suicide attempter group. Examination of individual factors comprising the total stress score revealed that suicide attempters were more likely to come from a broken home, more likely to report frequent parental quarrels and frequent disagreements with parents, and more likely to perceive their parents' characters negatively than were controls. When comparisons of the suicide attempt group classified on the basis of lethality of attempt were made, neither the incidence of early loss nor ratings of childhood stress differed among the groups. In addition, no differences in depression rating scores emerged when suicide attempters with and without parental loss were compared.

Two studies of early loss and early life experiences were conducted by Adam and his colleagues.[17,18] In the first, the authors compared 98 suicide attempters with matched controls from a sample of consecutive admissions to a New Zealand general hospital emergency department.[17] A significantly higher prevalence of parental loss among the suicide attempters was found, especially loss due to divorce or separation. Nearly half of the group had lost one or both of their parents before the age of 15 as compared with less than 25% of the control subjects. In addition, nearly all of the attempted suicide group (91%) came from a family environment rated as unstable or chaotic as compared with less than half of the control subjects. Between-group differences in family stability remained significant even when only subjects from intact homes were compared.

In their second study, Adam and his associates compared suicidal ideation and behavior in a group of 75 students presenting to a university mental health clinic who had a history of parental loss before the age of 16 to a matched student control group attending the clinic without a history of such loss.[18] Significantly more suicidal ideation characterized the early-loss group, and significantly more had made suicide attempts compared to the controls. Suicidal behavior was most marked in the early-loss group where such loss resulted in long-term disruption of family stability. Conversely, suicidal behavior was minimal in the early-loss group when family stability was maintained.

Personality

Pallis and Jenkins compared the Eysenck Personality Inventory scores of 124 suicide attempters categorized on the basis of seriousness of intent and as recurrent or not.[19] Two differences emerged from their analyses: male suicide attempters with low intent had higher scores on the extraversion-impulsivity subscale than did males with high intent; and recurrent attempters of both sexes had higher neuroticism scores than did first-time attempters.

Pallis and Birtchnell examined the clinical and derived subscale scores on the Minnesota Multiphasic Personality Inventory in three matched groups of psychiatric patients—42 serious suicide attempters, 42 nonserious suicide attempters, and 126 nonsuicidal controls.[20] They found no differences between serious attempters and controls on any of the measures. Nonserious attempters, on the other hand, showed higher levels of dependency, hostility, and unconventionality than did either of the other two groups, with deviations being most marked in nonserious male attempters.

Goldney, in a study of locus of control and suicidal behavior, compared the externality scores of his sample of 110 young female suicide attempters to those of 25 young female control subjects.[21] Suicide attempters had significantly higher externality scores than did controls. Within the attempter group, however, highly lethal attempts were associated with lower levels of externality. In addition, externality scores were found to correlate with ratings of childhood stress, but not depression scores.

Luscomb and his associates also compared locus of control scores in their sample of suicidal and nonsuicidal male psychiatric patients.[12] They found no differences between the two groups in levels of externality.

Finally, Banki and Arato included measures of personality among other, biochemical measures in their study of suicide attempters.[22] Comparisons of Marke-Nyman Temperament Scale (MNT) scores were made in a group of 19 female psychiatric patients who had attempted suicide, a group of 43 nonsuicidal female psychiatric patients, and a group of 70 normal female controls. Suicide attempters scored significantly higher on stability (a measure of emotional distance or introversion) and significantly lower on validity (a neuroticism-type measure) than did either of the other two groups. No differences were found on solidity (a measure of impulsivity). In contrast to previous reports, deviations in personality were most pronounced in violent suicide attempters.

COMPLETED SUICIDE

Life Events

The role of life events in completed suicide has been studied both retrospectively and prospectively. Dorpat and Ripley obtained information on 114 consecutive suicides from official records and from interviews with relatives.[4] They found that the occurrence of serious physical and psychiatric illness and the recent loss of a loved one were factors reported to have contributed significantly to the suicides in a large percentage of their subjects.

Hagnell and Rorsman[23] reported on the stressful life events occurring to the 28 suicides in the longitudinal Lundby study. Each suicide subject was matched with two normal controls and one natural death from the study and information obtained from official and study records and from interviews with relatives. Acute psychiatric illness was the most prominent life event preceding suicide. In addition, more of the suicides as compared to controls had experienced undesirable life events in the year prior to their death. Such events included humiliating experiences, particularly in the areas of work and legal, object loss, and change of residence.

In another prospective study of psychiatric patients, Borg and Stahl compared a group of 34 patients who had committed suicide in a two-year period to a control group of nonsuicidal psychiatric patients matched for age, sex, diagnosis, and patient status.[24] The suicide group had a significantly higher percentage of "nonmarrieds" than did controls. In addition, in a greater percentage of suicides, loss of a key person by death (but not by divorce or separation) had been judged a significant precipitating factor in their psychiatric disorder.

Finally, Murphy and his associates found that in a study of 50 unselected alcoholic suicides, 26% had experienced the loss of a close, interpersonal relationship within the six weeks prior to their death.[25]

Early Loss

In a study of the family backgrounds of 88 suicides, Dorpat and his colleagues found that 50% had come from broken homes and that more than 20% had experienced death of a parent before the age of 18.[13] A recent study by Roy also investigated early loss in completed suicides. Comparing matched groups of manic depressive patients, 13 who suicided and 13 controls, he found that more than half of the suicide group (7 of 13) had experienced early parental loss either through death, divorce, or separation, whereas only 1 of the controls had experienced such loss.[26]

Personality

To date, no research has been conducted to study the personalities of completed suicides using formal psychometric instruments.

DISCUSSION

Several psychosocial risk factors for suicidal behavior have been identified in the literature reviewed. As is true in most areas of suicide research, the literature relating psychosocial factors and completed suicide is more sparse and not as rigorous methodologically as that on attempted suicide. However, except in the area of personality where no studies employing formal psychometric measures are available on completed suicides, psychosocial risk factors for completed and attempted suicide appear to be similar—the occurrence of negative life events, particularly loss events, lack of social support, and a history of early loss or chaotic childhood environment. A comparison of psychosocial risk factors for completed and attempted suicide is presented in TABLE 3.

The results of studies of life events and suicidal behavior, taken as a whole, strongly suggest that the occurrence of negative life events plays a significant precipitating role in both attempted and completed suicide. Foremost among suicide-related events are interpersonal losses and most notably when more than one event occurs within a six-month period. Further, with regard to suicidal behavior in depressives, the continued occurrence of negative events after onset of the episode may be critical to the precipitation of such behavior. Lack of social supports—including living alone and lacking an intimate confidant—appears to be a significant indirectly contributing factor, most likely acting as a mediating factor to reduce the suicide risk associated with undesirable life events (as, conversely, the loss of such support may act as a precipitating factor).

Early loss of one or both parents also appears to represent a predisposing psychosocial risk factor for suicidal behavior in adulthood, particularly when such loss results in long-term disruption of family stability. As such, a history of early loss and/or a childhood home environment characterized by instability may act to increase vulnerability to suicidal behavior when faced with stressful life events in adulthood. However, since early loss has also been found to be a risk factor for depressive disorders and since a significant percentage of suicide completers and attempters evidence depressive symptomatology prior to the act, it is not clear whether there is a direct relationship between early loss and suicidal behavior or if this relationship is moderated by the presence of a depressive disorder. Goldney's finding that depression ratings did not differ between suicide attempters with and without early loss does not rule out the possibility that early loss increases vulnerability to depression which, in turn, increases vulnerability to suicidal behavior.[16] The studies by Crook and Raskin[14] and Roy,[26] which demonstrate higher percentages of suicidal and suiciding depressives experiencing early loss as compared to nonsuicidal depressives, do suggest specificity to suicidal behavior. However, in light of the inconsistent findings, overall, in this area of research, further replication of these findings is needed to establish the nature of the association between early loss/childhood environment and suicidal behavior.

Few investigations of personality and suicidal behavior using objective, standardized instruments have been undertaken, and those that have are limited in their generalizability due to methodological problems. Chief among these is the possible confounding of depressive—or distressed—state with personality traits. Virtually all

TABLE 3. Psychosocial Factors in Suicide Attempters and Completers

	Suicide Attempters	Suicide Completers
Life events	Increased in 6-12 months prior to attempt.	Increased in year prior to death.
	Interpersonal loss and other "undesirable" events most commonly reported.	Interpersonal loss and other "undesirable" events most commonly reported.
	Decreased social support.	Decreased social support.
Early loss	Increased early loss especially due to divorce and separation.	Increased early loss.
	Increased unstable family environment.	?
Personality	More deviant in "low"-intent attempters.	?

investigators of personality and attempted suicide have administered personality instruments in close proximity to the attempt, a time when most subjects are likely to be suffering some degree of distress and, quite possibly, evidencing symptoms of depression. In view of the fact that depressive symptomatology has been demonstrated to have a profound influence on personality assessments,[27,28] the validity of personality measures obtained in studies of attempted suicide is seriously called into question. Added to this is the problem that no two studies in this area have employed the same personality measures and, thus, findings have not to date been replicated. Nonetheless, one finding that clearly emerges from the available literature is that the personalities of suicide attempters with low intent are, in general, more deviant than those of suicide attempters with high intent. To date, there are no empirical data to support the notion that personality deviance contributes to either serious suicide attempts or completed suicide.

Several problems related to sample selection characterize this psychosocial research on suicidal behavior. First, inasmuch as most studies on the psychosocial correlates of suicidal behavior have been conducted on suicide attempters, obtained results cannot be assumed to generalize to suicide completers. Second, heterogeneity of attempter samples, particularly with regard to lethality and seriousness of attempts, reduces the comparability and replicability of findings. Finally, control groups selected for comparison frequently have not been matched to attempter samples on relevant characteristics, most notably presence of psychiatric disorder, thereby calling into question the specificity of findings to suicide attempters.

It is clear from existing studies that no one psychosocial factor is either necessary or sufficient for the commission of a suicidal act. Many suicides are attempted and completed by persons who have experienced no recognizable "life event," who have no history of childhood loss, and who have the support of a confidant. Likewise, "life events" occur to all of us—many who have no supportive confidant, and many who have been raised by a single parent—and the vast majority make no attempt, let alone complete suicide. There is a need for future research to provide information concerning the interaction of psychosocial and other risk factors for suicide. In addition, there is a need for a more systematic progression of investigatory efforts designed to fill in the many gaps in our knowledge. By taking a systematic, multifactorial approach which combines epidemiologic, psychosocial, and biochemical measures with more rigorous research design, a broader base of understanding may be established regarding the determinants of suicide and suicidal behavior.

REFERENCES

1. BARRACLOUGH, B., J. BUNCH, B. NELSON & P. SAINSBURY. 1974. A hundred cases of suicide: clinical aspects. Br. J. Psychiatry 125: 355-373.
2. BREED, W. 1963. Occupational mobility and suicide among white males. Am. Sociol. Rev. 28: 179-188.
3. DORPAT, T. L. & H. S. RIPLEY. 1960. A study of suicide in the Seattle area. Comp. Psychiatry 1: 349-359.
4. DORPAT, T. L. & H. S. RIPLEY. 1967. The relationship between attempted suicide and committed suicide. Comp. Psychiatry 8: 74-79.
5. HAGNELL, O., J. LANKE & B. RORSMAN. 1981. Suicide rates in the Lundby study: mental illness as a risk factor for suicide. Neuropsychobiology 7: 248-253.
6. ROBINS, E., G. E. MURPHY, R. H. WILKINSON, S. GASSNER & J. KAYES. 1959. Some clinical considerations in the prevention of suicide based on a study of 134 successful suicides. Am. J. Public Health 49: 888-899.
7. SANBORN, D. E., C. J. SANBORN & P. CIMBOLIC. 1974. Occupation and suicide. Dis. Nerv. Syst. 35: 7-12.
8. SHEPHERD, D. M. & B. M. BARRACLOUGH. 1980. Work and suicide: an empirical investigation. Br. J. Psychiatry 136: 469-478.
9. WEISSMAN, M. M. 1974. The epidemiology of suicide attempts, 1960 to 1971. Arch. Gen. Psychiatry 30: 737-746.
10. PAYKEL, E. S., B. A. PRUSOFF & J. K. MYERS. 1975. Suicide attempts and recent life events: a controlled comparison. Arch. Gen. Psychiatry 32: 327-333.
11. SLATER, J. & R. A. DEPUE. 1981. The contribution of environmental events and social support to serious suicide attempts in primary depressive disorder. J. Abnorm. Psychol. 90: 275-285.
12. LUSCOMB, R. L., G. A. CLUM & A. T. PATSIOKAS. 1980. Mediating factors in the relationship between life stress and suicide attempting. J. Nerv. Ment. Dis. 168: 644-650.
13. DORPAT, T. L., J. K. JACKSON & H. S. RIPLEY. 1965. Broken home and attempted and completed suicide. Arch. Gen. Psychiatry 12: 213-216.

14. CROOK, T. & A. RASKIN. 1975. Association of childhood parental loss with attempted suicide and depression. J. Consult. Clin. Psychol. **43:** 277.
15. MORGAN, H. G., C. J. BURNS-COX, H. POCOCK & S. POTTLE. 1975. Deliberate self-harm: clinical and soci-economic characteristics of 368 patients. Br. J. Psychiatry **127:** 564-574.
16. GOLDNEY, R. D. 1981. Parental loss and reported childhood stress in young women who attempt suicide. Acta Psychiatr. Scand. **64:** 34-59.
17. ADAM, K. S., A. BOUCKOMS & D. STREINER. 1982. Parental loss and family stability in attempted suicide. Arch. Gen. Psychiatry **39:** 1081-1085.
18. ADAM, K. S., J. G. LOHRENZ, D. HARPER & D. STREINER. 1982. Early parental loss and suicidal ideation in university students. Can. J. Psychiatry **27:** 275-281.
19. PALLIS, D. J. & J. BIRTCHNELL. 1977. Seriousness of suicide attempt in relation to personality. Br. J. Psychiatry **130:** 253-259.
20. PALLIS, D. J. & J. S. JENKINS. 1977. Extraversion, neuroticism, and intent in attempted suicides. Psychol. Rep. **41:** 19-22.
21. GOLDNEY, R. D. 1982. Locus of control in young women who have attempted suicide. J. Nerv. Ment. Dis. **170:** 198-201.
22. BANKI, C. M. & M. ARATO. 1983. Amine metabolism, neuroendocrine findings, and personality dimensions as correlates of suicidal behavior. Psychiatry Res. **10:** 253-261.
23. HAGNELL, O. & B. RORSMAN. 1980. Suicide in the Lundby study: a controlled prospective investigation of stressful life events. Neuropsychobiology **6:** 319-332.
24. BORG, E. S. & M. STAHL. 1982. A prospective study of suicides and controls among psychiatric patients. Acta Psychiatr. Scand. **65:** 221-232.
25. MURPHY, G. E., J. W. ARMSTRONG, S. L. HERMELE, J. R. FISCHER & W. W. CLENDENIN. 1979. Suicide and alcoholism: interpersonal loss confirmed as a predictor. Arch. Gen. Psychiatry **36:** 65-69.
26. ROY, A. 1984. Suicide in recurrent affective disorder patients. Can. J. Psychiatry **29:** 319-322.
27. HIRSCHFELD, R. M. A., G. L. KLERMAN, P. J. CLAYTON, M. B. KELLER, P. MACDONALD-SCOTT & B. H. LARKIN. 1983. Assessing personality: effects of the depressive state on trait measurement. Am. J. Psychiatry **140:** 695-699.
28. LIEBOWITZ, M. R., F. STALLONE, D. L. DUNNER & R. F. FIEVE. 1979. Personality features of patients with primary affective disorder. Acta Psychiatr. Scand. **60:** 214-224.

Hopelessness as a Predictor of Eventual Suicide

AARON T. BECK

*Department of Psychiatry
University of Pennsylvania
Room 602
133 South 36th Street
Philadelphia, Pennsylvania 19104*

Clinicians are often faced with the awe-inspiring problem of assessing and predicting a person's suicide potential. The decision has important treatment implications as well as social and legal consequences. If the assessment is incorrect, its implications may be traumatic or even tragic. For these reasons, there is a pressing need for valid assessment techniques that enable early recognition of high-risk suicidal individuals. Recognition of variables associated with high suicidal risk is important for early intervention and appropriate treatment.

CLASSIFICATION

Adequate assessment presupposes the utilization of an adequate system of classification. In view of the pressing need for such a system, a task force of the National Institute of Mental Health (NIMH) Center for Studies of Suicide Prevention developed a tripartite system consisting of suicidal ideation, suicide attempt, and completed suicide.[1] Each category was further categorized (as appropriate) according to suicidal intent, lethality of attempt, and method (see TABLE 1).

ASSESSMENT OF SUICIDAL RISK

With the appropriate distinctions between suicidal ideators and suicide attempters, it is possible to consider the development of procedures to assess suicidal risk. Numerous strategies have been employed in the past. For summaries and critical reviews of these attempters, the reader is referred to Beck *et al.*,[2] Brown and Sheran,[3] and Lester.[4,5]

The most widespread means of trying to predict suicidal behaviors has involved the use of demographic variables generally derived from the study of completed suicides. However, as Lester has pointed out,[5] demographic variables are of limited utility. Although it is useful to know that a divorced male over 40 years of age shares important demographic characteristics with completed suicides, the clinician is faced with the question of what the likelihood is that *this* particular individual may kill himself or be a high suicide risk at *this* particular time. In other words, the degree of specificity of such scales is extremely low and such a formula will identify a huge number of people who are not at risk at all.

In treatment settings, probably the most widespread procedures to assess suicidal risk have involved formal or informal clinical judgment. Attempts to quantify clinical judgment have typically employed bipolar rating scales of severity of the suicide attempt, which specify either the medical consequences of the attempt or the psychiatric seriousness of the case.

A major weakness of many of the retrospective studies is that data are collected *after* the suicide attempt or completed suicide. Although such studies add to the knowledge of suicidal behaviors, they are of limited use to the clinician or practitioner who has to make treatment decisions.

In view of the factors outlined above, there is a clear need for a new approach in

TABLE 1. Classification of Suicidal Behaviors

I. Suicide ideation
  Thinking, planning
  Impulse or desire
  A. Intent to die
    High, medium, low, none

II. Suicide attempt
  A. Intent
  B. Lethality
  C. Method

III. Completed suicide
  A. Intent
  B. Method

assessing suicidal risk, and thus, we constructed scales that would be applicable to suicide ideators and attempters and thus could be in prospective studies.

Suicide ideators are defined as individuals who admit to thoughts of or contemplation of suicide; specifically, thoughts of wishing to terminate one's life. The ideation may or may not involve actual planning or mental rehearsal of a suicidal act. Furthermore, suicidal ideators are distinguished from attempters by the fact that they have not yet fully implemented a suicide plan or engaged in any clear-cut act that may result in actual physical damage and thus qualify as a suicide attempt. Suicide ideation may be inferred from overt suicidal behavior and communications, except for overt acts classifiable under suicide attempts. Thus, this category includes suicide threats, suicide preoccupations, and expressions of the wish to die as well as indirect indicators of suicide planning. This definition is essentially the same one as that proposed by a task force assembled in 1971 by the Center for Studies of Suicide Prevention. A scale (Scale for Suicidal Ideation)[6] was developed to measure suicidal intent among ideators by assessing the various components of intent, such as intensity and pervasiveness of the wish to die, degree of planning, etc. A similar scale was developed to measure the degree of intent involved in an actual suicide attempt (Suicide Intent Scale).[7]

HOPELESSNESS AND SUICIDE

A number of papers by Beck and his collaborators reported that hopelessness is a key psychological factor in suicidal behaviors. Among hospitalized suicidal patients, hopelessness, or pervasive negative expectations, has been found to be a significant predictor of severity of suicidal intent among suicide attempters,[8,9] as well as the extent of suicidal ideation or risk.[10] It has also been reported that higher levels of hopelessness are associated with "escape or surcease" motives for a suicide attempt, while lower levels of hopelessness correlate with "manipulative" motives.[11] These empirical findings substantiate conventional beliefs that attribute suicide attempts to an individual's desire to escape from an apparently insoluble problem. They also strengthen previous professional observations on the importance of hopelessness in suicidal behaviors.[12]

Hopelessness is just one aspect of the clinical picture that a clinician weighs in gauging a patient's suicide potential. Other factors include previous suicidal attempts, family history of suicide, and substance abuse. Persons seriously planning a suicide attempt may, and often do, deny any suicidal intent. Nevertheless, a series of studies summarized by Bedrosian and Beck[13] has supported the presence of strong positive relationships among hopelessness, depression, and a variety of suicidal behaviors; hopelessness repeatedly emerged as a more powerful correlate than depression of suicidal intent.

Recently in a 10-year prospective follow-up study of 165 patients hospitalized with suicidal ideation, Beck *et al.* reported that the Hopelessness Scale (HS) was a very powerful indicator of eventual suicide.[14] Of the 11 patients who eventually committed suicide, 10 (90.9%) had HS scores greater than 9. Only one patient who eventually committed suicide had previously received an HS score below 10; the false-negative rate was, therefore, 9.1%. The mean HS score was significantly higher in the suicide group (mean = 13.27, standard deviation = 4.43) than in the nonsuicide group (m = 8.94, SD = 6.05) [t (163) = 2.33, p < 0.05].

Since the selection of the cutoff point in the hospitalized sample was designed to minimize the false-negative rate, a cross-validation study of a different group using the same cutoff scores was indicated. To ascertain how effectively the HS would identify eventual suicides in an outpatient sample, we examined the records of 2174 patients evaluated at the Center for Cognitive Therapy between 1976 and 1985. Of the 10 who eventually committed suicide, 9 (90.0%) had HS scores of 10 or above. The false-negative rate was 10.0%. Of the 2164 patients who did not commit suicide, 1137 (52.5%) had HS scores of 10 or above. The sensitivity rate for true suicides was 90.0%, and the specificity rate for true nonsuicides was 47.5% (1027/2164). A cutoff score of 17+ identified a "high-risk group" in which the proportion of suicides (7/286 or 2.4%) was 15 times greater than in the rest of the sample of clinic patients (3/1888 or 0.16%).

The HS scores were substantially higher in the outpatients who eventually committed suicide; their actual scores were 20, 19, 19, 18, 18, 17, 12, 11, 10, and 9. The mean HS scores for the outpatient suiciders and nonsuiciders were 17.43 (SD = 2.79) and 9.84 (SD = 5.48), respectively. The mean HS score of the suiciders was significantly higher than the mean HS score of the outpatient nonsuiciders [t (2172) = 4.48, p < 0.001, two-tailed test].

Both the long-term prospective follow-up study reported by Beck et al.[14] and the "constructive replication" described above indicate that the choice of appropriate HS cutoff scores can be effective in identifying those patients who do and do not eventually commit suicide. Only one patient in the inpatient study and one in the outpatient study was classified as a false negative according to the HS cutoff criterion of 10 or above.

It should be noted that the use of the terms "false negatives" and "false positives" may not be completely appropriate in the present context. Generally, these terms are applied when a specific test is able or not able to demonstrate the presence or absence of a known disease, such as diabetes or tuberculosis. However, the HS estimates the *potential* for fatal suicide attempts and not the behavior itself. Moreover, many high HS scores may continue at risk for suicide even though they have not yet made a fatal attempt. In interpreting the results of the present studies, hopelessness may best be construed as a risk factor—perhaps analogous to a history of smoking or elevated blood pressure as predispositional factors in heart disease. Since HS scores will fluctuate from time to time, the best test of the relationship between hopelessness and suicide would be to determine HS scores immediately prior to a fatal suicide attempt.

Why does hopelessness serve as such a powerful predictor of eventual suicide? We believe that the intensity of hopelessness displayed during one depressive episode is indicative of the level that emerges in future episodes. Hopelessness may constitute a stable schema incorporating negative expectancies which are very resistant to change in psychiatric patients. Therefore, hopelessness is an important clue that should alert clinicians to long-term suicide potential. Finally, it should be emphasized that a comprehensive assessment of suicidal risk should include, in addition to HS scores, such known predictors of suicide as a high level of suicide ideation, a history of previous suicide attempts, a family history of suicide, alcohol and drug abuse, and relevant demographic factors such as age, sex, and race. The inclusion of such factors in a "suicide potential index" should substantially reduce the number of "false positives" and possibly increase "true positives."

ALCOHOLISM AMONG SUICIDE ATTEMPTERS

A 10-year prospective study was carried out to clarify predictors of suicide in suicide attempters admitted to the psychiatric services of two general hospitals. The scores of the Beck Depression Inventory (BDI) were moderately high among the suicide attempters shortly after their index unsuccessful suicide attempt. However, their hopelessness scale score (8.6) was somewhat less than that among suicide ideators at an outpatient clinic. The suicide intent scale score was slightly greater among those who eventually died of suicide than among those who did not die by suicide. This difference, however, was not significant.

The important finding was that a history of alcohol abuse was highly predictive (p < 0.001) of eventual suicide among the 472 attempters who received detailed alcohol histories on admission to the hospital. Eighteen (72%) out of the 25 patients who eventually killed themselves had a history of alcoholism.

Of 161 alcoholic suicide attempters, 18 (11.2%) eventually committed suicide. Of the 311 nonalcoholics, 7 (2.2%) eventually committed suicide. Thus, the probability of eventual suicide was approximately five times greater among those attempters who were alcoholics than among those attempters who were not alcoholics.

This study thus targets a particular high-risk group, namely, alcoholic attempters. Since the follow-up study extended for only 5 to 10 years, it seems probable that the percentage of eventual suicides in the alcoholic suicide attempters could be substantially higher.

SUICIDE RISK AMONG PATIENTS IN TREATMENT

A review of the literature shows that a surprisingly high proportion of suicides among previously treated patients had been seen by a mental health professional just prior to the fatal suicide attempt. A study by Roy of 90 suicides at the Clarke Institute of Psychiatry in Toronto between July 1968 and June 1979 has direct bearing on this point.[15] Of the 75 outpatient suicides (most of whom had been previously treated as inpatients), 58% had seen a psychiatrist within the previous week. Of the previously hospitalized patients, 44% of the suicides occurred within a month of discharge. More striking, 15 of the 90 suicides occurred while the patients were inpatients at the institute.

A relatively short time lag between treatment and suicide is underscored in the case of the nine patients who had received electroconvulsive therapy (ECT) for depression in their last episode of contact. Four of these committed suicide while still inpatients. Of the nine suicides in this group, eight had completed a course of ECT and suicided a mean of 1.96 months after completion (range 123.8 months).

What are the implications of Roy's study? It shows that the vast majority of suicides were being treated at the time of their fatal suicide attempt or had only recently broken off contact. Patients who continued to be seen in psychiatric treatment should be considered the pool from which the high suicide risk patients are identified. Since these patients are already receiving scrutiny, all that would be required once the high risk is established—by means of the Depression Inventory, Hopelessness Scale, past history of suicide attempt, alcoholism, etc.— would be close monitoring during the period of time when the scores on, say, the Depression Inventory and Hopelessness Scale remain high.

Further, the mental health professionals should use whatever tools are in their own armamentarium to focus in on reducing the individual's hopelessness, whether this might be by social intervention, antidepressant drug, or cognitive therapy. In a clinical trial, cognitive therapy was shown to have a direct effect on hopelessness scores, which changed more rapidly in cognitive therapy patients than in patients who received only antidepressant medication.[16]

COGNITIVE THERAPY FOR HOPELESSNESS

Over the years, cognitive therapy (CT) has been developed in response to the need for an effective and short-term treatment approach to depression. The techniques and assumptions of CT have been described in detail by Beck, and Beck et al.[17,18] CT has been found to lead to a more rapid reduction of hopelessness than antidepressant drugs do.

In brief, CT is based on the postulate that the cognitive factors are of central importance in the development and perpetuation of depressive reactions. Moreover, it is assumed that some of the salient and dramatic symptoms of depressive syndromes (e.g., reduced interest and motivation, suicidal wishes) are the logical concomitants or consequences of the cognitive factors.

The depressed patient's cognitive set is characterized by a negative self-concept and a pervasively pessimistic view of the world and the future. He tends to be preoccupied with issues of rejection, loss, or deprivation. The various errors of thinking, described by Beck,[18] including overgeneralization, magnification, and selective attention for negative experiences, all contribute to the patient's conclusion that life is hopeless and that suicide may be an appropriate solution for his problems.

The goal of CT is to alter the maladaptive interpretations and beliefs that the patient employs to guide his behavior. In the course of CT the patient's negative cognitions and misconceptions are monitored and elucidated. Both semantic and behavioral techniques are employed to question the validity or basis of such cognitions and their supporting belief systems. The patient is an active participant in his own treatment and recovery. He is an active collaborator within the therapy sessions and continues his participation through the execution of homework assignments. Ultimately, CT aims to give the depressed patient some degree of mastery over the way he thinks and teaches him to substitute and employ reasonable and useful ways of evaluating himself and the world.

Negative cognitions that convey the patient's hopelessness and consequent suicidal wishes have been found to be amenable to questioning and modification, e.g.: "Nothing will ever work out for me," "What's the use of going on, I just can't see living my life without Margot," "I might as well be dead since I'm of no more use to anybody." The therapist helps the patient scrutinize the validity and usefulness of such cognitions and question the belief systems that support them. Is the statement a reasonable one? Is it based on factual evidence, is it based on a distortion of evidence, or is it simply a belief? What are alternate ways of evaluating the same event or problem; are there different ways of formulating the difficulty at hand? What are the behavioral and effective *consequences* of alternate formulations or more reasonable attitudes?

Clinical experience suggests that elucidation and modification of the hopeless attitude that underlies the depressed patient's suicidal wishes leads to an attenuation of the wish to kill oneself. Thus, future research should focus not only on the early identification of high-risk suicidal patients but also on their responsiveness to early intervention with techniques such as cognitive therapy.

REFERENCES

1. BECK, A. T., J. H. DAVIS, C. J. FREDERICK, *et al.* 1973. Classification and nomenclature. *In* Suicide Prevention in the Seventies. H. L. P. Resnik & B. C. Hathorne, Eds.: 7-12. National Institute of Mental Health Center for Studies of Suicide Prevention. Rockville, Md.
2. BECK, A. T., H. L. P. RESNIK & D. LETTIERI, Eds. 1974. The Prediction of Suicide. Charles Press. Bowie, Md.
3. BROWN, T. R. & T. J. SHERAN. 1972. Suicide prediction: a review. Life Threat. Behav. 2: 67-98.

4. LESTER, D. 1970. Attempts to predict suicidal risk using psychological tests. Psychol. Bull. **74:** 1-17.
5. LESTER, D. 1974. Demographic versus clinical prediction of suicidal behaviors: a look at some issues. *In* The Prediction of Suicide. A. T. Beck, H. L. P. Resnik & D. Lettieri, Eds.: 71-84. Charles Press. Bowie, Md.
6. BECK, A. T., M. KOVACS & A. WEISSMAN. 1979. Assessment of suicidal intention: the scale for suicide ideation. J. Consult. Clin. Psychol. **47:** 343-352.
7. BECK, A. T., I. HERMAN & D. SCHUYLER. 1974. Development of suicidal intent scales. *In* The Prediction of Suicide. A. T. Beck, H. L. P. Resnik & D. Lettieri, Eds.: 45-56. Charles Press. Bowie, Md.
8. BECK, A. T., M. KOVACS & A. WEISSMAN. 1975. Hopelessness and suicidal behavior; an overview. J. Am. Med. Assoc. **234:** 1146-1149.
9. MINKOFF, K., E. BERGMAN, A. T. BECK & R. BECK. 1973. Hopelessness, depression and attempted suicide. Am. J. Psychiatry **130:** 455-459.
10. KOVACS, M., A. T. BECK & A. WEISSMAN. 1975. Hopelessness: an indicator of suicidal risk. Suicide **5:** 98-103.
11. KOVACS, M., A. T. BECK & A. WEISSMAN. 1975. The use of suicidal motives in the psychotherapy of attempted suicides. Am. J. Psychother. **29:** 363-368.
12. SHNEIDMAN, E. S. 1973. Suicide. *In* Encyclopedia Brittanica. 14th edit. **21:** 383-385. William Benton. Chicago, Ill.
13. BEDROSIAN, R. C. & A. T. BECK. 1979. Cognitive aspects of suicidal behavior. Suicide Life Threat. Behav. **2:** 87-96.
14. BECK, A. T., R. A. STEER, M. KOVACS & B. GARRISON. 1985. Hopelessness and eventual suicide: a 10-year prospective study of patients hospitalized with suicidal ideation. Am. J. Psychiatry **142**(5): 559-563.
15. ROY, A. 1982. Risk factors for suicide in psychiatric patients. Arch. Gen. Psychiatry **39:** 1089-1095.
16. RUSH, A. J., A. T. BECK, M. KOVACS, *et al.* 1982. Comparison of the effects of cognitive therapy and pharmacotherapy on hopelessness and self-concept. Am. J. Psychiatry **139:** 862-866.
17. BECK, A. T., A. J. RUSH, B. F. SHAW & G. EMERY. 1979. Cognitive Therapy of Depression. Guilford Press. New York, N.Y.
18. BECK, A. T. 1967. Depression: Clinical, Experimental, and Theoretical Aspects. Harper and Row. New York, N.Y.

Genetics of Suicide

ALEC ROY

*National Institute of Alcohol Abuse and Alcoholism
Building 10, Room 3B-19
9000 Rockville Pike
Bethesda, Maryland 20892*

Suicide, like so much else in psychiatry, tends to run in families. Ernest Hemingway committed suicide by shooting himself with a shotgun, so did his father, and so did his brother. There are three lines of evidence that suicide runs in families. Firstly, many families have now been reported where more than one family member has committed suicide.[1-5] Secondly, some general population studies of suicide have found an excess of suicide among family members. Farberow and Simon reported that among 100 suicide victims, 6 had a parent who had killed themselves,[6] a rate more than 88 times the expected rate. Thirdly, studies of psychiatric patients have shown that a family history of suicide is not uncommon and that suicidal behaviors are found more commonly among those patients who have a family history of suicide.[7-10] For example, in my study significantly more patients with a family history of suicide had themselves attempted suicide than had patients without such a family history (TABLE 1).[11] Also, a family history of suicide was found significantly more often among the manic-depressive than the other patients ($p < 0.0001$) (TABLE 2).

However, there is some controversy about what interpretation to give to the fact that suicide runs in families. The great majority of suicide victims are suffering from a psychiatric disorder with affective disorder, alcoholism, and schizophrenia being the disorders most commonly found.[12-14] Genetic factors play a part in the etiology of these psychiatric disorders, and thus in this way they clearly play a part in suicide. However, controversy comes in the suggestion that there may be a genetic component to suicide independent of the genetic transmission of depression, alcoholism, and schizophrenia.[15] Thus, the purpose of the remainder of this paper is to examine this suggestion critically by examining relevant studies.

TWIN STUDIES

The strongest evidence for the genetic transmission of manic-depression and schizophrenia is that the concordance rate for these psychiatric disorders is substantially higher among identical twins, who share the same genes, than it is among fraternal twins who only share 50% of their genes.[16] Thus, if the propensity to commit suicide were genetically transmitted, concordance for suicide should be found more among identical than fraternal twins. And, indeed, that is the case. Haberlant, in 1967, pooled the data from twin studies from different countries.[17,18] At that time there were 149 sets of twins reported where one twin was known to have committed suicide. Among

TABLE 1[a]

	Second- or First-Degree Relative Suicided		No Family History of Suicide	
Diagnostic Group	Number (%) Attempted	Number of Attempts	Number (%) Attempted	p
Schizophrenia	15/33 (45.4)	28	150/1114 (13.5)	<0.0001
Unipolar	13/32 (41.6)	24	50/372 (13.4)	<0.0001
Bipolar	22/58 (37.9)	48	56/405 (13.9)	<0.0001
Depressive neurosis	26/47 (55.3)	45	221/715 (30.9)	<0.0001
Personality disorder	33/48 (68.8)	89	328/1048 (31.3)	<0.0001
Alcohol	3/7 (42.9)	3	42/147 (28.5)	NS
Others	6/18 (33.3)	15	378/1801 (21.0)	NS
Total	118/243 (48.6)	252	1225/5602 (21.8)	<0.0001

[a] A consecutive series of 5845 inpatients admitted to the Clarke Institute between January 1974 and June 1981. Patients, by diagnostic group, who attempted suicide comparing those with a family history of suicide with those without such a history. Published from Reference 11 with the permission of *Archives of General Psychiatry*.

them there were 9 sets of twins where both twins were known to have committed suicide and all of these 9 sets were identical twins (TABLE 3).

However, 4 of these 9 monozygotic twin sets concordant for suicide came from the Danish Psychiatric Twin Register and their case histories revealed that in 3 of them the twins were also concordant for manic-depressive disorder.[19,a] Another of these 9 monozygotic twins sets, initially reported by Kallman et al.,[20,21] were also concordant for schizophrenia. Since Haberlandt's review, Zair has reported a 10th pair of identical twins who both committed suicide.[22] Again there was an association with affective disorder, as both twins had killed themselves during a depressive episode and both of their parents, and a grandmother, had also been treated for depression.

Approximately 1 in 250 live births is an identical twin and between 0.5% and 1% of all deaths are due to suicide. Thus, it is somewhat surprising that only 10 pairs of monozygotic twins concordant for suicide have been reported in the 173 years since the first report of suicide in twins.[23] Also, in 5 of these 10 twin pairs it is well documented that the twins were concordant for either depression or schizophrenia. Thus, twin data provide evidence for the genetic transmission of suicide but are not a very strong source of support for the idea that there may be a genetic transmission of suicide independent of psychiatric disorder.

THE IOWA 500 STUDY

The 30- to 40-year follow-up study of the 685 selected psychiatric patients and surgical controls admitted to hospital in Iowa City between 1934 and 1944 revealed

[a] Four of these 9 sets of twins have been reported twice. They are included in Haberlandt's 1967 review[18] and have also been reported in detail in 1970 by Juel-Nielsen and Videbech.[19]

that there had been 30 suicides—29 among the 525 psychiatric patients (5.5%) and 1 among the 160 controls (0.6%) (p < 0.001).[24,25] In 1983, Tsuang reported the follow-up study of the 5721 first-degree relatives.[26] That study also highlights the strong association between suicide and psychiatric disorder. Tsuang found that the risk of suicide in the relatives of psychiatric patients (2.3%) was nearly eight times greater than the risk among the relatives of the surgical controls (p < 0.01). Furthermore, the relatives of patients who committed suicide had a four times greater risk of committing suicide themselves than did the relatives of patients who did not commit suicide (7.9% vs. 2.1%, p < 0.05) (TABLE 4). Although these findings support "the presence of a genetic element in suicide,"[26] the study involved patients with known psychiatric disorder and was not designed to examine the possibility of an independent genetic transmission of suicide. Also, it is noteworthy that the suicide risk was highest for the relatives of depressed patients (p < 0.01). Similarly, the increased suicide risk for relatives of patients who had committed suicide was confined to the relatives of the bipolar and unipolar patients who committed suicide (TABLE 4). As the risk of affective disorder is significantly higher among the relatives of manic-depressives, it could be that these interesting findings in relation to suicide are reflecting the genetic transmission of depression. The increased suicide risk among the relatives of depressed patients who committed suicide could be related to the genetic transmission of the severity of depression.[27,28] Hopefully further papers will report on the psychiatric history and mental state at the time of suicide of the relatives who committed suicide.

ADOPTION STUDIES

The strongest evidence for the possibility that suicidal behavior may be genetically transmitted independently of psychiatric disorders comes from the Danish Adoption Studies of Schulsinger, Kety, Wender, and Rosenthal.[15,29] The Psykologisk Institut has a register of the 5483 adoptions that occurred in greater Copenhagen between 1924 and 1947. A screening of the register of causes of death revealed that 57 of these adoptees committed suicide. They were matched with adopted controls for sex, age, social class of the adopting parents, and time spent both with their biological relatives

TABLE 2[a]

Diagnostic Group	Number of Patients	Number of Patients with a Family History of Suicide
Manic-depression	867	90 (10.4%)
All other patients without a primary affective disorder diagnosis	4216	106 (2.5%)
p < 0.0001		

[a] Among a consecutive series of 5845 psychiatric inpatients admitted to the Clarke Institute significantly more of the manic-depressive patients than the patients without a primary affective disorder diagnosis had a family history of suicide. Patients with a primary diagnosis of depressive neurosis were excluded.

TABLE 3. Suicide in Twins[a]

Type of Twins	Number of Twin Pairs	Number of Twin Pairs where Both Twins Committed Suicide (%)
Identical	51	9 (17.7%)
Fraternal	98	0 (0%)
p < 0.0001		

[a] Based on Haberlandt, 1967.[18]

and in institutions before being adopted. Searches of the causes of death revealed that 12 of the biological relatives of these 57 adopted suicides had themselves committed suicide compared with only 2 of the biological relatives of the 57 adopted controls (p < 0.01). None of the adopting relatives had committed suicide (TABLE 5).

However, Schulsinger *et al.* also investigated whether or not any of these 12 biological relative suicides had ever had a psychiatric hospitalization or were known alcoholics. Six of these 12 biological suicide relatives of the adopted suicide victims had such a psychiatric history. Schulsinger *et al.* comment that the fact that this was not known for the other 6 does not exclude the possibility that they too may have had psychiatric disorders. The 6 biological relative suicides with a known psychiatric history, compared with the 6 without such a history, also had significantly more biological relatives with a known psychiatric disorder (p < 0.01).[15] Thus, although Schulsinger *et al.* believe that this adoption study suggests that there may be a genetic component for suicide independent of psychiatric disorders, half of the 12 biological relative suicides of the adopted suicides had a psychiatric disorder.

In another study this group compared the 71 adoptees known to have suffered from depressive disorder with 71 matched adopted controls.[29,30] Significantly more of the adoptees with depression, than their matched controls, had a biological relative who had committed suicide (TABLE 6). Again, this study shows that there is a genetic component to suicide, but the family history of suicide in these depressive adoptees may represent the genetic transmission of depressive disorder. TABLE 7 reviews studies of manic-depressive patients where family history is reported and shows that 303 of the total of 2563 manic-depressive patients (11.8%) had a family history of suicide. Two of these studies also investigated the relative who committed suicide. Stenstedt

TABLE 4. Iowa 500 Study—Summary of Morbidity Risks of Suicide in Patients and Their First-Degree Relatives

Diagnostic Group	Patients n	BZ	MR(%)	Relatives n	BZ	MR(%)	Relatives of Suicides n	BZ	MR(%)
Schizophrenia	8	125	6.4	9	746	1.2	0	23	0.0
Mania	6	62	9.7	7	458	1.5	3	32	9.4
Depression	5	173	8.7	39	1144	3.4	6	59	10.2
Control	1	97	1.0	2	672	0.3	0	7	0.0

[a] n is number of suicides; BZ is age-adjusted number of relatives exposed to risk of suicide; MR is morbidity risk. Taken from Tsuang.[26] Published with permission of the *Journal of Clinical Psychiatry*.

TABLE 5. Copenhagen Adoption Study—Incidence of Suicide in the Relatives of Adoptees Who Committed Suicide and Their Controls[a]

Adoptees	Biological Relatives	Adoptive Relatives
57 adoptees died by suicide	12/269 (4.5%)	0/148 (0%)
57 matched control adoptees	2/269 (0.7%)	0/150 (0%)
	$p < 0.01$	

[a] From Schulsinger et al.[15] and published by permission of Dr. Kety.

reported that 19 of the 26 first-degree relatives in his study who committed suicide themselves had manic-depressive disorder.[31] Pitts and Winokur found that the great majority of the first-degree relative suicides in their study were also diagnosed as having affective disorder.[33] Most of the data about psychiatric disorder in the Copenhagen studies have come from discharge diagnoses from a variety of institutions.[15] Hopefully future reports will present more details about the psychiatric histories of the suicides and their relatives.

CONCLUSION

It is clear that suicide runs in families. The question is, what is being transmitted? No doubt in some suicide victims what is transmitted is not a genetic factor but a psychological one—identification with a role model of suicide as one possible "solution" to intolerable psychological pain. However, the Copenhagen adoption studies show beyond a doubt that there are genetic factors in suicide and the Iowa 500 and other studies show that a family history of suicide is associated with the major psychiatric disorders. The question then becomes the interesting one raised by Schulsinger et al. of whether "there is a special etiology of suicide independent of the affective disorders, the alcoholism, the schizophrenias, and other conditions associated with suicide."[15] Having examined the currently available evidence from twin and

TABLE 6. Copenhagen Adoption Study—Incidence of Suicide in the Relatives of Adoptees Who Have Suffered a Depressive Illness and Their Controls[a]

Adoptees	Biological Relatives	Adoptive Relatives
71 adoptees with depression	15/407 (3.7%)	1/187 (0.5%)
71 matched control adoptees	1/360 (0.3%)	2/171 (1.2%)
	$p < 0.01$	

[a] From Schulsinger et al.[29] and Wender et al.[30] and published by permission of Dr. Kety.

adoption studies, this reviewer, in respect to that particular question, would have to bring in the Scottish verdict of "not proven"—because many of the suicides in these studies are associated with psychiatric disorder.

However, recent studies suggest that this question might well be reformulated, as suggested by Kety, to ask whether there is "a genetic factor favoring suicide which may operate additively with depression or other major psychosis."[40] In this respect Asberg et al. found that among 68 depressed patients, significantly more of the patients with low levels of the serotonin metabolite 5-hydroxyindoleacetic acid (5-HIAA) had attempted suicide than did those in the high cerebrospinal fluid (CSF) 5-HIAA mode,[41] leading to the proposal that low CSF 5-HIAA levels may be associated with suicidal behavior. Since then other studies in personality-disordered,[42-45] schizophrenic,[46,47] and depressed patients[48,49] have also reported an association between low levels of CSF 5-HIAA and aggressive and suicidal behavior, though there have also been some negative reports.[50-52]

TABLE 7. Family History of Suicide in 11 Studies of Manic-Depressive Patients

Study	Number of Manic-Depressive Patients	Number and Percent of Manic-Depressive Patients with a Family History of Suicide
Stendstedt, 1952[31]	216	26 (12.0%)
Leonhard et al., 1962[32]	84	14 (16.7%)
Pitts and Winoker, 1964[33]	365	25 (6.8%)
Perris, 1966[34]	277	48 (17.3%)
Brodie and Leff, 1971[35]	30	3 (10%)
Mendlewicz et al., 1972[36]	60	14 (23%)
Dunner et al., 1975[37]	68	3 (4.4%)
Johnson et al., 1979[38,a]	50	16 (32%)
Roy, 1983[11,a]	867	90 (10.4%)
Tsuang, 1983[26]	315	46 (14.6%)
Roy, 1985[39,a]	231	18 (7.8%)
Total	2563	303 (11.8%)

[a] Studies reporting suicide in both first- and second-degree relatives. All the other studies report suicide in first-degree relatives only.

When we recently examined the biological correlates of suicidal behavior among a group of depressed inpatients, we found that the depressed patients who attempted suicide, compared with those who had not, had the combination of low CSF levels of the dopamine metabolite homovanillic acid (HVA) and nonsuppression on the dexamethasone suppression test (DST).[52] Both of these biological measures have been claimed to be indicators of melancholia[53] (and reviewed by Post).[54] One might speculate that patients with severe depressive illness who commit suicide may "choose" to do so as an escape from the intolerable psychological pain that is associated with melancholia. The strongest, and most replicated, evidence that low CSF levels of 5-HIAA are associated with suicidal behavior comes from studies of personality-disordered patients.[43-46] Thus it may be that there are several biological substrates to the multidetermined act that is suicide.[55] In the Copenhagen study the adopted suicide victims without a history of psychiatric disorder may represent a subgroup of personality-disordered individuals who have a genetic predisposition to abnormality of their serotonin system which, at times of stress, renders them vulnerable to impulsive suicidal behavior—as suggested by Schulsinger[15] and Kety.[40]

REFERENCES

1. WOOD, J. & A. URQUHART. 1901. A family tree illustrative of insanity and suicide. J. Ment. Sci. **47:** 764-767.
2. SHAPIRO, L. 1935. Suicide: psychopathology and familial tendency. J. Nerv. Ment. Dis. **81:** 547-553.
3. SMITH, P. 1912. Psychoses occurring in twins. N.Y. State J. Med.: 1268-1272.
4. LOWENBERG, R. D. 1941. Suicide in twins. J. Nerv. Ment. Dis. **93:** 182-184.
5. SWANSON, D. W. 1960. Suicide in identical twins. Am. J. Psychiatry **116:** 934-935.
6. FARBEROW, N. & M. SIMON. 1969. Suicide in Los Angeles and Vienna: an intercultural study of two cities. Public Health Rep. **84:** 389-403.
7. TSUTSUMI, S., S. TSUJINO, K. TSUDA, et al. 1967. A study on suicides in families of psychotic. In Clinical Genetics in Psychiatry. H. Mitsuda, Ed. Osaka Medical College. Osaka, Japan.
8. STENGEL, E. 1964. Suicide and Attempted Suicide. Viking Penguin Inc. New York, N.Y.
9. MURPHY, G. & R. WETZEL. 1982. Family history of suicidal behaviour among suicide attempters. J. Nerv. Ment. Dis. **170:** 86-90.
10. ROY, A. 1982. Risk factors for suicide in psychiatric patients. Arch. Gen. Psychiatry **39:** 1089-1095.
11. ROY, A. 1983. Family history of suicide. Arch. Gen. Psychiatry **40:** 971-974.
12. ROBINS, E., G. MURPHY, R. WILKINSON, et al. 1959. Some clinical observations in the prevention of suicide based on a study of 134 successful suicides. Am. J. Public Health **49:** 888-889.
13. DORPAT, T. & H. RIPLEY. 1960. A study of suicide in the Seattle area. Compr. Psychiatry **1:** 349-359.
14. BARRACLOUGH, B., J. BUNCH, B. NELSON, et al. 1974. A hundred cases of suicide. Clinical aspects. Br. J. Psychiatry **125:** 355-373.
15. SCHULSINGER, R., S. KETY, D. ROSENTHAL, et al. 1979. A family study of suicide. In Origins, Prevention and Treatment of Affective Disorders. M. Schou & E. Stromgren, Eds.: 277-287. Academic Press Inc. New York, N.Y.
16. TSUANG, M. 1977. Genetic factors in suicide. Dis. Nerv. Syst. **38:** 498-501.
17. HABERLANDT, W. 1965. Der Suizid als Genetisches Problem (Zwillings-und Familien analyse). Anthropol Anz. **29:** 65-89.
18. HABERLANDT, W. 1967. Aportacion a la genetica del suicidio. Folia Clin. Int. **17:** 319-322.
19. JUEL-NIELSEN, N. & T. VIDEBECH. 1970. A twin study of suicide. Acta Genet. Med. Gemellol **19:** 307-310.
20. KALLMAN, F. & M. ANASTASIO. 1947. Twin studies on the psychopathology of suicide. J. Nerv. Ment. Dis. **105:** 40-55.
21. KALLMAN, F., J. DEPORTE, E. DEPORTE & L. FEINGOLD. 1949. Suicide in twins and only children. Am. J. Hum. Genet. **2:** 113-126.
22. ZAW, K. 1981. A suicidal family. Br. J. Psychiatry **189:** 68-69.
23. WILLIAMS, S. 1812. (As cited in Reference 4.)
24. WINOKUR, G. & M. T. TSUANG. 1975. The Iowa 500: suicide in manic depression and schizophrenia. Am. J. Psychiatry **132:** 650-651.
25. TSUANG, M. T. 1978. Suicide in schizophrenics, manics, depressives and surgical controls. A comparison with general population suicide mortality. Arch. Gen. Psychiatry **35:** 153-155.
26. TSUANG, M. 1983. Risk of suicide in the relatives of schizophrenics, manics, depressives, and controls. J. Clin. Psychiatry **44:** 396-400.
27. JUEL-NIELSEN, N. 1979. Suicide risk in manic depressive disorders. In Origins, Prevention

and Treatment of Affective Disorders. M. Schou & E. Stromgren, Eds.: 269-276. Academic Press, Inc. New York, N.Y.
28. BERTELSEN, A., B. HARVALD & M. HAUGE. 1977. A Danish twin study of manic-depressive disorders. Br. J. Psychiatry 130: 330-351.
29. SCHULSINGER, F., S. KETY, D. ROSENTHAL, et al. 1981. A family study of suicide. Read before a meeting of the Third World Congress of Biological Psychiatry, Stockholm, Sweden.
30. WENDER, P., S. KETY & F. SCHULSINGER. Unpublished data.
31. STENDSTEDT, A. 1952. A study in manic-depressive psychosis. Acta Psychiatr. Scand. Suppl. No. 79.
32. LEONHARD, D., I. KORFF & H. SCHULZ. 1962. Temperaments in the families of monopolar and bipolar psychoses. Psychiatr. Neurol. 143: 416-434.
33. PITTS, F. & G. WINOKUR. 1964. Affective disorder. III. Diagnostic correlates and incidence of suicide. J. Nerv. Ment. Dis. 139: 176-181.
34. PERRIS, C. 1966. A study of bipolar (manic-depressive) and unipolar recurrent depressive psychoses. Acta Psychiatr. Scand. Suppl. No. 194.
35. BRODIE, K. & M. LEFF. 1971. Bipolar depression—a comparative study of patient characteristics. Am. J. Psychiatry 127: 1086-1090.
36. MENDLEWICZ, J., R. FIEVE & J. RAINER. 1972. Manic depressive illness—comparative study of patients with and without a family history. Br. J. Psychiatry 120: 523-530.
37. DUNNER, D., E. GERSHON & F. GOODWIN. 1976. Heritable factors in the severity of affective illness. Biol. Psychiatry 11: 31-42.
38. JOHNSON, G. F. & G. HUNT. 1979. Suicidal behavior in bipolar manic-depressive patients and their families. Compr. Psychiatry 20: 159-164.
39. ROY, A. 1985. Family history of suicide in manic-depressive patients. J. Affective Dis. 8: 187-189.
40. KETY, S. 1986. Genetic factors in suicide. In Suicide. A. Roy, Ed. Williams and Wilkins. Baltimore, Md.
41. ASBERG, M., L. TRASKMAN & P. THOREN. 1976. 5-HIAA in the cerebrospinal fluid: a biochemical suicide predictor? Arch. Gen. Psychiatry 33: 1193-1197.
42. BROWN, G., F. GOODWIN, J. BALLENGER, et al. 1979. Aggression in humans correlates with cerebrospinal fluid amine metabolites. Psychiatry Res. 1: 131-139.
43. BROWN, G., M. EBERT, P. GOYER, D. JIMERSON, W. KLEIN, W. BUNNEY & K. GOODWIN. 1982. Aggression, suicide and serotonin: relationship to CSF amine metabolism. Am. J. Psychiatry 1982. 139: 741-746.
44. LINNOILA, M., M. VIRKKUNEN, M. SCHEININ, et al. 1983. Low cerebrospinal fluid 5-hydroxyindoleacetic acid concentration differentiates impulsive from nonimpulsive violent behavior. Life Sci.: 2609-2614.
45. LIDBERG, L., J. TUCK, M. ASBERG, G. SCALIA-TOMBA & L. BERTILSSON. 1985. Homicide, suicide and 5-HIAA. Acta Psychiatr. Scand. 71: 230-236.
46. NINAN, P., D. VAN KAMMEN, M. SCHEININ, et al. 1984. Cerebrospinal fluid 5-HIAA in suicidal schizophrenic patients. Am. J. Psychiatry 141: 566-569.
47. VAN PRAAG, H. 1983. CSF 5-HIAA and suicide in non-depressed schizophrenics. Lancet: 977-978.
48. AGREN, H. 1980. Symptom patterns in unipolar and bipolar depression correlating with monoamine metabolites in the cerebrospinal fluid. II. Suicide. Psychiatry Res. 3: 225-236.
49. VAN PRAAG, H. 1982. Depression suicide and metabolism of serotonin in the brain. J. Affect. Disord. 4: 275-290.
50. ROY-BYRNE, P., R. POST, D. RUBINOW, et al. 1983. CSF 5-HIAA and personal and family history of suicide in affectively ill patients: a negative study. Psychiatry Res. 10: 263-274.
51. ROY, A., P. NINAN, A. MAZONSON, D. PICKAR, D. VAN KAMMEN, M. LINNOILA & S. PAUL. 1985. CSF monoamine metabolites in chronic schizophrenic patients who attempt suicide. Psychol. Med. 15: 335-340.
52. ROY, A., H. AGREN, D. PICKAR, M. LINNOILA, A. DORAN, N. CUTLER & S. PAUL. Reduced cerebrospinal fluid concentrations of homovanillic acid and homovanillic acid to 5-hydroxyindoleacetic acid ratios in depressed patents: relationship to suicidality and dexamethasone nonsuppression. Am. J. Psychiatry. (In press.)

53. CARROL, B., M. FEINBERG & O. GREDEN, et al. 1981. A specific laboratory test for the diagnosis of melancholia: standardization, validation and clinical utility. Arch. Gen. Psychiatry **38:** 15.
54. POST, R., J. BALLENGER & G. GOODWIN. 1980. Cerebrospinal fluid studies of neurotransmitter function in man and depressive illness. *In* Neurobiology of Cerebrospinal Fluid J. Wood, Ed. (Chapter 47). Plenum press. New York, N.Y.
55. ROY, A. 1985. Suicide: a multidetermined act. *In* Self-Destructive Behavior. Psychiatr. Clin. North Am.: 243-250.

Prospective Studies of Suicide and Mortality in Psychiatric Patients

DONALD W. BLACK AND GEORGE WINOKUR

Department of Psychiatry
University of Iowa College of Medicine
500 Newton Road
Iowa City, Iowa 52242

In earlier papers,[1-4] we described the Iowa Record Linkage Study and our findings. In this prospective study, a list of all patients admitted to our hospital over a 10-year period was linked to Iowa death certificates for the same period. We found excessive deaths during the follow-up but this was limited to the first two years; the excess mortality affected both men and women, and most psychiatric diagnostic categories (we had created 10). When a breakdown of death causes was done, we found that during the entire follow-up natural deaths were excessive in women and both accidents and suicides were excessive for both sexes. During the first two years of follow-up, however, natural deaths, accidental deaths, and suicides were excessive for men and women.

We have now completed an analysis of suicides, accidental deaths, and natural deaths by follow-up time and diagnosis. This study will demonstrate early risk by diagnostic group.

METHODS

The Iowa Record Linkage Study is described in detail elsewhere.[1-4] Briefly, 5412 patients admitted to our hospital between January 1, 1972 and December 31, 1981 were electronically matched by computer against Iowa death certificates for the same period. Three hundred and thirty-one patients had died during follow-up. Each patient was assigned a single diagnosis based on a hierarchical and shortened list of 10 diagnostic categories derived from ICD-9.[5] We developed a program that reviewed a patient's clinical diagnosis made by the ward psychiatrists and picked the one with the highest priority in the hierarchy. They were, in order, organic mental disorders, schizophrenia (and paranoia), acute schizophrenia, affective disorders, depressive neuroses, neuroses, alcohol and drug abuse, psychophysiologic disorders or special symptoms, adjustment disorders, and personality and sexual disorders. Follow-up ranged from 0-10 years but averaged 4.27 years for men and 4.20 years for women.

To compare the observed number of deaths with the expected, we adjusted for age, sex, and follow-up time among the patients by computing mortality tables specific for these factors with the use of vital statistics and census data for Iowa. Expected and observed rates were tested by chi square analysis based on Freeman-Tukey deviates. Follow-up time was considered as either less than two years, or greater than two years.

Cause-specific deaths were classified as either accidental (ICD-9 E800-949, 970-999), suicide (ICD-9 E950-969), or natural (all other death codes).

Standardized mortality ratios (SMRs) were calculated and represent the ratio of observed to expected mortality. Men and women were combined for this analysis.

RESULTS

Suicides

Of 68 suicides, 54 (79.4%) occurred during the first two years of follow-up. Suicide throughout follow-up was significantly excessive, but a comparison of SMRs shows a near eightfold increase during the first two years compared with follow-up beyond two years. All diagnoses were initially at risk for suicide except organic mental disorders and psychophysiologic disorders or special symptoms; after two years, only persons with affective disorders or schizophrenia remained at risk.

Accidents

Of 38 accidental deaths, 19 (50%) occurred during the first two years of follow-up. Accidental deaths are significant throughout follow-up, but a comparison of SMRs shows a twofold increase during the first two years of follow-up compared with follow-up beyond two years. During the first two years, those with organic mental disorders, personality disorders, and alcohol and other drug abuse were at increased risk, while after, only those with personality disorders and psychophysiologic disorders or special symptoms remained at risk.

Natural Deaths

Of 225 natural deaths, 115 (51%) occurred during the first two years of follow-up, significantly in excess of expected. Patients at risk included those with organic mental disorders, schizophrenia, alcohol and other drug abuse, and psychophysiologic disorders or special symptoms. After two years, no increase of natural deaths was found.

DISCUSSION

The first two years of follow-up have emerged as a period of great risk for psychiatric patients for early death by both natural and unnatural causes. Although

TABLE 1. Suicides (Men and Women)

Diagnosis	<2 Years Follow-up			>2 Years Follow-up		
	Observed	Expected	Observed/Expected	Observed	Expected	Observed/Expected
Organic mental disorders	1	0.14	7.25	0	0.28	0
Schizophrenia	10	0.13	76.92[c]	4	0.24	16.67[b]
Acute schizophrenia	4	0.05	80.00[b]	1	0.10	10.00
Affective disorder	19	0.28	67.85[c]	3	0.50	6.00[a]
Depressive neuroses	3	0.05	60.00[b]	2	0.11	18.18
Neuroses	3	0.06	50.00[b]	2	0.11	18.18
Alcohol and other drug abuse	6	0.10	60.00[c]	0	0.22	0
Adjustment reactions	3	0.06	50.00[b]	0	0.15	0
Psychophysiologic disorders or special symptoms	0	0.02	0	0	0.08	0
Personality disorders	5	0.16	31.25[c]	2	0.38	5.26
Total	54	1.05	51.43[c]	14	2.17	6.45[c]

[a] $p < 0.05$.
[b] $p < 0.01$.
[c] $p < 0.001$.

TABLE 2. Accidental Deaths (Men and Women)

Diagnosis	<2 Years Follow-up			>2 Years Follow-up		
	Observed	Expected	Observed/Expected	Observed	Expected	Observed/Expected
Organic mental disorders	4	0.84	4.76[a]	1	1.32	0.76
Schizophrenia	1	0.70	1.42	2	1.19	1.68
Acute schizophrenia	2	0.26	7.69	1	0.47	2.13
Affective disorders	1	1.17	0.85	2	2.17	0.92
Depressive neuroses	1	0.26	3.85	1	0.48	2.08
Neuroses	1	0.23	4.35	0	0.51	0
Alcohol and other drug abuse	4	0.51	7.84[a]	1	0.94	1.06
Adjustment reactions	1	0.36	2.78	2	1.03	1.94
Psychophysiologic disorders or special symptoms	0	0.12	0	3	0.30	10.00[a]
Personality disorders	4	0.91	4.50[a]	6	1.83	3.28[a]
Total	19	5.36	3.54[c]	19	10.24	1.86[b]

[a] $p < 0.05$.
[b] $p < 0.01$.
[c] $p < 0.001$.

TABLE 3. Natural Deaths (Men and Women)

Diagnosis	<2 Years Follow-up			>2 Years Follow-up		
	Observed	Expected	Observed/Expected	Observed	Expected	Observed/Expected
Organic mental disorders	46	13.61	3.16[c]	35	29.73	1.28
Schizophrenia	10	2.90	3.44[b]	5	7.10	0.70
Acute schizophrenia	5	1.93	2.59	6	4.96	1.21
Affective disorder	22	19.24	1.14	33	42.08	0.78
Depressive neuroses	6	2.92	2.05	10	7.77	1.29
Neuroses	5	2.11	2.37	3	4.66	0.64
Alcohol and other drug abuse	10	3.59	2.79[a]	7	9.82	0.71
Adjustment reactions	3	2.31	1.30	3	7.23	0.42
Psychophysiologic disorders or special symptoms	3	0.57	5.26[a]	3	1.79	1.67
Personality disorders	5	4.04	1.24	5	13.96	0.35
Total	115	53.42	2.15[c]	110	134.42	0.82

[a] $p < 0.05$.
[b] $p < 0.01$.
[c] $p < 0.001$.

unnatural causes carry risk throughout follow-up, excessive natural death seems to be confined to this early period of follow-up. Mortality was striking in the first two years of follow-up, when 54 (79.4%) suicides, 19 (50%) accidental deaths, and 115 (51.1%) natural deaths occurred. In comparison, we had expected 1.05 (32.6%) suicides, 5.36 (34.6%) accidental deaths, and 53.42 (28.4%) natural deaths.

Earlier work is consistent with our findings of increased risk for mortality early in follow-up, particularly from unnatural causes.[6-10] For example, Rorsman found in a six-year follow-up study increased risk during all years for all cause mortality, but particularly during the first two when 83 (31.9%) deaths occurred but only 34 (21.5%) had been expected.[6] Innes and Millar,[7] Hoenig and Hamilton,[8] and Tsuang and Woolson[9] have also found excess mortality to be confined to the early follow-up period.

Persons in all diagnostic categories were at increased risk for suicide except for those with organic mental disorders and psychophysiologic disorder or special symptoms. (The latter group was comprised primarily of these with eating disorders.) Although the literature is clear in demonstrating that those with organic mental disorders are at comparatively little risk for suicide,[3,11,12] less is known about the risk for suicide of those with eating disorders.[13] After two years follow-up, those with affective disorders and schizophrenia remained at risk, but not those with other disorders. The reason for this may be the smaller numbers of deaths in other disorders. Alternatively, suicide risk continuing throughout follow-up may suggest that schizophrenia and affective disorder are more pernicious.

Interestingly, accidental deaths were significant among patients with organic mental disorders, personality disorders, and alcohol and other drug abuse. This is not unexpected, for clearly the impairment of cognition, judgment, or coordination found in organic states and intoxicated persons or the anger, impulsivity, and resulting inattention found in those with personality disorders could lead to an accident with lethal consequences. There is considerable literature on the interaction of these factors with accidents.[14,15] There is no obvious reason why those with psychophysiologic disorders or special symptoms are at risk for accidental death late in follow-up. This may represent a statistical fluke, but should be explored, if replicated.

A significant excess of natural deaths was confined to those with organic mental disorders and schizophrenia, to alcohol and drug abusers, and to those with psychophysiologic disorders or special symptoms. These findings are consistent with our experience and not particularly surprising. Those with organic disorders are known to suffer high rates of physical illness and experience death from natural causes;[16] alcohol and drug abusers may easily suffer the physical consequences of their behavior and develop malnutrition, peptic ulcers, pancreatitis, or other physical disorders.[17] Those with psychophysiologic disorders and special symptoms (e.g., eating disorders) are also known to suffer the medical consequences of their behavior, and develop malnutrition, electrolyte imbalance, or cardiac abnormalities.[18] There is less consensus in the literature about the relationship between schizophrenia and physical illness, but the disorder has been linked to increased mortality from gastrointestinal cancer and cardiovascular and infectious diseases.[19] That our findings make intuitive sense and confirm the literature adds to their validity.

What do these findings mean? First, tertiary care psychiatric patients who require hospitalization are at great risk for death early in follow-up. These patients form a special subgroup of psychiatric patients, and results may not be generalizable to other groups. Why these persons are subject to death soon after discharge is problematic. It may be that these patients have more severe physical or psychiatric illnesses, or had inadequate treatment, inadequate hospitalization with premature discharge, or a combination of these.

To some extent, the clustering of deaths within two years may represent an artificial finding because of the now commonplace "revolving door" phenomenon, whereby chronic mental patients return to hospital for frequent but relatively brief stays and so are rarely more than two years from discharge. There may be merit to this argument as approximately 75% of our patients had prior hospitalizations and could possibly be considered "revolving door" patients. It would be interesting to see if the deaths that occurred early after follow-up involved the "revolving door" patients, but unfortunately our program did not allow us to check this.

That many of our patients died prematurely from natural causes would suggest to some degree an interaction of both medical and psychiatric disorders. Naturally, the combination of a physical illness with a psychiatric disorder would increase the likelihood that a patient would be admitted for hospitalization, particularly in a tertiary care facility. Both illnesses presenting together increase the "social burden" that a patient carries, so that these persons are more likely to present for admission or be referred by a local physician for admission. The early deaths of these persons may suggest either that the mental illness is hastening the advance of a physical illness through either neglect, poor nutrition, inadequate follow-up, poor treatment compliance, and so on, or that the mental illness has created a new psychiatric disorder (e.g., major depression) or exacerbated an existing one. These issues are difficult to tease apart, but in a related paper we compared the 115 patients who had died within two years to 111 age- and sex-matched controls who had not.[20] We concluded that those dying of natural causes suffered significantly more physical disorders than did the controls, and had reason to die a natural death. On the other hand, those who died from unnatural causes were no more likely than controls to have physical illness and, in essence, died as a result of their psychiatric disorder.

In this and earlier papers,[1-4] we have emphasized the importance of risk for early death that psychiatric patients are subject to, because of its obvious clinical importance. If a psychiatric patient is at greater risk early after discharge (that is, within the first two years), then it is incumbent on the physician to assess the patient for early symptoms of a recurrence of illness, or an exacerbation of illness, and adjust treatment accordingly. In patients with physical disorders in addition to mental disorders, the physician should be aware of the risk for natural death. Being aware of which patient might be at risk for either a natural or unnatural death, then, assumes great importance.

SUMMARY

Mortality in a psychiatric population was studied. During the first two years following hospital discharge, natural deaths, accidental deaths, and suicide were excessive. After two years, suicide and accidental deaths continued to be excessive, but not natural deaths. Diagnostic categories were linked to cause-specific deaths. Clinical implications were discussed.

REFERENCES

1. BLACK, D. W., G. WARRACK & G. WINOKUR. 1985. Excess mortality among psychiatric patients: the Iowa Record Linkage Study. JAMA 253: 58-61.

2. BLACK, D. W., G. WARRACK & G. WINOKUR. 1985. The Iowa Record Linkage Study I. Suicides and accidental deaths among psychiatric patients. Arch. Gen. Psychiatry **42:** 71-77.
3. BLACK, D. W., G. WARRACK & G. WINOKUR. 1985. The Iowa Record Linkage Study II. Excess mortality among patients with organic mental disorders. Arch. Gen. Psychiatry **42:** 78-81.
4. BLACK, D. W., G. WARRACK & G. WINOKUR. 1985. The Iowa Record Linkage Study III. Excess mortality among patients with "functional" disorders. Arch. Gen. Psychiatry **42:** 82-88.
5. 1980. International Classification of Disease. Ninth revision. 2nd edit. Vol. 1. U.S. Department of Health and Human Services. Washington, D.C.
6. RORSMAN, G. 1974. Mortality among psychiatric patients. Acta Psychiatr. Scand. **50:** 354-375.
7. INNES, G. & W. M. MILLAR. 1976. Mortality among psychiatric patients. Scott. Med. J. **15:** 143-148.
8. HOENIG, J. & M. W. HAMILTON 1966. Mortality in psychiatric patients. Acta Psychiatr. Scand. **42:** 349-361.
9. TSUANG, M. T. & R. F. WOOLSON. 1977. Mortality in patients with schizophrenia, mania, depression, and surgical conditions. Br. J. Psychiatry **130:** 162-166.
10. MILES, C. 1977. Conditions predisposing to suicide: a review. J. Nerv. Ment. Dis. **164:** 231-246.
11. EASTWOOD, M. R., S. STIASNY, H. M. R. MEIER & C. M. WOOGH. 1982. Mental illness and mortality. Compr. Psychiatry **23:** 377-385.
12. BARRACLOUGH, B., J. BUNCH, B. NELSON & P. SAINSBURY. 1974. A hundred cases of suicide. Br. J. Psychiatry **125:** 355-373.
13. VIESSELMAN, J. O. & M. ROIG. 1985. Depression and suicidality in eating disorders. J. Clin. Psychiatry **46:** 118-124.
14. NOYES, P. 1985. Auto accidents related to psychiatric impairment. Psychosomatics: 569-596.
15. SCHAFFER, J. W., W. N. TOWNS, C. W. SCHMIDT, et al. 1974. Social adjustment profiles of fatally injured drivers. Arch. Gen. Psychiatry **30:** 508-511.
16. ANANTH, J. 1983. Physical illness and psychiatric disorders. Compr. Psychiatry **44:** 42-46.
17. BERGLUND, M. 1984. Mortality in alcoholics related to clinical state at first admission. Acta Psychiatr. Scand. **70:** 407-416.
18. SEIDENSTICKEN, J. F. & M. TZAGOURNIS. 1968. Anorexia nervosa—clinical features and long-term follow-up. J. Chron. Dis. **21:** 361-367.
19. TSUANG, M. T., K. PERKINS & J. C. SIMPSON. 1983. Physical diseases in schizophrenic and affective disorder. J. Clin. Psychiatry **44:** 42-46.
20. WINOKUR, G. & D. W. BLACK. Psychiatric and medical diagnoses as risk factors for mortality in psychiatric patients: a case control study. Am. J. Psychiatry. (In press.)

Postmortem Monoamine Receptor and Enzyme Studies in Suicide[a]

J. JOHN MANN,[b] P. ANNE McBRIDE,[b] AND MICHAEL STANLEY[c,d]

[b]*Laboratory of Psychopharmacology*
Department of Psychiatry
Cornell University Medical College
1300 York Avenue
New York, New York 10021

[c]*Departments of Psychiatry and Pharmacology*
Wayne State University School of Medicine
Lafayette Clinic
951 East Lafayette
Detroit, Michigan 48207

Measurement of absolute levels of amines and their metabolites in postmortem human brain tissue provides only limited information as to the functional status of these systems. Postmortem delay, the agonal process, drugs, age, gender, seasonal and diurnal effects may all influence amine levels.[1-4] Moreover it has been proposed, since a substantial proportion of the biogenic amines are actually in storage pools and not immediately available for amine release and transmission, that the ratio of metabolite to amine level is a better guide to functional activity. Two alternative approaches to the assessment of neuronal activity are the measurement of postsynaptic binding indices and the assay of biosynthetic enzyme activity.[5,6] This paper will address the application of these methods in the area of postmortem brain research in suicide.

PRESYNAPTIC POSTMORTEM STUDIES OF NEUROCHEMICAL INDICES IN SUICIDE

Initial postmortem neurochemical studies in suicide measured levels of serotonin (5-HT) and/or 5-hydroxyindoleacetic acid (5-HIAA) in the brain stem. The results are shown in TABLE 1. It is clear that some but not all studies reported modestly lower levels of 5-HIAA and/or 5-HT in the frontal cortex or brain stem regions of suicide victims.[7-13]

Results of the few published studies of levels of the catecholamines norepinephrine (NE) and dopamine (DA) in suicide victims[7,10,11] have tended to be negative (see TABLE 2). The absence of systematic data on metabolite levels, together with the fact

---

[a]These studies were supported by Public Health Service grant MH 40210 to Dr. Mann.
[d]Present affiliation: Departments of Psychiatry and Pharmacology, Columbia University and New York State Psychiatric Institute, 722 West 168th Street, New York, N.Y. 10032.

TABLE 1. Levels of Serotonin and 5-Hydroxytryptamine in Postmortem Brain Tissue from Suicide Victims versus Controls

Study	Brain Stem 5-HT	Brain Stem 5-HIAA	Frontal Cortex 5-HT	Frontal Cortex 5-HIAA	Other Regions 5-HT	Other Regions 5-HIAA
Pare et al.[7]	↓11%	NC[a] (↓13%)	—	—	—	—
Shaw et al.[8]	↓11%	—	—	—	—	—
Lloyd et al.[9]	—	NC	—	—	—	—
Bourne et al.[10]	NC	↓28%	—	—	—	—
Beskow et al.[11]	—	↓26%	NC	↓43%	NC	NC
Stanley et al.[12]	—	—	NC	NC	—	—
Owen et al.[13]	—	—	—	↓28%	—	—

[a] Greater assay variance in the control group and half the sample size may have contributed to the lack of statistical significance for the difference in 5-HIAA levels.

that only one of these studies reported results in frontal cortex and none assayed the brain stem, makes it impossible to draw meaningful conclusions about the role of catecholamines in suicide.

POSTMORTEM MONOAMINE RECEPTOR BINDING STUDIES IN SUICIDE

The development in the late 1970s of methods that permitted the reliable assay of neurotransmitter receptors in brain tissue offered a new approach for examining the question of aminergic function in suicide. Destruction of the serotonergic neurons at the level of the raphe nuclei by chemical or electrolytical methods has been found in animal studies to increase the number (or up regulate) postsynaptic 5-HT$_2$ binding sites.[14] Conversely, increasing intrasynaptic levels of 5-HT by chronic administration of 5-HT reuptake inhibitors reduces the number of (or down regulates) 5-HT$_2$ binding sites.[15,16] These sites are labeled by 5-HT antagonist drugs such as mianserin and ketanserin, and most antipsychotics including spiroperidol and haloperidol. Similarly beta-adrenergic receptors can be regulated by the same mechanisms. Reduction of

TABLE 2. Postmortem Brain Levels of Catecholamines and Metabolites in Suicide Victims Versus Controls

Study	Brain Stem NE	Brain Stem DA	Frontal Cortex NE	Frontal Cortex DA	Frontal Cortex HVA[a]	Other Regions NE	Other Regions DA	Other Regions HVA
Bourne et al.[10]	NC	—	—	—	—	—	—	—
Pare et al.[7]	—	—	—	—	—	NC	NC	—
Beskow et al.[11]	—	—	—	—	↑100%	NC or ↓75%[b]	NC	NC

[a] HVA is homovanillic acid.
[b] Putamen. Statistically nonsignificant lower levels were also found in hypothalamus (31%) and caudate (40%).

noradrenergic transmission by 6-hydroxydopamine treatment in animals results in up regulation of the beta$_1$-subtype of adrenergic receptors,[17] and chronic administration of NE-reuptake inhibitors down regulates beta$_1$-adrenergic receptors.[17] Thus, assay of the 5-HT$_2$ and the beta-adrenergic receptor populations may offer an important insight into the level of functional activity in the serotonergic and noradrenergic systems in suicide. Some of the results of our pilot studies[18-20] in this area are summarized in TABLE 3. These data indicate a 28% increase in the number of 5-HT$_2$ binding sites and a 73% increase in beta-adrenergic binding. Since about 50% of cortical beta-adrenergic receptors are of the beta$_1$-subtype, the considerable increase in beta-adrenergic binding in the suicide victims probably involves largely the beta$_1$-subtype.

Dr. Stanley will describe elsewhere in this volume the details of presynaptic serotonergic receptor binding studies using ^{3}H-imipramine as the ligand. These studies indicate fewer imipramine binding sites in the frontal cortex of suicide victims,[12] a finding indicative of fewer functional presynaptic serotonergic nerve terminals.

Thus, taken together these results are consistent with a state of reduced serotonergic (fewer presynaptic ^{3}H-imipramine receptors and an increased number of 5-HT$_2$ postsynaptic receptors) and noradrenergic (an increased number of postsynaptic beta$_1$-receptors) activity in suicide victims. Other investigators have also reported increased 5-HT$_2$ binding[13] and beta-adrenergic binding[21] in frontal cortex in suicide victims although results from another laboratory were not in agreement with the beta-adrenergic receptor findings.[22] Most of the studies included too few samples to permit meaningful statistical analysis. Nevertheless these exciting preliminary findings indicate that postmortem receptor binding studies represent a very promising and informative approach for assessing aminergic function in the central nervous system (CNS).

POSTMORTEM BIOGENIC AMINE METABOLIC ENZYME STUDIES IN SUICIDE

The study of monoamine biosynthetic and degradative enzymes as a guide to transmitter turnover and neuronal activity has barely been applied in the area of suicide research. TABLE 4 summarizes the pertinent literature. Results from three laboratories are in agreement that monoamine oxidase (MAO) enzyme kinetics are

TABLE 3. Postmortem Serotonin$_2$ and Beta-Adrenergic Binding in the Frontal Cortex of Suicide Victims Compared to Matched Controls

		Percent of Control Values in Suicide Group
Serotonin$_2$[a]	B_{max}	128%[c]
	K_D	100%
Beta adrenergic binding[b]		173%[d]

[a] ^{3}H-Spiroperidol saturation binding isotherm.
[b] (^{125}I) Iodopindolol binding at 45 pM concentration.
[c] < 0.05 contrast with controls (two-tailed Wilcoxon paired-sample test or one-tail Mann-Whitney test).
[d] p < 0.05 Mann-Whitney Test.

TABLE 4. Postmortem Studies of Biogenic Amine Synthetic and Degradative Enzymes in Suicide

Study	MAO A	MAO B	COMT[c]	Tyrosine hydroxylase	Dopamine-B-hydroxylase
Grote et al.[a,23]	NC	NC	NC	NC or ↑219%	NC
Gottfries et al.[24]	NC	NC	—	—	—
Mann & Stanley[b,24]	NC	NC	—	—	—

[a] Assayed 28 brain regions in 4-10 brain samples/group.
[b] Assayed enzyme kinetics V_{max} and K_D.
[c] COMT is catechol-O-methyltransferase.

unaltered in suicide.[23-25] In contrast, there is only one reported investigation of other relevant enzymes[23] and that study involved a very small sample of controls and suicide victims. Clearly studies of both enzyme kinetics as well as immunohistochemical studies are urgently needed and may provide valuable biochemical data and perhaps permit neuroanatomical localization of the neurochemical changes associated with suicide. The studies of Grote et al. (1974) indicate that there may be important differences in enzyme activity that are specific for certain brain regions only.[23] For example, substantial increases were reported in the suicide group in tyrosine hydroxylase (TH) activity in basal ganglia areas such as substantia nigra, head of the caudate nucleus, putamen, and in the red nucleus, but no differences were apparent in cerebral cortex, hippocampal gyrus, mesencephalon tegmentum, as well as in whole brain homogenate.

VIOLENCE OF SUICIDE ATTEMPT, AGGRESSION, AND SEROTONERGIC STUDIES

It has been suggested on the basis of studies of cerebrospinal fluid (CSF) levels of 5-HIAA[26,27] that the reduction in serotonergic activity correlates with degree of violence of suicide attempts. An examination of postmortem studies from this perspective is shown in TABLE 5. It is clear that insufficient data are currently available on the relationship between the violence of the suicide attempt and the biochemical indices studied to permit any definite conclusions. Investigators either failed to address this question or the study population died predominantly by either violent or nonviolent means of suicide. This issue remains to be addressed by future studies of postmortem tissue.

A second important finding made in studies of levels of CSF 5-HIAA has been an association between aggressive, impulsive behavior and low CSF 5-HIAA.[28] Such studies have yet to be carried out in postmortem brain tissue. Thus, lowered levels of serotonergic activity may contribute to the violent and impulsive aspects of suicidal behavior. It is not clear why this behavior is inwardly directed in some individuals in the form of suicidal acts and outwardly directed in other individuals (aggression towards others). Coexistent changes in other neurotransmitter systems such as the noradrenergic or dopaminergic systems may determine the direction of the violent impulsive act. For example, our postmortem findings suggest the presence of reduced noradrenergic activity in suicide victims and other laboratories have suggested that increased noradrenergic activity is associated with aggression. This hypothesis has profound theoretical and treatment implications and invites urgent study.

The magnitude of the serotonin or imipramine receptor changes in suicide is much greater than that reported for levels of 5-HT or 5-HIAA. It is not clear whether this is because of regional differences (frontal cortex versus brain stem); the fact that the receptor studies were carried out in patients dying by violent suicide while most patients included in studies of 5-HT and 5-HIAA levels died by nonviolent methods; or differences in the sensitivity of these various indices to changes in serotonergic functional status. Future postmortem studies are required to address these important questions more systematically.

TABLE 5. Postmortem Neurochemical Studies in Violent and Nonviolent Suicide

Proportion of Nonviolent Suicides	5-HT	5-HIAA	NE	5-HT$_2$ Binding	^{3}H-Imipramine Binding
Beskow et al[11] 12/23 (did not distinguish from violent)	—	↓26%	NC	—	—
Bourne et al.[10] 21/23	NC	↓28%	NC (2/23 with violent attempt had low NE (↓39%) versus 21/23 nonviolent)	—	—
Pare et al.[7] 26/26	↓11%	↓13%	NC	—	—
Shaw et al.[8] 24/28	↓11% 4/28 did not differ	—	—	—	—
Stanley et al.[12] 0/9	—	—	—	—	↓44%
Stanley & Mann[19] 0/11	—	—	—	↑44%	—

NEUROCHEMICAL SPECIFICITY OF CORRELATES OF SUICIDAL BEHAVIOR

A final comment should be made about the biochemical selectivity or specificity of the postmortem neurochemical correlates of suicide. Most work has concentrated on the serotonergic system. A confluence of postmortem studies,[10,19,20] CSF studies,[26–29] and neuroendocrine challenge tests[30,31] has pointed toward an association between reduced serotonergic activity and suicidal behavior. However other investigators including our own laboratory have reported alterations in indices of adrenergic function such as increased beta-adrenergic binding[20,21] and lower norepinepephrine/epinephrine ratios in urine.[32,33] These data suggest involvement of the noradrenergic system. In contrast we and others have reported no differences in cholinergic binding in the frontal cortex of suicide victims[34,35] suggesting that the cholinergic system may be spared, although clearly more complete studies of this system are necessary since cholinergic muscarinic binding does not appear to be altered in Alzheimer's disease where degeneration of cholinergic neurons and loss of choline acetyltransferase activity have been demonstrated. Therefore, a wider range of neurotransmitter systems need to be studied to permit a determination of the *neurochemical specificity* of the changes associated with suicidal behavior. Finally the combination of pre- and postsynaptic measures may assist in localizing the reason for altered neural transmission to the pre- or postsynaptic region.

TREATMENT IMPLICATIONS

Antidepressants produce changes in the opposite direction on precisely the same monoaminergic receptor systems that are altered in suicide victims.[16] It is therefore reasonable to hypothesize that this effect may account for both the *antidepressant* and *antisuicidal* action of these compounds. Since suicidal behavior is seen in nondepressive syndromes, antidepressant drugs are potentially effective for the suicidal component of nondepressive psychiatric syndromes. This hypothesis is explored in detail elsewhere in this volume.

ACKNOWLEDGMENTS

The technical assistance of Ms. Joan Chin contributed to this work.

REFERENCES

1. SPOKES, E. G. S. 1979. An analysis of factors influencing the measurements of dopamine, noradrenaline, glutamate decarboxylase and choline acetylase in human post-mortem brain tissue. Brain 102: 333-346.
2. CARLSSON, A., R. ADOLFSSON, S. M. AQUILONIUS, C. G. GOTTFRIES, L. ORELAND, L. SVENNERHOLM & B. WINBLAD. 1980. Biogenic amines in human brain in normal aging, senile dementia and chronic alcoholism. *In* Ergot Compounds and Brain Function: Neuroendocrine and Neuropsychiatric Aspects. M. Goldstein *et al.*, Eds.: 295-304. Raven Press. New York, N.Y.
3. ALLEN, S. J., J. S. BENTON, M. J. GOODHARDT, E. A. HAAN, N. R. SIMS, C. C. T. SMITH, J. A. SPILLANE, D. M. BOWEN & A. N. DAVISON. 1983. Biochemical evidence of selective nerve cell changes in normal aging human and rat brain. J. Neurochem. 41: 256-265.
4. MANN, J. J., C. PETITO, P. A. MCBRIDE, M. STANLEY, J. CHIN & A. PHILOGENE. 1984. Age and gender effects upon amine receptors and MAO in postmortem human brain tissue. *In* Clinical and Pharmacological Studies in Psychiatric Disorders. G. D. Burrows & T. R. Norman, Eds. John Libbey & Co. London, England.

5. CREESE, I., D. R. BURT & S. H. SNYDER. 1976. Dopamine receptor binding predicts clinical and pharmacological potencies of antischizophrenic drugs. Science 192: 481-483.
6. REIS, D. J., R. A. ROSS & T. H. JOH. 1977. Changes in the activity and amount of enzymes synthesizing catecholamines and acetylcholine in brain, adrenal medulla and sympathetic ganglia of aged rat and mouse. Brain Res. 136: 465-474.
7. PARE, C. M. B., D. P. H. YOUNG, K. PRICE & R. S. STACEY. 1969. 5-Hydroxytryptamine, noradrenaline, and dopamine in brainstem, hypothalamus, and caudate nucleus of controls and of patients committing suicide by coal-gas poisoning. Lancet ii: 133-135.
8. SHAW, D. M., E. F. CAMPS & E. G. ECCLESTON. 1967. 5-Hydroxytryptamine in the hindbrain of depressive suicides. Br. J. Psychiatry 113: 1407-1411.
9. LLOYD, K. G., I. J. FARLEY, J. H. N. DECK, et al. 1974. Serotonin and 5-hydroxyindoleacetic acid in discrete areas of brainstem of suicide victims and control patients. In Serotonin: New Vistas. E. Costa, G. L. Gessa & M. Sandler, Eds.: 387-398. Raven Press. New York, N.Y.
10. BOURNE, H. R., W. E. BUNNEY, JR., R. W. COLBURN, J. M. DAVIS, D. M. SHAW & A. J. COPPEN. 1968. Noradrenaline, 5-hydroxytryptamine, and 5-hydroxyindoleacetic acid in hindbrains of suicidal patients. Lancet ii: 805-808.
11. BESKOW, J., C. G. GOTTFRIES, B. E. ROOS & B. WINBLAD. 1976. Determination of monoamine and monoamine metabolites in the human brain: postmortem studies in a group of suicides and a control group. Acta Psychiatr. Scand. 53: 7-20.
12. STANLEY, M., I. MCINTYRE & S. GERSHON. 1983. Postmortem serotonin metabolism in suicide victims. Abstr. Annual Meeting, American College of Neuropsychopharmacology.
13. OWEN, F., A. J. CROSS, T. J. CROW, J. F. W. DEAKIN, I. N. FERRIER, R. LOFTHOUSE & M. POULTER. Brain 5-HT$_2$ receptors and suicide. Lancet ii: 1256.
14. BRUNNELLO, N., D. M. CHUANG & E. COSTA. 1982. Different synaptic location of mianserin and imipramine binding sites. Science 215: 1112-1115.
15. PEROUTKA, S. J. & S. H. SNYDER. 1980. Long-term antidepressant treatment decreases spiroperidol-labelled serotonin receptor binding. Science 210: 88-90.
16. STANLEY, M. & J. J. MANN. 1984. Suicide and serotonin receptors. Lancet i: 349.
17. MINNEMAN, K. P., M. D. DIBNER, B. B. WOLFE & P. B. MOLINOFF. B$_1$- and B$_2$-adrenergic receptors in rat cerebral cortex are independently regulated. Science 204: 866-868.
18. STANLEY, M., J. J. MANN & S. GERSHON. 1983. Alterations in pre- and post-synaptic serotonergic neurons in suicide victims. Psychopharmacol. Bull. 19: 684-687.
19. STANLEY, M. & J. J. MANN. 1983. Serotonin-2 binding sites are increased in the frontal cortex of suicide victims. Lancet i: 214-216.
20. MANN, J. J., M. STANLEY, P. A. MCBRIDE & B. S. MCEWEN. Increased serotonin$_2$ and beta$_1$-adrenergic receptor binding in the frontal cortex of suicide victims. Arch. Gen. Psychiatry. (In press.)
21. ZANKO, M. T. & A. BIEGON. 1983. Increased B adrenergic receptor binding in human frontal cortex of suicide victims. Abstr. Annual Meeting, Society of Neuroscience, Boston, Mass.: 719.
22. MEYERSON, L. R., L. P. WENNOSLE, M. S. ABEL, et al. 1982. Human brain receptor alterations in suicide victims. Pharmacol. Biochem. Behav. 17: 159-163.
23. GROTE, S. S., S. G. MOSES, E. ROBINS, R. W. HUDGENS & A. B. CRONINGER. 1974. A study of selected catecholamine metabolizing enzyme: a comparison of depressive suicides and alcoholic suicides with controls. J. Neurochem. 23: 791-802.
24. GOTTFRIES, C. G., L. ORELAND, A. WIBERG & B. WINBLAD. 1975. Lowered monoamine oxidase activity in brains from alcoholic suicides. J. Neurochem. 25: 667-673.
25. MANN, J. J. & M. STANLEY. 1984. Postmortem monoamine oxidase enzyme kinetics in the frontal cortex of suicide victims and controls. Acta Psychiatr. Scand. 69: 135-139.
26. TRASKMAN, L., M. ASBERG, L. BERKILSSON & L. SJOSTRAND. 1981. Monoamine metabolites in CSF and suicidal behavior. Arch. Gen. Psychiatry 38: 631-636.
27. VAN PRAAG, H. M. 1983. CSF 5-HIAA and suicide in non-depressed schizophrenics. Lancet ii: 977-978.
28. BROWN, G. L., F. K. GOODWIN & W. E. BUNNEY, JR. 1982. Human aggression and suicide: their relationship to neuropsychiatric diagnoses and serotonin metabolism. In Serotonin in Biological Psychiatry. B. T. Ho et al., Eds.: 287-307. Raven Press. New York, N.Y.

29. AGREN, H. 1980. Symptom patterns in unipolar and bipolar depression correlating with monoamine metabolites in the cerebrospinal fluid. II. Suicide. Psychiatry Res. **3:** 225-236.
30. MELTZER, H. Y., R. PERLINE, B. J. TRICOU, M. LOWY & A. ROBERTSON. 1984. Effect of 5-hydroxytryptophan on serum cortisol levels in major affective disorders. Arch. Gen. Psychiatry **41:** 379-387.
31. LINKOWSKI, P., J. P. VAN WETTERE, M. KERKHOFS, H. BRAUMAN & J. MENDLEWICZ. 1983. Thryotrophin response to thyereostimulin in effectively ill women: relationship to suicidal behavior. Br. J. Psychiatry **143:** 401-405.
32. OSTROFF, R., E. GILLER, K. BONESE, E. EBERSOLE, L. HARKNESS & J. MASON. 1982. Neuroendocrine risk factors of suicide. Am. J. Psychiatry **139:** 1323-1325.
33. PRASAD, A. 1984. Neuroendocrine differences between violent and nonviolent parasuicide. Abstr. Annual Meeting Collegium Internationale Neuropsychopharmacologium: 64. Jerusalem, Israel.
34. STANLEY, M. 1984. Cholinergic receptor binding in the frontal cortex of suicide victims. Am. J. Psychiatry **141:** 1432-1436.
35. KAUFMAN, C. A., J. C. GILLIN, T. O'LAUGHLIN, *et al.* 1983. New Res. Abstr., Annual Meeting American Psychiatric Association: 65.

Serotonin and Serotonergic Receptors in Suicide

MICHAEL STANLEY,[a] J. JOHN MANN,[b] AND LEE S. COHEN[c]

[a]*Departments of Psychiatry and Pharmacology*
Columbia University and
New York State Psychiatric Institute
722 West 168th Street
New York, New York 10032

[b]*Department of Psychiatry*
Cornell University Medical College
1300 York Avenue
New York, New York 10021

[c]*Department of Psychiatry*
Columbia University
722 West 168th Street
New York, New York 10032

Biochemical parameters are currently under investigation in postmortem research to assess their role in suicidal behavior. Most notable among these studies are examinations of the serotonergic system. This research has included work on serotonin (5-HT), and 5 hydroxyindoleactic acid (5-HIAA) levels in suicide victims compared with controls. Examination of receptor studies in this system include [^{3}H]imiprimine binding sites and 5-HT binding sites.

Postmortem suicide studies typically measured 5-HT and 5-HIAA in brain stem areas where serotonin cell bodies are concentrated in the raphe nuclei. In those studies where information was available, approximately 50% of the suicide victims carried a diagnosis of major depressive episode; the remaining cases carried diagnoses of alcohol abuse, adjustment disorder with depressed mood, schizophrenia or a personality disorder,[1-4] suggesting that the altered 5-HT and 5-HIAA levels were primarily associated with suicidal behavior rather than depression per se.

Postmortem biochemical measures of various neurotransmitters in suicide victims compared to controls indicate five studies showing decreases in measures of 5-HT,[4-8] three studies showing decreases in 5-HIAA levels,[8-10] five studies showing no change in 5-HIAA levels,[5,6,9-11] and two studies showing no change in 5-HT levels[2,9] (see TABLE 1). Our group also examined the ratio of 5-HIAA to 5-HT to estimate turnover rates in suicide victims as compared to controls and found no significant differences.[9] The findings on 5-HIAA and 5-HT levels are summarized in TABLE 1. In general these studies have indicated decreased levels of 5-HT and 5-HIAA in the brain stems of suicide victims. In contrast to the findings in brain stem, no significant changes are seen with regard to 5-HT and 5-HIAA levels in the cortices of suicide victims compared with controls.

Possible reasons that have been posited to explain these inconsistent findings are that neurotransmitters have been shown to be acutely affected by drug effects,[12,13] postmortem interval,[9-14] temperature,[15] and regional concentration differences in brain dissection.[16] In contrast to biogenic amines, which are responsive to the above acute influences, examination of receptors that change in response to chronic but not acute treatment may serve as better indicators of a system's steady state immediately prior to death. The experimental support for this contention is supplied by research showing serotonergic receptor change in response to chronic but not acute exposure to antidepressants.[17] In addition, there has been no significant correlation between 5-HT$_2$ receptors and postmortem interval, although 5-HT$_1$ receptors are negatively correlated with this parameter.[18] Receptor studies may therefore give more accurate results.

Imipramine binding has been shown in animal experiments to be associated with presynaptic serotonergic nerve terminals.[19] These binding sites have been characterized in platelets and various regions of the brain. Some of the additional experimental evidence linking imipramine binding with 5-HT is that (1) radioautography studies

TABLE 1. Postmortem Neurotransmitter and Metabolite Studies in Completed Suicides

Study	Neurochemical Findings
Shaw et al.[7]	↓ Brain stem 5-HT
Bourne et al.[43]	↓ Brain stem 5-HIAA
Pare et al.[6]	↓ Brain stem 5-HT
	No change in brain stem 5-HIAA
Lloyd et al.[5]	↓ Brain stem 5-HT
	No change in brain stem 5-HIAA
Gillin et al.[8]	↓ Hypothalamus 5-HT
	↓ Nucleus acumbens 5-HIAA
Korpi et al.[4]	↓ Hypothalamus 5-HT
Beskow et al.[3]	↓ 5-HIAA in brain stem
Owens et al.[11]	No change in 5-HIAA levels in frontal cortex
Crow et al.[10]	No change in 5-HIAA levels in frontal cortex
Cochrane et al.[2]	No change in brain 5-HT
Stanley et al.[9]	No change in 5-HIAA or 5-HT levels in frontal cortex

of [^{3}H]imipramine binding sites show distribution similar to serotonergic terminals;[20] (2) chemical and electrolytic lesions of the Raphe nucleus cause a significant reduction in serotonin level and in the number of imipramine binding sites;[19] (3) the use of an irreversible ligand results in reduced [^{3}H]imipramine binding and serotonin uptake;[21] (4) the potency of antidepressant drugs to inhibit serotonin uptake is significantly correlated with their potency to inhibit [^{3}H]imipramine binding;[22] (5) serotonin is the only neurotransmitter known to inhibit [^{3}H]imipramine binding;[23-24] and (6) there is a similar pharmacologic profile between brain and platelet [^{3}H]imipramine binding sites.[25]

Initial studies of imipramine binding in the platelets of patients with major depressive episode have indicated decreases in the number of binding sites.[26] The combined association of imipramine binding with 5-HT function as well as the significant reduction in binding density in depressives suggests a possible alteration in imipramine binding in suicide victims since approximately 50% of these people carry a diagnosis of major depressive episode.

To test this hypothesis, our group examined imipramine binding in the brains of suicide victims and controls.[27] In this study there were no significant differences between the two groups with respect to age, sex, or postmortem interval. Additionally, the mode of suicide studied in the suicides and controls was of a sudden and violent nature.

Our findings indicate a significant reduction in the number of imipramine binding sites (B_{max}) with no difference in binding affinity (K_d).

These results are consistent with the accumulating evidence suggesting the involvement of 5-HT in suicide. Specifically, reduced imipramine binding (associated with presynaptic terminals) may be indicative of reduced 5-HT release and would be in agreement with those reports of reduced postmortem levels of 5-HT and 5-HIAA in suicides cited above.

TABLE 2. Postmortem Receptor Studies of Suicide Victims

Study	Neurochemical Findings
Stanley et al.[27]	↓ ³H-Imipramine binding in cortex
Paul et al.[28]	↓ ³H-Imipramine binding in hypothalamus
Perry et al.[30]	↓ ³H-Imipramine binding[a] in cortex
Crow et al.[10]	↓ ³H-Imipramine binding in cortex
Meyerson et al.[31]	↑ ³H-Imipramine binding in cortex
Stanley and Mann[32,33]	↑ 5-HT₂ binding in cortex
Owen et al.[11]	↑ 5-HT₂ binding in cortex[b]
Crow et al.[10]	No change in 5-HT₂ binding in cortex
Stanley[40]	No change in muscarinic cholinergic receptor binding in cortex
Kaufman et al.[41]	No change in muscarinic cholinergic receptor binding in cortex
Meyerson et al.[31]	↑ Muscarinic cholinergic receptor binding in cortex
Zanko and Biegon[46]	↑ Beta-receptor binding in cortex
Mann and Stanley[45]	↑ Beta-receptor binding in cortex
Meyerson et al.[21]	No change in beta-receptor binding in cortex

[a] Depressed patients dying of natural causes.
[b] Increased but not significantly.

Several studies on imipramine binding have shown significant decreases in this parameter in completed suicides[10,28,29] and in depressed patients who died from natural causes.[30] One study, however, indicated increased imipramine binding in completed suicides[31] (see TABLE 2).

In addition to examining presynaptic receptor sites, our group has also studied postsynaptic 5-HT binding sites using ³H-spiroperidol (specifically 5-HT₂ receptors).[32,33]

A significant increase in the number of 5-HT₂ binding sites (B_{max}) with no change in binding affinity (K_d) was found. These patients committed sudden, violent suicide, i.e., gunshot wound, jumping from height, hanging, and were compared to controls matched for age, sex, and postmortem interval. This is consistent with an up regulation of this site in response to previously mentioned decreases in levels of 5-HT, 5-HIAA, and [³H]imipramine binding sites.

The finding of increased numbers of 5-HT$_2$ (postsynaptic) binding sites in the frontal cortex of suicide victims supports the involvement of 5-HT in suicidal behavior. A study in nonmedicated suicide victims compared to controls has also indicated increases in 5-HT$_2$ binding with no difference in 5-HT$_1$ receptors, with one study showing no change in 5-HT$_1$ or 5-HT$_2$ receptors[10] (see TABLE 2). Previously mentioned research indicates that chronic antidepressant treatment decreases the number of 5-HT$_2$ receptors; therefore the increase in these binding sites in suicide victims is not treatment related.

We may postulate from the above data that the serotonergic system is altered in suicide victims as evidenced by changes in 5-HT and 5-HIAA levels, and [^{3}H]imipramine and 5-HT binding sites as compared to controls.

Other neurotransmitter system receptors have also been examined in relation to suicide. It has been postulated that muscarinic cholinergic receptors may be related to affective disorders.[34] The characterization of muscarinic cholinergic receptors with the reversible muscarinic antagonist 3 quinuclidinyl benzilate (QNB) has been used in studies of both animal and human samples of brain specimens.[35] Because of the high incidence of suicide among affectively disordered patients[36-38] and because of a preliminary report indicating an increased density of QNB binding sites in a small sample of suicide victims,[39] our group has examined this receptor more extensively.

We examined muscarinic cholinergic receptor binding in the frontal cortex of suicide victims and controls matched for age, sex, and postmortem interval.[40] There were no significant differences between the groups in either the number of binding sites (B_{max}) or their relative affinity (K_d). Another recent study[41] is in agreement with our findings of no difference in muscarinic cholinergic binding between suicides and controls. One study reported increases in muscarinic cholinergic receptor binding.[31]

Suicidal behavior has also been investigated via examination of the adrenergic system by examining cerebrospinal fluid (CSF) 3 methoxy-4-hydroxyphenylglycol (MHPG) levels in suicide attempters, where two studies have shown lowered MHPG[3,42] and three studies showed no difference in MHPG levels.[6,43,44]

Our group examined β-adrenergic receptor binding in the frontal cortex of suicide victims as compared with controls matched for sex and postmortem interval.[45] The results of this study indicate a significant increase in beta-adrenergic receptor binding in the suicide victims. These data on increased beta-adrenergic receptor binding in suicide victims compared to controls have been confirmed by one recent study,[46] while another study has shown no change in beta-receptor binding.[31]

Preliminary studies indicate that more than one neurotransmitter system may be related to suicidal behavior. These interrelationships may hold additional promise for our understanding of this behavior and may contribute to improved treatment techniques.

REFERENCES

1. SHAW, D. M., F. E. CAMPS & E. G. ECCLESTON. 1967. 5 Hydroxytryptamine in the hindbrain of depressive suicides. Br. J. Psychiatry 113: 1407-1411.
2. COCHRANE, E., E. ROBINS & S. GROTE. 1976. Regional serotonin levels in brain: a comparison of depressive suicides and alcoholic suicides with controls. Biol. Psychiatry 11(3): 283-294.
3. BESKOW, J., C. G. GOTTFRIES, B. E. ROOS & B. WINDLAND. 1976. Determination of monoamine and monoamine metabolites in the human brain: postmortem studies in a group of suicides and in a control group. Acta Psychiatr. Scand. 53: 7-20.

4. KORPI, E. R., J. E. KLEINMAN, S. J. GOODMAN, et al. 1983. Serotonin and 5-hydroxyindoleacetic acid concentration in different brain regions of suicide victims: comparison in chronic schizophrenia patients with suicide as cause of death. Paper presented at the meeting of the International Society for Neurochemistry, Vancouver, Canada, July 14.
5. LLOYD, K. G., I. J. FRALEY, J. H. N. DECK & O. HORNYKIEWICZ. 1974. Serotonin and 5-hydroxyindoleacetic acid and discrete areas of the brainstem of suicide victims and control patients. Adv. Biochem. Psychopharmacol. 2: 387-397.
6. PARE, C. M. B., D. P. H. YEUNG, K. PRICE & R. S. STACEY. 1969. 5-Hydroxytryptamine, noradrenaline, and dopamine in brainstem, hypothalamus, and caudate nucleus of controls and of patients committing suicide by coal-gas poisoning. Lancet: 133-135.
7. SHAW, D. M., F. E. CAMPS & E. G. ECCLESTON. 1967. 5-Hydroxytryptamine in the hindbrain of depressive suicides. Br. J. Psychiatry 113: 1407-1411.
8. GILLIN, J. C., et al. Muscarinic receptor density in skin fibroblasts and autopsied brain tissue in affective disorder. Ann. N.Y. Acad. Sci. (This volume.)
9. STANLEY, M., I. MCINTYRE & S. GERSHON. 1983. Postmortem serotonin metabolism in suicide victims. Paper presented at the American College of Neuropsychopharmacology Meeting, Puerto Rico.
10. CROW, T. J., A. J. CROSS, S. J. COOPER, et al. 1984. Neurotransmitter receptors and monoamine metabolites in the brains of patients with alzheimer-type dementia and depression and suicides. Neuropharmacology 23(12B): 1561-1569.
11. OWENS, F., A. J. CROSS, T. J. CROW, J. F. W. DEAKIN, I. N. FERRIER, R. LOFTHOUSE & M. POULTER. 1983. Brain 5-HT$_2$ receptors and suicide. Lancet ii: 1256.
12. ASHCROFT, G. W., R. C. DOW, C. M. YATES & I. A. PULLAR. 1976. Significance of lumbar CSF metabolite measurements in affective illness. In CNS and Behavioral Pharmacology. J. Tuomisto & M. K. Paasonen, Eds. 3: 277-284. University of Helsinki, Finland.
13. WALINDER, J., A. SKOTT, A. CARLSSON, et al. 1976. Potentiation of the antidepressant action of clomipramine by tryptophan. Arch. Gen. Psychiatry 33: 1384-1389.
14. STANLEY, M. Unpublished data.
15. VAN WIJKIM, M. & J. KORF. 1981. Postmortem changes of 5 hydroxytryptamine and 5 hydroxyindoleacetic acid in mouse brain and their prevention by pargyline and microwave irradiation. Neurochem. Res. 6: 425-430.
16. MCINTYRE, I. M. & M. STANLEY. 1984. Postmortem and regional changes of serotonin, 5 hydroxyindoleacetic acid and tryptophan in brain. J. Neurochem. 42(6): 1588-1592.
17. PEROUTKA, S. J. & S. H. SNYDER. 1980. Regulation of serotonin (5HT$_2$) receptors labeled with [^{3}H]spiroperidol by chronic treatment with antidepressant amitriptyline. Pharmacol. Exp. Ther. 215: 582-587.
18. MANN, J. J., C. PETITO, M. STANLEY, et al. Amine receptor binding and monoamine oxidase activity in postmortem human brain tissues: effect of age, gender and postmortem delay. (Submitted for publication.)
19. BRUNELLO, N., D. M. CHUANG & F. COSTA. 1982. Different synaptic location of mianserin and imipramine binding sites. Science 215: 1112-1115.
20. BEIGON, A. & T. C. RAINBOW. 1983. Distribution of imipramine binding sites in the rat brain studied by quantitative autoradiography. Neurosci. Lett. 37(3): 209-214.
21. REHAVI, M., Y. ITTAH, K. L. PRICE, et al. 1981. 2-Nitroimipramine: a selective irreversible inhibitor of [^{3}H]serotonin uptake and [^{3}H]imipramine binding in platelets. Biochem. Biophys. Res. Commun. 99: 954.
22. PAUL, S. M., M. REHAVI, P. SKOLNICK, et al. 1981. Depressed patients have decreased binding of tritiated imipramine to platelet serotonin "transporter." Arch. Gen. Psychiatry 38: 1315-1317.
23. PAUL, S. M., M. REHAVI, K. C. RICE, et al. 1981. Does high affinity [^{3}H]imipramine binding label serotonin reuptake sites in brain and platelet? Life Sci. 28: 2753-2760.
24. LANGER, S. T., C. MORET, R. RAISMAN, et al. 1980. High affinity [^{3}H]imipramine binding in rat hypothalamus: association with uptake of serotonin but not of norepinephrine. Science 210: 1133-1135.
25. RELAUI, M., S. M. PAUL, P. SKOLNICLE & F. K. GOODWIN. 1980. Demonstration of specific high affinity binding sites for [^{3}H]imipramine in human brain. Life Sci. 26: 2273-2279.

26. LANGER, S. F. & R. RAISMAN. 1983. Binding of [^{3}H]imipramine and [^{3}H]desipramine as biochemical tools for studies in depression. Neuropharmacology 22: 407-413.
27. STANLEY, M., J. VIRGILIO & S. GERSHON. 1982. Tritiated imipramine binding sites are decreased in the frontal cortex of suicides. Science 216: 1337-1339.
28. PAUL, S. M., M. REHAVI, P. SKOLNICK & F. K. GOODWIN. 1984. High affinity binding of antidepressants to a biogenic amine transport site in human brain and platelet; studies in depression. In Neurobiology of Mood Disorders. R. M. Post & J. C. Bellinger, Eds.: 845-853. Williams and Wilkins. Baltimore, Md.
29. CROW, T. Personal communication.
30. PERRY, E. K., E. F. MARSHALL, G. BLESSED, B. E. TOMLINSON & R. H. PERRY. 1983. Decreased imipramine binding in the brains of patients with depressive illness. Br. J. Psychiatry 1412: 188-192.
31. MEYERSON, L. R., L. P. WENNOGLE, M. S. ABEL, J. COUPET, A. S. LIPPA, C. E. RAUH & B. BEER. 1982. Human brain receptor alterations in suicide victims. Pharmacol. Biochem. Behav. 17: 159-163.
32. STANLEY, M. & J. J. MANN. 1983. Increased serotonin-2 binding sites in frontal cortex of suicide victims. Lancet: 214-216.
33. STANLEY, M., J. J. MANN & A. GERSHON. 1983. Alterations in pre and post synaptic serotonergic neurons in suicide victims. Psychopharmacol. Bull. 4: 684-687.
34. NADI, N. S., J. I. NURNBERGER, JR. & E. S. GERSHON. 1984. Muscarinic cholinergic receptors on skin fibroblasts in familial affective disorder. N. Engl. J. Med. 311: 225-230.
35. YAMAMURA, H. I. & S. H. SNYDER. 1974. Muscarinic cholinergic binding in rat brain. Proc. Nat. Acad. Sci. USA 71: 1725-1729.
36. DORPAT, T. L. & H. S. RIPLEY. 1960. A study of suicide in the Seattle area. Compr. Psychiatry 1: 349-359.
37. BARRACLOUGH, B., J. BUNCH, B. NELSON, et al. 1974. A hundred cases of suicide: clinical aspects. Br. J. Psychiatry 125: 355-373.
38. ROBINS, E., G. E. MURPHY, R. H. WILKINSON, et al. 1959. Some clinical considerations in the prevention of suicide based on a study of 134 successful suicides. Am. J. Public Health 49: 888-899.
39. MEYERSON, L. R., L. P. WENNOGLE, M. S. ABEL, et al. 1982. Human brain receptor alterations in suicide victims. Pharmacol. Biochem. Behav. 17: 159-163.
40. STANLEY, M. 1984. Cholinergic receptor binding in the frontal cortex of suicide victims. Am. J. Psychiatry 141(11): 1432-1436.
41. KAUFMAN, C. A., J. C. GILLIN, T. O'LAUGHLIN & J. E. KLEINMAN. 1984. Muscarinic binding in suicides. Psychiatry Res. 12: 47-55.
42. AGREN, H. 1980. Symptom patterns in unipolar and bipolar depression correlating with monoamine metabolites in the cerebrospinal fluid. II. Suicide. Psychiatry Res. 3: 325-336.
43. BOURNE, H. R., W. E. BUNNEY, JR., R. W. COLBURN, J. M. DAVIS, D. M. SHAW & A. J. COPPEN. 1968. Noradrenaline, 5-hydroxytryptamine, and 5-hydroxyindoleacetic acid in the hindbrains of suicidal patients. Lancet: 805-808.
44. ORELAND, L., A. WIBERG, M. ASHBURG, L. TRASKMAN, K. SJOSTAND, P. THOREN, L. BERTILSSON & G. TYBRING. Platelet MAO activity in postmortem human brain tissue. In Clinical and Pharmacological Studies in Psychiatric Disorders. G. D. Burrows & T. R. Norman, Eds. John Libey & Co., Ltd. London, England. (In press.)
45. MANN, J. J., M. STANLEY, P. A. MCBRIDE & B. MCEWEN. Increased serotonin and beta adrenergic receptor binding in the frontal cortex of suicide victims. (Unpublished manuscript.)
46. ZANKO, M. T. & A. BIEGON. 1983. Increased β adrenergic receptor binding in human frontal cortex of suicide victims. Abstr., Annual Meeting, Society for Neuroscience, Boston, Mass.: 719.

Postmortem Neurochemical Studies in Depression

I. N. FERRIER,[a,b] I. G. McKEITH,[b] A. J. CROSS,[c]
E. K. PERRY,[d] J. M. CANDY,[a] AND R. H. PERRY[a,d]

[a]*MRC Neuroendocrinology Unit*
Newcastle General Hospital
Westgate Road
Newcastle upon Tyne NE4 6BE, United Kingdom

[b]*Department of Psychiatry*
University of Newcastle
Newcastle upon Tyne NE1 8AH, United Kingdom

[c]*Department of Physiology*
University of Manchester
Manchester M13 9PT, United Kingdom

[d]*Department of Neuropathology*
Newcastle General Hospital
Westgate Road
Newcastle upon Tyne NE4 6BE, United Kingdom

INTRODUCTION

The delineation of monoamine neurotransmitter systems in the brain and the observation that drugs affecting these systems can alter both pathological and normal mood represent circumstantial evidence suggesting a disturbance of neurotransmitter function in the major affective disorders. Current neurochemical hypotheses of major affective illnesses are based on the observation that reserpine, which depletes brain serotonin (5-HT),[1] noradrenaline (NA),[2] and dopamine (DA),[3] is associated with the development of depression in a substantial number of subjects.[4] These observations, together with some data on the neurochemical effects of antidepressants, have led to the noradrenaline deficit[5] and serotonin deficit[6] hypotheses of depression. More recently, the clinical observation of a delayed response to antidepressant therapy has led to the suggestion that an alteration in receptor function leads to depression[7] and may account for the therapeutic effect of antidepressant treatments.[8] Indirect evidence that supports these various hypotheses has been found in a series of studies of monoamines and metabolites in urine and cerebrospinal fluid (CSF)[9] and in some neuroendocrine studies,[10] but results are not always consistent and are open to various interpretations. More direct evidence of a putative neurochemical disturbance in depression may be provided by studies of postmortem tissue (which have proved valuable in the case of some neuropsychiatric conditions, e.g., Parkinson's disease, Alzheimer's disease). This paper describes such a study and also discusses some of the problems associated with autopsy studies.

Early postmortem studies used material collected from cases who had committed suicide, and examined the serotonin hypothesis. Shaw et al. (1967) reported a reduction in 5-HT concentrations in hindbrain in 11 cases of suicide said to have been previously depressed.[11] Pare et al. (1969) replicated this finding[12] but three subsequent studies have failed to do so,[13-15] although the percentage of suicide cases with confirmed depression in these latter studies was rather low. In some, but not all, of these studies, concentrations of 5 hydroxyindoleacetic acid (5-HIAA—the principal metabolite of 5-HT) were normal which mitigates against the serotonin deficit hypothesis of depression. Indeed, in a recent study of 20 suicide victims, 10 of whom had been "definitely" or "probably" depressed prior to death, a significant increase in 5-HIAA was noted in the hippocampus.[16] A similar but nonsignificant increase was noted in hippocampus in a small study of suicide cases[13] and in a study of depressed cases.[17]

Postmortem studies of suicide and/or depression have failed to reveal consistent abnormalities in the catecholamines (NA and DA) or their metabolites. Three groups have examined DA concentrations in a large number of brain regions and found no differences from controls.[12,14,18] The DA metabolite homovanillic acid (HVA) was similarly unchanged in a study of suicide cases.[14] However, in a group of depressed brains included in a collaborative Newcastle/London (United Kingdom) study (Cross et al., 1983),[17] a significant increase in HVA in hippocampus was noted—a result discussed in more detail later. Concentrations of NA and its major metabolite 3-methoxy-4-hydroxyphenylgycol (MHPG) have been found to be normal in most brain areas in postmortem studies of depression.[18,19]

Changes in receptor binding following antidepressant and electroconvulsive therapy (ECT) administration have been documented,[8] although reports are not always consistent. Evidence for corresponding changes in receptor binding in brain tissue from cases of depression and/or suicide have therefore been sought. Some promising leads have been reported but again there is a lack of consistent findings. β-Adrenergic receptors are "down regulated" by antidepressant treatments,[8] but a study of suicide cases[20] and a small number of depressed cases[21] revealed no alteration in their binding. A recent autoradiographic study of β-receptors in drug-free cases of violent suicide revealed a qualitative increase in receptor density in cortex,[22] and this requires further evaluation. Muscarinic cholinergic receptors were increased in one study of suicide victims[20] but not in another[23] and not in a small group of depressives.[24] In this latter group of depressives, a reduction in α_1 adrenergic binding was noted in hippocampus, but not in occipital cortex, and α_2 receptors were unchanged.[21]

Serotonergic receptors have been classified on the basis of their pharmacological properties into 5-HT$_1$ and 5-HT$_2$ receptors.[25] Using ^{3}H-LSD as a ligand (which binds to both 5-HT$_1$ and 5-HT$_2$ receptors), Crow et al. reported no difference in serotonin receptor binding between depressed patients and controls either in hippocampus or frontal cortex.[21] In a group of suicide cases, Stanley and Mann (1983) demonstrated an increased binding of 5-HT$_2$ receptors.[26] However, this result was not replicated in a recent study of 20 suicide cases.[16] Differences in the clinical material and/or drug therapy of these cases may account for these differences. Most animal experiments suggest that 5-HT$_2$ receptor binding is decreased by antidepressant medication.[27] Similar controversy exists in the case of imipramine binding sites (probably 5-HT recognition sites)[28] in suicide and/or depression. Myerson et al. (1982) found an increase in these sites in a group of suicide cases,[20] whereas Cooper et al. (1985) reported no changes in similar material[16] and both Stanley et al. and Perry et al. reported a decrease in suicide and depressed cases respectively.[29,30]

γ-Aminobutyric acid (GABA) receptor binding has been reported as normal in depression[21] and in a group of suicide cases with a confirmed history of depression,[31] but these studies differed in their findings on benzodiazepine receptor binding. Crow *et al.* (1984) reported no change in ^{3}H-diazepam binding in frontal cortex,[21] but Cheetham *et al.* (1985) reported an increase in ^{3}H-flunitrazepam binding in the same area.[31] The different methods employed may account for this disparity which could also be explained by different drug histories of the groups studied.

Thus postmortem studies have failed to generate evidence of a consistent abnormality in depression and provide no direct support for any current neurochemical hypotheses of affective illness. There has been a reliance on using brains from suicide victims as material to investigate affective illness—a strategy with several drawbacks. Suicide cases are frequently poorly documented and the immediate precedents of the incident are often uncertain. Drug overdoses (sometimes preceded by variable drug intake) are common. If drugs are excluded as the cause of death (due to the possible influences of them on neurochemical measures), then violent causes of death become overrepresented. Such cases may be distinct in terms of personality and/or neurochemistry. Several studies have indicated that a relatively low proportion of suicide victims have had a *definite* depressive episode (40 and 15% respectively).[32,16] In a series of 100 consecutive suicides in one geographical area of Newcastle, United Kingdom, 33 had a psychiatric past history of whom only 20 had a clear-cut major depressive illness (RDC criteria—F. Hassanyeh, personal communication). On the other hand, depressed cases dying of natural causes do not often die in hospital and may therefore miss detection. Such patients with a history of affective disorders may be euthymic at death and it is an open question as to whether recovered depressives are likely to show any biochemical ("trait") changes. Patients with depression who die of natural causes are often old, and this raises the additional difficulty of associated neuropsychiatric and other physical conditions. The problems of diagnosis and of drug therapy may further confound the interpretation of postmortem neurochemical findings. Nevertheless in view of the substantial difficulties of using suicide cases as a method of investigating affective illness (outlined above), brains from documented depressed patients remain one of the best approaches.

A collection of brains from depressed patients dying in local hospitals has been under way in Newcastle for several years. Data from this group have been reported elsewhere[17,21,23,30]—the main findings included raised HVA, a reduction in α_1 receptors, and a decrease in imipramine binding in the hippocampus but the remaining metabolites and receptors were normal in this and other areas. The collection of brains from patients with affective disorder has since enlarged, and it was appropriate to repeat some of these measures selecting more clinically defined subgroups from the larger available cohort.

MATERIALS AND METHODS

Postmortem Material

Cases

An outline of the cases used is given in TABLE 1. Thirty patients dying whose case-note diagnosis included that of depression were considered for the study. Fourteen were excluded on a variety of grounds including the presence of other significant

TABLE 1. Clinical Characteristics of Cases Studied[a]

Group	No.	Sex	Age (years)	DSM III Diagnosis	Melancholia?	Psychotic?	Newcastle Score	Last Recorded Mental State	Antidepressants
Major affective disorder	9	5 F 4 M	75 ± 6	8 MDD (6 recurrent) 1 ? bipolar	8 definite 1 ?	3/9	6 (±3-+10)	mean 2 weeks 5 MDD 2 normal 2 uncertain	1 none 3 > 1/12 4 < 1/12 1 uncertain
Dysthymic disorder	7	6 F 1 M	81 ± 5	7 dysthymic disorder	0	0	0 (−1-+4)	mean 2 weeks 4 depressed mood 3 normal	2 none 3 > 1/12 1 < 1/12 1 uncertain
Controls	6	5 F 1 M	76 ± 6	no psychiatric disorder	—	—	—	—	none

[a] Means ± standard deviation. MDD = major depressive disorder.

psychiatric conditions (e.g., dementia, alcoholism, recent cerebrovascular accidents, and paranoid psychosis). Psychiatric case notes with adequate mental state examinations were available on the remaining 16 cases. Most cases died in hospital, and only in 1 case was there even a possibility of deliberate self-harm as a cause of death. In 14 of the 16 cases a detailed mental state was available within four weeks of death.

The criteria of the *Diagnostic and Statistical Manual* of the American Psychiatric Association (DSM III) were applied to the case notes. Eight of the cases were given a diagnosis of major depressive disorder (MDD) and one of bipolar disorder. In five of these cases the MDD was present within 4 weeks of death. In the three remaining cases the last episode of affective disturbance had occurred 8 weeks, 12 weeks, and four years previously. Seven cases were given a DSM III diagnosis of dysthymic disorder. Mental state assessment was available on all of these cases within 4 weeks of death. In four the mood was adjudged to be depressed but not of sufficient severity to classify a major depressive episode. The three remaining cases were considered to be euthymic in the period prior to death. Six control cases were included, all of whom had received a thorough clinical assessment revealing no history of psychiatric or neurological illness. A global assessment of cognitive functioning[33] (the 37-item mental test score) was available for most of the cases and was not in the range suggestive of dementia. Brains with significant neuropathological change of Alzheimer's disease were excluded.

Drugs

An outline of the antidepressant medication of these cases is given in TABLE 1. For the purposes of this analysis both monamine oxidase inhibitors and tricyclics were denoted as antidepressants. A substantial proportion of the patients either had never received antidepressants or had not received them for a month prior to death; and there were 4 such patients in the major affective disorder group. Seven of the 16 depressed patients had received neuroleptic drugs (usually in low doses) in the period prior to death, and most were taking them at the time of death.

ECT

Four of the patients in the major affective disorder groups and two of the patients in the dysthymic group had received ECT. No patient had received ECT in the month prior to death.

Brain Samples

Tissue samples were removed at autopsy as previously described[34] from Brodmann area 10 (frontal) of the cerebral cortex of the left hemisphere and stored at −70°C.

Delay between death and autopsy was similar in the groups studied. {Major affective disorder:- 28 ± 4 hours [mean ± standard error of the mean (SEM)], dysthymic disorder:- 30 ± 11 hours, controls:- 28 ± 9 hours}.

Neurochemical Techniques

Adrenergic Receptor Binding

Tissue homogenates were prepared as previously described.[35] Beta receptor binding was measured according to a modification of the method of Cash et al.[36] using ^{3}H-dihydroalprenolol (DHA) at a concentration of 2.5 nM. Nonspecific binding was defined as that displaced by 1 µM propranolol. Alpha receptor binding was measured using ^{3}H-prazosin at a concentration of 2 nM according to the method of Cash et al.[36] Nonspecific binding was defined as that displaced by 1 µM phentolamine. Alpha$_2$ receptor binding was measured by application of the method of Pimoule et al.[37] ^{3}H-RX781094 was used at a concentration of 4 nM, and nonspecific binding defined by 1 µM phentolamine. All of these assays were incubated at room temperature for 30 minutes and filtered using a cell harvester.[35]

Antidepressant Binding

Antidepressant binding was assessed using a modification of the method of Mellerup et al.[38] with ^{3}H-paroxetine at a final concentration of 1 nM and nonspecific binding defined with 10 µM imipramine. Incubation was at room temperature for two hours.

5-HT Receptor Subtype Binding

Tissue was homogenized in 10 volumes of 0.32 M sucrose which was centrifuged at 5000 rpm for 10 minutes and the pellet discarded (see Reference 39). The supernatant was centrifuged at 17,000 rpm for 10 minute and the pellet was resuspended in 10 volumes of tris-HCl (pH 7.7) and centrifuged for a further 10 minutes at 17,000 rpm. The pellet was resuspended in 40 volumes of buffer and stored at −40°C.

5-HT$_1$ receptors were measured by a modification of the method of Peroutka and Synder[27] using 2.0 nM ^{3}H-5-HT. Nonspecific binding was defined as that displaced by 10^{-6} M unlabeled 5-HT. 5-HT$_2$ receptor binding was measured by a modification of the method of Leysen et al.[40] ^{3}H-Ketanserin was used at a concentration of 2 nM, and nonspecific binding defined as that displaced by 10^{-6} M unlabeled ketanserin.

5-HIAA

5-HIAA was measured by high-performance liquid chromatography with electrochemical detection using a modification of the method of Kilts et al.[41]

Statistics

All assays were performed blindly and independently. Comparisons between groups were made using Students' t-test (two-tailed) or, where data were not normally distributed, by the Mann-Whitney U test (two-tailed).

RESULTS

Adrenergic Receptors

Results for α_1, α_2, and β receptor binding in the three groups studied are shown in TABLE 2. There was no significant difference between the groups on any of these measures. Alpha$_1$ receptors were nonsignificantly increased in the major affective disorder group (see TABLE 2) and this increase was more marked, but not significantly, in those five patients who had symptoms of MDD in the month before death [134 ± 4 compared to controls 111 ± 13 (fmol ligand bound, means $\pm$ SEM) $p < 0.1$]. There was no significant difference in α_1 receptor binding between those patients with MDD who had not received antidepressant drugs in the month before death (120 ± 10, $n=4$) compared with those who had (143 ± 18, $n=4$). Alpha$_2$ receptors were not significantly different in the groups studied (TABLE 2) or in those patients with recent MDD symptoms (126 ± 15) compared to controls (116 ± 21). There was a nonsignificant elevation in α_2 receptors in those MDD patients who had not received medication in the month before death (144 ± 13) compared to those MDD patients who had (109 ± 9). Beta receptors were unchanged, and no effect of recent medication or recent depression was apparent.

Antidepressant Binding

Results for paroxetine binding are shown in TABLE 3. No significant differences were noted. In those patients with MDD with no antidepressant medication in the last month ($n=4$) there was a nonsignificant decrease in paroxetine binding sites (69 ± 15) compared with controls (80 ± 11) but the decrement was due to a single patient with a low value.

TABLE 2. Adrenergic Receptors in Frontal Cortex in Depressed Subgroups and Controls[a]

Group	Number	α_1 Receptors (fmol ^{3}H-parazosin bound/mg protein)	α_2 Receptors (fmol ^{3}H-RX 781094 bound/mg protein)	β Receptors (fmol ^{3}H-DHA bound/mg protein)
Major affective disorder	9	130 ± 10	119 ± 11	85 ± 8
Dysthymic disorder	7	121 ± 12	130 ± 13	91 ± 9
Controls	6	111 ± 10	115 ± 8	86 ± 11

[a] Results expressed as means ± SEM. No significant differences.

TABLE 3. Serotonergic Receptors in Frontal Cortex in Depressed Subgroups and Controls[a]

Group	Number	5-HT$_1$ Receptors[b] (fmol ^{3}H-5-HT bound/mg protein)	5-HT$_2$ Receptors[b] (fmol ^{3}H-ket bound/mg protein)	Paroxetine Sites (fmol ^{3}H-parox bound/mg protein)
Major affective disorder	9	47 ± 15(7)	103 ± 19	75 ± 7
Dysthymic disorder	7	34 ± 7	68 ± 12	83 ± 8
Controls	6	31 ± 7	75 + 14	80 ± 9

[a] Results expressed as means ± SEM. Sample numbers in parentheses if different from group. No significant differences.
[b] I.G. McKeith, 1985.[39]

5-HT Receptor Subtypes

Results are shown in TABLE 3. No significant differences were noted although there was a nonsignificant tendency for 5-HT$_1$ and 5-HT$_2$ receptor binding to be higher in the major affective disorder group compared to both dysthymic disorder patients and controls. In the case of 5-HT$_2$ binding this trend was more marked if patients depressed in the immediate period prior to death were compared to controls (131 ± 19 cf. 96 ± 27) but this difference did not reach statistical significance. No effects of antidepressant medication were discernable.

5-HIAA

No significant differences were noted between the three clinical groups studied. There was a tendency for lower 5-HIAA levels in frontal cortex in those patients with major affective disorder [0.48 ± 0.09 fmoles/mg wet tissue (mean ± SEM)] and those with dysthymic disorders (0.47 ± 0.16) compared to controls (0.95 ± 0.27), but the variability was too large and the numbers too small for this to reach statistical significance. 5-HIAA was significantly lower ($p < 0.05$, Mann-Whitney U test) in those patients off drugs (for at least a month) at death (0.27 ± 0.07) compared to those on drugs at, or immediately prior to, death (0.65 ± 0.09) and to controls (FIGURE 1).

DISCUSSION

The results of postmortem studies designed to examine the neurochemistry of depression (outlined in the Introduction) have not provided consistent evidence to support any neurochemical hypothesis. It is conceivable that this may be related to the problems inherent in using suicide brains. However, the present study, in which only brains from patients with a definite depressive history were included, has provided only limited support for one of the currently held neurochemical theories of affective illness.

In the present study there was a trend toward significant increase in 5-HT$_2$ receptors and a decrease in 5-HIAA particularly in those patients with evidence of a major depressive episode in the month before death. There was a significant reduction in 5-HIAA in those patients who were not taking antidepressant drugs at death compared with those who were. Adrenergic receptors (α_1, α_2, and β) were unchanged as was antidepressant binding. More complex statistical analysis of these data is in progress, particularly to examine for the effects of age and postmortem delay.

The reduction in 5-HIAA noted in the patients not on medication in the present study is of considerable interest. Since 5-HIAA is the principal metabolite of 5-HT, its concentration is thought to reflect 5-HT turnover. Reduced 5-HIAA in suicide victims has been found in hindbrain in studies by Bourne et al.[42] and by Beskow et al.,[14] but in the latter case this result was thought to reflect a postmortem delay effect. Normal 5-HIAA concentrations in suicide brain have been found in other studies.[12,13]

Recently, Cooper et al. found a significant increase in 5-HIAA in hippocampus in suicide cases.[16] In a previous smaller study of depressed brains 5-HIAA was found to be normal in hippocampus.[17] Reduced 5-HIAA has been found in CSF in several[43,44] but not all[45] studies of depression and particularly in patients with suicidal intent.[46] There is clearly a need for larger postmortem studies of depressed cases and for 5-HIAA measurements in a wider range of brain areas.

The observation that 5-HIAA levels were higher in depressed patients taking antidepressant medication compared with drug-free cases merits further examination.

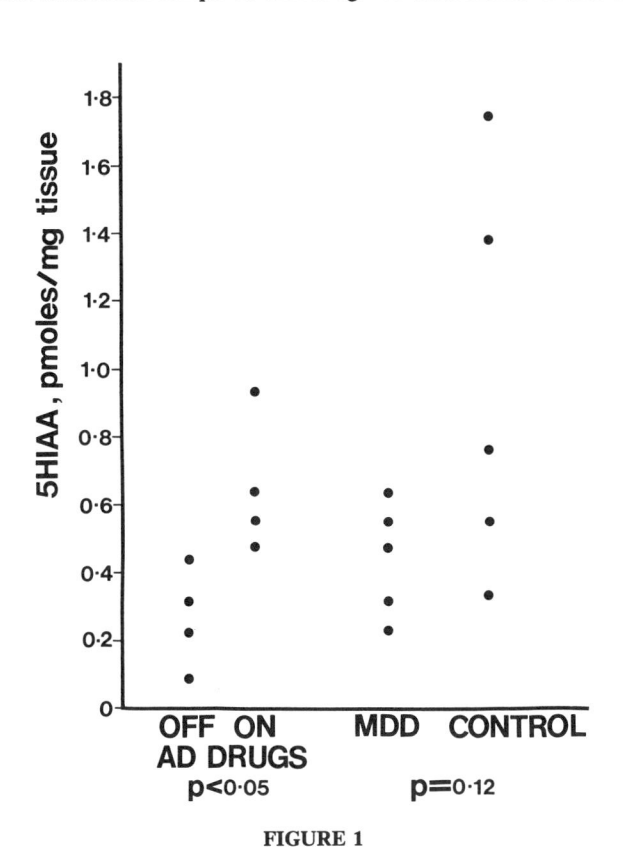

FIGURE 1

The effects of long-term antidepressant medication on 5-HIAA levels in rat brain are variable (see Charney et al. for review)[8] and, in man, it appears that antidepressant medication reduces CSF 5-HIAA[47] but the relationship of these findings to central 5-HIAA levels in man is unclear.

Previous studies on imipramine binding sites in suicide brains in frontal cortex have suggested both an increase[20] and a decrease.[29] A previous report from Newcastle suggested a decrease in these sites in depression in hippocampus.[30] In the present study, on a larger, more clinically defined population of depressives, no change in paroxetine sites was noted in frontal cortex. Paroxetine may be a more selective ligand for the putative 5-HT uptake site.[38] No change was noted in those patients with clear-cut major depressive episodes just prior to death, suggesting that changes in 5-HT uptake sites are unlikely to be of etiological significance for depression although further studies, including a reinvestigation of the hippocampus, are indicated.

Adrenergic receptors in frontal cortex were found to be unchanged in the present study, in disagreement with the decrease in α_1 receptors in hippocampus reported in depression by Crow et al.[21] The different area and/or different ligands employed in these studies may perhaps account for this disparity. The normality of α_2 receptors in depression in the present studies argues against their role in depression which has been suggested by neuroendocrine studies reporting a blunted growth hormone response to clonidine (an α_2 agonist) in depression.[10] A more extensive study of α_2 receptors including an examination of the hypothalamus and Scatchard analysis is indicated before finally ruling out this possibility. Beta receptors were unchanged in this study and no effect of antidepressant medication was seen, thus questioning the interesting possibility that an increase in receptor numbers underlies depression.

HVA measurements are not yet available from the brains of this series and will appear elsewhere.[39] Review of the patients' medication revealed that significant numbers had received neuroleptics prior to death—probably as nonspecific sedation for agitation. The finding of increased HVA in the hippocampus in a smaller number of these depressed brains[17] may therefore be a drug effect, since HVA rises when dopamine receptors are blocked.

In summary, this study provides tentative support for the serotonin deficit hypothesis of depression[6] with reduced 5-HIAA levels and a tendency for increased 5-HT$_2$ receptors perhaps as an adaptive response to decreased 5-HT turnover. It is suggested that suicide brains are not ideal material for investigating etiological theories of depression and brains from patients with a recent history of major depression are the best material. Such cases should be collected and more extensively studied perhaps on a multicenter basis. The negative aspects of this study should not preclude further studies using other methods and investigating other brain areas. Neuropeptide analyses may be worth conducting although initial studies from our group are unpromising[48,49] (and unpublished data, Perry et al.). The demonstration of serotonin receptors in the living brain has recently been reported,[50] and the application of this and similar scanning techniques to psychiatric disease such as depression may well be the best way to proceed.

ACKNOWLEDGMENTS

We wish to thank the psychiatrists and pathologists who helped in the collection of these brains, particularly Drs. Andrew Fairbairn and Gary Blessed. Our thanks are also due to the Medical Research Council, Professor James Edwardson, the Nuffield Foundation, and to Dr. E. Marshall, Mr. W. Kennedy, and Prof. Donald Eccleston.

REFERENCES

1. PLETSCHER, A., P. A. SHORE & B. B. BRODIE. 1956. Serotonin as a mediator of reserpine action in the brain. J. Pharmacol. **116:** 84-89.

2. HOLZBAUER, M. & M. VOGT. 1956. Depression by reserpine of the noradrenaline concentration in the hypothalamus of the cat. J. Neurochem. **1:** 8-11.
3. BERTLER, A. 1961. Effect of reserpine on the storage of catecholamines in brain and other tissues. Acta Physiol. Scand. **51:** 75-83.
4. FREISS, E. 1954. Mental depression in hypertensive patients treated for long periods with large doses of reserpine. N. Engl. J. Med. **251:** 1006-1008.
5. SCHILDKRAUT, J. J. & S. S. KELY. 1967. Biogenic amines and emotion. Science **156:** 21-30.
6. COPPEN, A. J. 1967. The biochemistry of affective disorders. Br. J. Psychiatry **113:** 1407-1411.
7. Medical Research Council, Brain Metabolism Unit. 1972. Modified amine hypothesis for the aetiology of affective illness. Lancet **ii:** 573-577.
8. CHARNEY, D. S., D. B. MENKES & G. R. HENINGER. 1981. Receptor sensitivity and the mechanism of action of antidepressant treatment—implications for the etiology and therapy of depression. Arch. Gen. Psychiatry **38:** 1160-1180.
9. JOHNSTONE, E. C. 1982. Affective disorder. *In* Disorder of Neurohumeral Transmission. T. J. Crow, Ed.: 255-286. Academic Press. London, England.
10. CHECKLEY, S. A. 1980. Neuroendocrine tests of monoamine function in man; a review of basic theory and the application to the study of depressive illness. Psychol. Med. **10:** 35-53.
11. SHAW, D. M., F. E. CAMPS & E. G. ECCLESTON. 1967. 5-Hydroxytryptamine in the hindbrain of depressive suicides. Br. J. Psychiatry **1113:** 1407-1411.
12. PARE, C. M. B., D. P. H. YEUNG, K. PRICE & R. S. STACEY. 1969. 5-Hydroxytryptamine, noradrenaline and dopamine in brainstem, hypothalamus and caudate nucleus of controls and of patients committing suicide by coal-gas poisoning. Lancet **11:** 133-135.
13. LLOYD, K. G., I. J. FARLEY, J. H. N. DECK & O. HORNYKIEWICZ. 1974. Serotonin and 5-hydroxindoleacetic acid in discrete areas of the brain stem of suicide victims and controls patients. Adv. Biochem. Psychopharmacol. **11:** 387-397.
14. BESKOW, J., C. G. GOTTFRIES, B. E. ROOS & B. WINBLAD. 1976. Determination of monoamines and monoamine metabolites in the human brain: post-mortem studies in a group of suicides and in a control group. Acta Psychiatr. Scand. **53:** 7-20.
15. COCHRAN, E., E. ROBINS & S. GROTE. 1976. Regional serotonin levels in brain: a comparison of depressive suicides and alcoholic suicides with controls. Biol. Psychiatry **3:** 283-294.
16. COOPER, S. J., F. OWEN, D. R. CHAMBERS, T. J. CROW, J. JOHNSTON & M. POULTER. 1986. Post-mortem neurochemical findings in suicide victims and depression: a study of the serotonergic system and imipramine binding in suicide victims. *In* The Biology of Depression. J. F. W. Deakin, Ed.: 53-71. Gaskell Press. Royal College of Psychiatrists. London, England.
17. CROSS, A. J., T. J. CROW, J. A. JOHNSON, E. K. PERRY, R. H. PERRY, G. BLESSED & B. E. TOMLINSON. 1983. Monoamine metabolism in senile dementia of Alzheimer type. J. Neurol. Sci. **60:** 383-392.
18. MOSES, S. G. & E. ROBINS. 1978. Regional distribution of norepinephrine and dopamine in brains of depressive suicides and alcoholic suicides. Psychopharmacol. Commun. **1:** 327-337.
19. RIEDERER, P., W. BIRKMAYER, D. SEEMAN & S. WINKFICH. 1980. 4-Hydroxy-3-methoxyphenylglycol as an index of brain noradrenaline turnover in endogenous depression. Acta Psychiatr. Scand. **61:** 251-257.
20. MEYERSON, L. R., L. P. WENNOGLE, M. S. ABEL, J. COUPET, A. S. LIPPA, C. E. RAUH & B. BEER. 1982. Human brain receptor alterations in suicide victims. Pharmacol. Biochem. Behav. **17:** 159-163.
21. CROW, T. J., A. J. CROSS, S. J. COOPER, J. R. W. DEAKIN, I. N. FERRIER, J. A. JOHNSON, M. H. JOSEPH, F. OWEN, M. POULTER, R. LOFTHOUSE, J. A N. CORSELLIS, D. R. CHAMBERS, G. BLESSED, E. K. PERRY, R H. PERRY & B. E. TOMLINSON. 1984. Neurotransmitter receptors and monoamine metabolites in the brains of patients with Alzheimer-type dementia and depression, and suicides. Neuropharmacology **23:** 1561-1569.
22. ZANKO, M. & A. BIEGON. 1983. Increased β-adrenoreceptor binding in frontal cortex of suicides. Soc. Neurosci. **9:** 210.5.

23. STANLEY, M. 1984. Cholinergic receptor binding in the frontal cortex of suicide victims. Am. J. Psychiatry **141**: 1432-1436.
24. PERRY, E. K. & R. H. PERRY. 1980. The cholinergic system in Alzheimer's disease. *In* Biochemistry of Dementia. P. J. Roberts, Ed.: 135-183. John Wiley. London, England.
25. PEROUTKA, S. J. & S. H. SYNDER. 1979. Multiple serotonin receptors: differential binding of ^{3}H-5 hydroxytryptamine, ^{3}H-lysergic acid diethylamide and ^{3}H-spiroperidol. Mol. Pharmacol. **16**: 687-699.
26. STANLEY, M. & J. J. MANN. 1983. Increased serotonin-2 binding sites in frontal cortex of suicide victims. Lancet **i**: 214-216.
27. PEROUTKA, S. J. & S. H. SYNDER. 1980. Long-term antidepressant treatment decreased spiroperidol-labelled serotonin receptor binding. Science **210**: 88-90.
28. SETTE, M., R. RAISMAN, M. BRILEY & S. Z. LANGER. 1981. Localisation of tricyclic antidepressant binding on serotonin nerve terminals. J. Neurochem. **37**: 40-42.
29. STANLEY, M., J. VIRGILLO & S. GERSHON. 1982. Tritiated imipramine binding sites are decreased in frontal cortex of suicides. Science **216**: 1337-1339.
30. PERRY, E. K., E. F. MARSHALL, G. BLESSED, B. E. TOMLINSON & R. H. PERRY. 1983. Decreased imipramine binding in the brains of patients with depressive illness. Br. J. Psychiatry **142**: 188-192.
31. CHEETHAM, S. C., M. R. CROMPTON, C. L. E. KATONA, R. W. HORTON, S. J. PARKER & G. P. REYNOLDS. 1985. GABA and benzodiazepine binding sites in the cortex of depressed suicide victims. Br. J. Pharmacol. **86**: 593P.
32. BARRACLOUGH, B., J. BUNCH, B. NELSON & P. SAINSBURY. 1974. A hundred cases of suicide: clinical aspects. Br. J. Psychiatry **125**: 355-373.
33. BLESSED, G., B. E. TOMLINSON & M. ROTH. 1968. The association between quantitative measures of dementia and of senile change in the cerebral grey matter of elderly subjects. Br. J. Psychiatry **114**: 797-811.
34. PERRY, E. K., M. CURTIS, D. J. DICK, J. M. CANDY, J. R. ATAK, C. A. BLOXHAM, G. BLESSED, A. FAIRBAIRN, B. E. TOMLINSON & R. H. PERRY. 1985. Cholinergic correlates of cognitive impairment in Parkinson's disease: comparisons with Alzheimer's disease. J. Neurol. Neurosurg. Psychiatry **48**: 413-421.
35. CROSS, A. J., T. J. CROW, I. N. FERRIER, J. A. JOHNSON, S. R. BLOOM & J. A. N. CORSELLIS. 1984. Serotonin receptor changes in dementia of the Alzheimer-type. J. Neurochem. **43**: 1574-1581.
36. CASH, R., R. RAISMAN, M. RUBERG & Y. AGID. 1985. Adrenergic receptors in frontal cortex in human brain. Eur. J. Pharmacol. **108**: 225-232.
37. PIMOULE, C., B. SCATTON & S. Z. LANDER. 1983. ^{3}H-RX1094: a new antagonist ligand labels α_2 adrenoreceptors in the rat brain cortex. Eur. J. Pharmacol. **95**: 79-85.
38. MELLERUP, E. T., P. PLENGE & M. ENGELSTOFT. 1983. High affinity binding of ^{3}H-imipramine and ^{3}H-paroxetine to human platelet membranes. Eur. J. Pharmacology **96**: 303-309.
39. MCKEITH, I. G. M.D. Thesis. University of Newcastle. Newcastle, United Kingdom. (In preparation.)
40. LEYSEN, J. E., C. J. E. NIEMEGEERS, J. M. VAN NUETEN & P. M. LADURON. 1982. ^{3}H-Ketanserin (R41 468) a selective ^{3}H ligand for serotonin (S$_2$) receptor binding sites: binding properties, brain distribution and functional role. Mol. Pharmacol. **21**: 301-314.
41. KILTS, C. D., G. R. BREESE & R. B. MAILMAN. 1981. Simultaneous quantification of dopamine, 5HT and four metabolically related compounds by means of reversed phase high performance liquid chromatography with electrochemical detection. J. Chromatogr. **225**: 347-357.
42. BOURNE, H. R., W. E. BUNNEY, R. W. COLBURN, J. M. DAVIS, J. N. DAVIS, D. M. SHAW & A. COPPEN. 1968. Noradrenaline, 5-hydroxytryptamine and 5-hydroxyindole acetic acid in hindbrains in suicidal patients. Lancet **ii**: 805-808.
43. ASHCROFT, G. W. & D. F. SHARMAN. 1960. 5-Hydroxyindoles in human cerebrospinal fluids. Nature **186**: 1050-1051.
44. ASBERG, M., L. BERTILSSON, B. MARTENSON, G-P. SCALIA-TOMBA, P. THOREN & L. TRASKMAN-BENDZ. 1984. CSF monoamine metabolites in melancholia. Acta Psychiatr. Scand. **69**: 201-219.
45. VESTERGAARD, P., T. SORENSEN, E. HOPPE, O. J. RAFELSON, C. M. YATES & N.

NICOLAOU. 1978. Biogenic amine metabolites in cerebrospinal fluid of patients with affective disorders. Acta Psychiatr. Scand. **58:** 88-96.
46. ASBERG, M., L. TRASKMAN & P. THOREN. 1976. 5HIAA in the cerebrospinal fluid: a biochemical suicide predictor. Arch. Gen. Psychiatry **33:** 1193-1197.
47. BOWERS, M. B. 1974. Amitriptyline in man: decreased formation of central 5-hydroxyindole acetic acid. Clin. Pharmacol. Ther. **15:** 90-92.
48. PERRY, R. H., G. J. DOCKRAY, R. DIMALINE, E. K. PERRY, G. BLESSED & B. E. TOMLINSON. 1981. Neuropeptides in Alzheimer's disease, depression and schizophrenia. A post-mortem analysis of vasoactive intestinal peptide and cholecystokinin in cerebral cortex. J. Neurol. Sci. **51:** 465-472.
49. BIGGINS, J. A., E. K. PERRY, J. R. MCDERMOTT, I. A. SMITH, R. H. PERRY & J. A. EDWARDSON. 1983. Post-mortem levels of thyrotrophin-releasing hormone and neurotensin in the amygdala in Alzheimer's disease, schizophrenia and depression. J. Neurol. Sci. **58:** 117-122.
50. WONG, D. F., H. N. WAGNER, N. F. DANNALS, J. M. LINKS, J. J. FROST, H. T. RAVERT, A. A. WILSON, A. E. ROSENBAUM, A. GJEDDE, K. H. DOUGLAS, J. D. PETRONIS, M. F. FOLSTEIN, J. K. T. TOUNG, D. BURNS & M. J. KUMAR. 1984. Effects of age on dopamine and serotonin receptors measured by positron tomography in the living human brain. Science **226:** 1393-1396.

Muscarinic Receptor Density in Skin Fibroblasts and Autopsied Brain Tissue in Affective Disorder[a]

J. CHRISTIAN GILLIN,[b] JOHN R. KELSOE, JR.,[b,c]
CHARLES A. KAUFMAN,[d] JOEL E. KLEINMAN,[d]
S. CRAIG RISCH,[b] AND DAVID S. JANOWSKY[b]

[b]*Department of Psychiatry (M003)*
University of California, San Diego
and San Diego Veterans Administration Medical Center
La Jolla, California 92093

[d]*Neuropsychiatry Branch*
Intramural Research Program
National Institute of Mental Health
St. Elizabeths Hospital
Washington, D.C. 20032

INTRODUCTION

In 1972, Janowsky *et al.* proposed the cholinergic-aminergic imbalance hypothesis of affective disorders.[1] According to this hypothesis, depression results from an increase in the ratio of central cholinergic to aminergic neurotransmission, whereas mania results from the opposite. The hypothesis was originally formulated largely on the basis of inferences of how therapeutic drugs alter mood. Most of the data that have been generated in subsequent years have been based upon pharmacological effects. The existing evidence is summarized extensively elsewhere.[2,3] At this point, it is sufficient to say that cholinomimetic agents (such as physostigmine and arecoline) have been reported to induce depressive-like mood changes in normals and to intensify these feelings in patients with depression. Furthermore, these drugs or ones with similar pharmacological effects can apparently reduce mania.

Likewise, attempts have been made to interpret known biological markers of depression in light of cholinergic-aminergic mechanisms. For example, short rapid eye movement (REM) sleep latency is a well-established state marker of moderate to severe depression.[4] Based upon both pharmacological and neurophysiological data that indicate that cholinergic neurotransmission induces and aminergic neurotransmission

---

[a]Supported by National Institute of Mental Health Grant MH 38738 and the Veterans Administration Medical Service.
[c]Present affiliation: Clinical Neuroscience Branch, Intramural Research Program, National Institute of Mental Health, Bethesda, Md. 20205.

delays REM sleep, it has been suggested that short REM latency could be consistent with the cholinergic-aminergic balance hypothesis.[5,6] For example, pretreatment with scopolamine induces sleep patterns in normal volunteers that are similar to those seen in depressives, i.e., short REM latency, elevated REM density, decreased total sleep time and sleep efficiency, and increased sleep latency.[7] These sleep alterations may result from up-regulated muscarinic receptors since prolonged treatment with scopolamine will increase muscarinic receptor density in rats.[8]

As Asnis et al. have shown, short REM latency is shorter in depressed patients with hypercortisolemia than those without hypercortisolemia.[9] This observation suggests that these two biological markers of depression—short REM latency and hypercortisolemia—may be associated or even caused by a common pathophysiological mechanism.

One of the commonly used tests of hypothalamic-pituitary-adrenal (HPA) activity is the dexamethasone suppression test (DST). An abnormal response of the DST has been shown to be another relatively sensitive if not entirely specific marker of some types of depression. DST "escape" is usually associated with short REM latency. It has been suggested that a cholinergic-aminergic balance may regulate secretion of CRF-ACTH-cortisol,[10,11] and that a pattern of "escape" on the DST reflects increased central cholinergic activity.[12,13]

TABLE 1. Estimated Muscarininc Receptor Density $(B_{max})^a$

	Suicides	Controls	Wilcoxon Two-Tailed
Cortex	185 ± 81	170 ± 66	$T = 20$, p > 0.05
Hypothalamus	122 ± 46	187 ± 99	$T = 14$, p > 0.05
Pons	77 ± 33	78 ± 56	$T = 17$, p > 0.05

[a] Results are in fmol/mg protein.

In addition, Risch et al. have pioneered a series of studies that indicate that depressed patients respond more vigorously to cholinomimetic agonists than do other psychiatric patients or controls.[14] For example, they show greater secretion of ACTH and prolactin, more vomiting, greater change in cardiovascular response, and more depressive-like mood changes to physostigmine.

In an attempt to establish cholinergic trait as well as cholinergic state markers for affective disorders, Sitaram et al. reported that bipolar patients both in remission and while ill entered REM sleep more rapidly following an intravenous infusion of arecoline during non-REM sleep than did controls [the so-called cholinergic REM induction test (CRIT)].[15] Recently, Sitaram et al. (presented at the Fourth International Congress of Biological Psychiatry, Philadelphia, September 1985) have presented preliminary evidence indicating that a "hypersensitive response" on the CRIT segregated within families in individuals with endogenous depression. Family members with endogenous depression were more likely to respond than those without affective illness. In addition, Sitaram and his colleagues reported that a rapid response differentiated primary major disorder, endogenous subtype, from primary anxiety disorder.[16]

Thus, there is considerable evidence in favor of the cholinergic-aminergic imbalance hypothesis, but most of it is indirect and inferential. Little evidence has been found that directly implicates abnormalities of the cholinergic or aminergic nervous systems in affective disorders. The fact that depressive mood can be induced by physostigmine in normals does not prove, of course, that clinical depression in patients results from cholinergic mechanisms. Likewise, the fact that REM latency can be shortened or cortisol secretion elevated in normals by cholinomimetic agonists does not prove that short REM latency and hypercortisolemia in depression are caused by overactivity of central cholinergic pathways.

This chapter relates our attempts to replicate two previously reported findings indicating an increased density of muscarinic receptors in patients with affective disorders, the first in brains of suicide victims,[17] the second in skin fibroblasts of patients with affective disorders.[18]

MUSCARINIC RECEPTOR BINDING IN BRAIN TISSUE FROM SUICIDES

In an attempt to measure muscarinic receptor density directly in the brains of patients with affective disorders, we obtained brain tissue from autopsied individuals who had committed suicide.[19] They were matched with nonsuicide controls for age, sex, postmortem interval (time from death until autopsy), and freezer time (time from autopsy to assay). Frontal cortex was compared in 10 pairs, hypothalamic tissue in 10 pairs, and pons in 8 pairs. Assays were performed blind.

Further details are provided in Kaufman et al.[19] Briefly, muscarinic receptor binding was performed according to the method of Snyder et al.[20] Two sets of triplicate tubes were incubated with ^{3}H-quinuclidinyl benzilate (QNB) (100 μl at 0.01-1.0 nM), one with atropine sulfate (100 μl 10^{-5}M). Binding was found to be saturable.

The results (see TABLE 1) showed no significant differences between suicides and controls in estimated number of muscarinic receptor binding. Estimates of receptor affinity (K_d) were also no different between suicides and controls for any of the three brain areas.

These results failed to replicate the previous report of Meyerson et al., who reported a 47% increase in muscarinic receptor density in cortex, with no change in receptor affinity, from suicides compared with homicide controls.[17]

The limitations of research in suicide victims should not be overlooked. The preexisting diagnoses of the subjects can be neither assumed nor verified through direct observation by the investigator. Only about 53% of suicides meet diagnostic criteria for major depression and only about 11% meet criteria for bipolar illness.[21] Uncertainty about the validity of the measurements will also remain for many reasons, such as cause and circumstances of death, influence of drugs or other treatments, confounding effects of other illnesses, differing methods of obtaining, handling, and storing tissues, and so forth.

IS THERE A MUSCARINIC RECEPTOR ON CULTURED SKIN FIBROBLASTS?

Cultured skin fibroblasts have been used as models of neuronal function in a variety of genetic neuropsychiatric illnesses. This peripheral tissue can be easily obtained through skin biopsy and cultured for up to six months or 20 generations. The cultured fibroblast manifests a number of characteristics similar to neurons, making it appealing as a possible peripheral model of neuronal function.[22-28] The fibroblast is cultured in a standardized environment, isolated from hormonal, dietary, drug, or other influences; abnormalities are, therefore, more likely to reflect genetic effects. For this reason, the cultured fibroblast is particularly useful in exploring generalized genetic trait markers.

Nadi *et al.* reported evidence for functional muscarinic receptors on cultured human adult skin fibroblasts.[18] Specific, high-affinity [^{3}H]-quinuclidinyl benzilate ([^{3}H]-QND) binding was displaced by several cholinergic drugs with relative affinities similar to those found in brain. Receptor up regulation occurred after atropine pretreatment, and adenylate cyclase was inhibited by several cholinergic agonists. Nadi *et al.* then applied the cultured fibroblast as a clinical cholinergic model and found an increased B_{max} for [^{3}H]-QNB in fibroblasts from patients with familial affective disorder.

We have attempted to replicate the findings of Nadi *et al.* regarding the presence of functional muscarinic receptors on cultured adult skin fibroblasts as well as the elevated receptor number in affective disorder.[29-31] Our initial experiments with [^{3}H]-QNB resulted in nonspecific binding eight times higher than specific binding at 800 pM, making meaningful Scatchard analysis impossible. As intracellular trapping of unbound [^{3}H]-QNB seemed a likely explanation for the high nonspecific binding, we undertook studies using another radioligand, [^{3}H]-N-methyl scopolamine ([^{3}H]-NMS). [^{3}H]-NMS has a much lower lipid solubility than [^{3}H]-QNB and is, therefore, less able to penetrate intact cells. As predicted, [^{3}H]-NMS reduced nonspecific binding nearly 100-fold, making meaningful Scatchard analysis possible in some, but not all, cell lines. Furthermore, even cell lines manifesting specific binding had B_{max} considerably lower than those reported by Nadi *et al.* for [^{3}H]-QNB.

In cell lines manifesting specific binding, [^{3}H]-NMS was displaced by the agonists arecoline and carbachol and the antagonists atropine and NMS, with relative affinities (atropine, NMS, arecoline, carbachol) similar to those seen in rat brain.[32] The nonmuscarinic drugs nicotine, hexamethonium, *d*-tubo cararine, *l*-propranolol, and serotonin showed no significant displacement of [^{3}H]-NMS at 10 μM.

These binding data suggest the presence of muscarinic receptors on some lines of cultured adult skin fibroblasts. Evidence of functional muscarinic response would confirm this. For this reason, we studied the response to carbachol of three biochemical processes known to be coupled to muscarinic receptors: inhibition of adenylate cyclase, stimulation of guanylate cycase, and stimulation of phosphoinositide hydrolysis. No significant functional response was found in any of five cell lines studied. Of note, some of the cell lines in each of these three experiments had shown high [^{3}H]-NMS specific binding. In summary, despite the binding data, we could find no functional evidence for the existence of muscarinic receptors.

Despite questions regarding its physiological significance, we have examined B_{max} for [^{3}H]-NMS in patients with affective disorder (16 unipolar, 14 bipolar) and 8 normal controls. No significant differences were found between normal controls and either bipolar or unipolar affective patients by parametric or nonparametric methods.

The question remains whether there really are receptors on cultured adult skin fibroblasts. Despite lack of functionality, the pharmacological specificity found in our displacement experiments argues for the presence of muscarinic receptors. If nonfunctional receptors are present, they may have been functional at one time but have become uncoupled from their effector mechanisms. Despite every effort to replicate the procedures of Nadi *et al.*, it remains possible that differences in culture or assay procedure could produce the observed differences in binding and function. Further basic and clinical studies are required to fully assess the utility of this proposed model.

Our difficulty in reliably measuring muscarinic receptors on adult skin fibroblasts has also been confirmed by other groups.[33] Indeed, Nadi and her associates have not been able to reproduce their original findings.[34]

DISCUSSION

Neither of these attempts to measure muscarinic receptors was successful in differentiating patients from controls. The problems in measuring muscarinic receptors on adult skin fibroblasts proved to be formidable. Most cells showed virtually no receptors and those that did, did so by binding characteristics rather than functional responses. In any case, no differences were found between patients and controls. These data, together with those of other groups, indicate that the adult skin fibroblast is not an appropriate model in which to draw inferences about central muscarinic receptor function and density at this time.

The failure to differentiate patients from controls by brain tissue measures could be interpreted as a blow to the cholinergic supersensitivity hypotheses of affective disorder, but it would be inappropriate to regard this finding as the final answer to these issues. First, the problems of autopsy studies have been alluded to already. Second, if affective disorder results from an imbalance between cholinergic-aminergic systems, measures of muscarinic receptor density could be irrelevant. These problems have been discussed elsewhere.[2-4] Third, neither the skin fibroblast nor the areas of the brain studied in this report are necessarily the correct locations to test these hypotheses.

If the arguments in favor of the cholinergic-aminergic imbalance hypothesis, outlined in the Introduction, are still valid, then further research on cholinergic mechanisms in affective disorder is still important and appropriate. The question is which research strategy to take at this time.

REFERENCES

1. JANOWSKY, D. S., M. K. EL-YOUSEF, J. M. DAVIS & H. J. SEKERKE. 1972. A cholinergic-adrenergic hypothesis of mania and depression. Lancet i: 632.
2. JANOWSKY, D. S., S. G. RISCH & J. C. GILLIN. 1983. Adrenergic-cholinergic balance and the treatment of affective disorders. Prog. Neuropsychopharmacol. Biol. Psychiatry 7: 297-307.
3. GILLIN, J. C., W. B. MENDELSON & N. SITARAM. 1982. Acetylcholine, sleep, and depression. Hum. Neurobiol. 11: 211-219.
4. GILLIN, J. C. & A. A. BORBELY. 1985. Sleep: a neurobiological window on affective disorders. Trends Neurosci. 8: 537-542.
5. SITARAM, N., J. I. NURNBERGER, E. S. GERSHON & J. C. GILLIN. 1983. Cholinergic regulation of mood and REM sleep: potential model and marker of vulnerability to affective disorder. Am. J. Psychiatry 139: 571.
6. MCCARLEY, R. 1982. REM sleep and depression: common neurobiological control mechanisms. Am. J. Psychiatry 139: 565-570.
7. GILLIN, J. C., N. SITARAM & W. C. DUNCAN. 1979. Muscarinic supersensitivity: a possible model for the sleep disturbance of primary depression? Psychiatry Res. 1: 17-22.
8. MAJOCHA, R. & R. J. BALDESSARINI. 1980. Increased muscarinic receptor binding in rat forebrain after scopolamine. Eur. J. Pharmacol. 67: 327-328.

9. ASNIS, G., U. HALBREICH, E. J. SACKAR, R. S. NATHAN, L. C. OSTROW, H. NOVACENKO, M. DAVIS, J. ENDICOTT & PUIG-ANTICH. 1983. Plasma cortisol secretion and REM period latency in adult endogenous depression. Am. J. Psychiatry 140: 750-753.
10. RISCH, S. C., N. KALIN, D. S. JANOWSKY, R. M. COHN, D. PICKAR & D. L. MURPHY. 1983. Co-release of ACTH and beta-endorphin immunoreactivity in human subjects in response to central cholinergic stimulation. Science 222: 77.
11. RISCH, S. C., D. S. JANOWSKY, J. C. GILLIN, J. L. RAUSCH, B. L. LOEVINGER & L. Y. HUEY. 1983. Muscarinic supersensitivity of anterior pituitary ACTH release in major depressive illness, adrenal cortical dissociation. Psychopharmacol. Bull. 19: 343-346.
12. RISCH, S. C., D. S. JANOWSKY & J. C. GILLIN. 1983. Muscarinic supersensitivity of anterior pituitary ACTH and beta-endorphin release in major depressive illness. Peptides 4: 789-792.
13. CARROLL, B. J., J. F. GREDEN, R. HASKETT, M. FEINBERG, A. A. ALBALA, F. I. MARTIN, R. T. RUBIN, B. HEATH, P. T. SHART & W. L. MCLEOD. 1979. Neurotransmitter studies of neuroendocrine pathology in depression. Acta Psychiatr. Scand. 280(Suppl. 1): 183.
14. RISCH, S. C., N. H. KALIN & D. S. JANOWSKY. 1981. Cholinergic challenges in affective illness: behavioral and neuroendocrine correlates. J. Clin. Pharmacol. 1: 186.
15. SITARAM, N., J. I. NURNBERGER, E. S. GERSON & J. C. GILLIN. 1982. Cholinergic regulation of mood and REM sleep: potential model and marker of vulnerability to affective disorder. Am. J. Psychiatry 139: 571.
16. JONES, D., S. KELWOLA, J. BELL, E. JACKSON & N. SITARAM. 1985. Cholinergic REM sleep induction response correlation with endogenous major depression subtype. Psychiatry Res. 14: 99-110.
17. MEYERSON, L. R., L. P. WONOGLE, M. S. ABEL, J. COUPET, L. S. LIPPA, E. C. RAUH & B. BEER. 1982. Human brain receptor alterations in suicide victims. Pharmacol. Biochem. Behav. 17: 159.
18. NADI, N. S., J. I. NURNBERGER & E. S. GERSHON. 1984. Muscarinic cholinergic receptors on skin fibroblasts in familial affective disorder. N. Engl. J. Med. 311: 225-230.
19. KAUFMAN, C. A., J. C. GILLIN, B. HILL, T. O'LAUGHLIN, I. PHILLIPS, J. E. KLEINMAN & R. J. WYATT. 1984. Muscarinic binding in suicides. Psychiatry Res. 12: 47-55.
20. SNYDER, S. H., K. J. CHANG, M. J. KUHAR & H. I. YAMAMURA. 1975. Biochemical identification of the mammalian muscarinic cholinergic receptor. Fed. Proc. 34: 1915.
21. BARRACLOUGH, B., J. BUNCH, B. NELSON & P. SAINSBURY. 1974. A hundred cases of suicide: clinical aspects. Br. J. Psychiatry 125: 355.
22. HASLAM, R. J. & S. GOLDSTEIN. 1974. Adenosine 3':5'-cyclic monophosphate in young and senescent human fibroblasts during growth and stationary phase in vitro. Biochem. J. 144: 253-263.
23. GRAY, P. N. & S. L. DANA. 1978. GABA synthesis by cultured fibroblasts obtained from persons with Huntington's disease. J. Neurochem. 33: 985-992.
24. SCHWARTZ, J. P. & X. O. BREAKEFIELD. 1980. Altered nerve growth factor in fibroblasts from patients with familial dysautonomia. Proc. Nat. Acad. Sci. USA 77: 1154-1158.
25. RIKER, D. K., R. M. ROTH & X. O. BREAKEFIELD. 1981. High affinity [^{3}H]-choline accumulation in cultured human skin fibroblasts. J. Neurochem. 36: 746-752.
26. MUNSON, R., B. WESTERMARK & L. BLASER. 1979. Tetrodotoxin-sensitive sodium channels in normal human fibroblasts and normal glia-like cells. Proc. Nat. Acad. Sci. USA 76: 6425-6429.
27. EDELSTEIN, S. B., C. M. CASTIGLIONE & X. O. BREAKEFIELD. 1978. Monoamine oxidase activity in normal and Lesch-Nyhan fibroblasts. J. Neurochem. 31: 1247-1254.
28. GROSHONG, R., R. J. BALDESSARINI, A. GIBSON, J. F. LIPINSKI, D. AXELROD & A. POPE. 1978. Activities of types A & B MAO and COMT in blood cells and skin fibroblasts or normal and chronic schizophrenic subjects. Arch. Gen. Psychiatry 35: 1198-1204.
29. KELSOE, J., JR., J. C. GILLIN, D. S. JANOWSKY, J. H. BROWN, S. C. RISCH & B. LUMKIN. 1985. Muscarinic receptor binding on human skin fibroblasts. N. Engl. J. Med. 312: 861-862.
30. KELSOE, J. R., JR., J. C. GILLIN, D. S. JANOWSKY, J. H. BROWN, S. C. RISCH & B. LUMKIN. 1986. Specific 3H-N Methylscopolamine binding without cholinergic function in cultured skin fibroblasts. Life Sci. 38(15): 1399-1408.

31. KELSOE, J. R., JR., J. C. GILLIN, D. DARKO, H. H. KALIR, S. C. RISCH & D. S. JANOWSKY. Muscarinic receptor binding in cultured skin fibroblasts from patients with affective disorders. (Submitted.)
32. YAMAMURA, H. I. & S. H. SNYDER. 1974. Muscarinic cholinergic binding in rat brain. Proc. Nat. Acad. Sci. USA **71:** 1725-1729.
33. LENOX, R. H., R. J. HITZEMANN, E. RICHELSON & J. R. KELSOE, JR. 1985. Failure to confirm muscarinic receptors on skin fibroblasts. N. Engl. J. Med. **312:** 861.
34. GERSHON, E. S., N. S. NADI, J. I. NURNBERGER, JR. & W. B. BERRETTINI. 1985. N. Engl. J. Med. **31:** 862. (Letter.)

The Serotonin Hypothesis of (Auto)Aggression

Critical Appraisal of the Evidence

H. M. VAN PRAAG, R. PLUTCHIK, AND H. CONTE

Department of Psychiatry
Albert Einstein College of Medicine
Montefiore Medical Center
1300 Morris Park Avenue
Bronx, New York 10461

DATA ON WHICH THE HYPOTHESIS IS BASED

The major biochemical abnormalities reported to be correlated with suicidal behavior are lowered concentration of 5-hydroxyindoleacetic acid (5-HIAA)—the major degradation product of serotonin (5-hydroxytryptamine, 5-HT)—in cerebrospinal fluid (CSF); increased secretion of cortisol; diminished cortisol suppression after dexamethasone; and blunted response of thyroid-stimulating hormone (TSH) after thyrotropin-releasing hormone (TRH). Most extensively studied is CSF 5-HIAA, and we will restrict our discourse to that variable. For a comprehensive review of the biology of suicide, we refer to another paper.[42]

Low CSF 5-HIAA has primarily been reported in depression by several though not all investigators (FIGURE 1). The likelihood of this finding was found to be greater in major depression than in other depression types; greater in the melancholic type than in other forms of major depression; greater in severe than in less severe melancholic depression; and greater in delusional than in nondelusional major depression. Probenecid studies have been more consistent than those measuring only baseline concentration. However the group that studied baseline 5-HIAA most extensively and carefully[5] has repeatedly reported the baseline 5-HIAA value to be decreased (FIGURE 2). The pertinent literature has been reviewed elsewhere.[13,45,64] Several authors reported low CSF 5-HIAA to persist after remission, at least in a substantial number of the patients, suggesting the state-character of this variable.[38,48,49]

5-HIAA in CSF is correlated to metabolism of 5-HT in the central nervous system (CNS).[28] Probenecid blocks the efflux of 5-HIAA from the CNS including CSF, and the accumulation of 5-HIAA in CSF after probenecid provides information on CNS 5-HT degradation. Low CSF baseline and postprobenecid 5-HIAA indicates decreased 5-HT metabolism.[48,49] This decrease could be a primary phenomenon, and related to diminished serotonergic activity[23,50] or, alternatively, a phenomenon secondary to a hyperactive serotonergic system, due to, say, hypersensitive postsynaptic receptors.[4] Which of the two hypotheses is the more plausible is still debated.

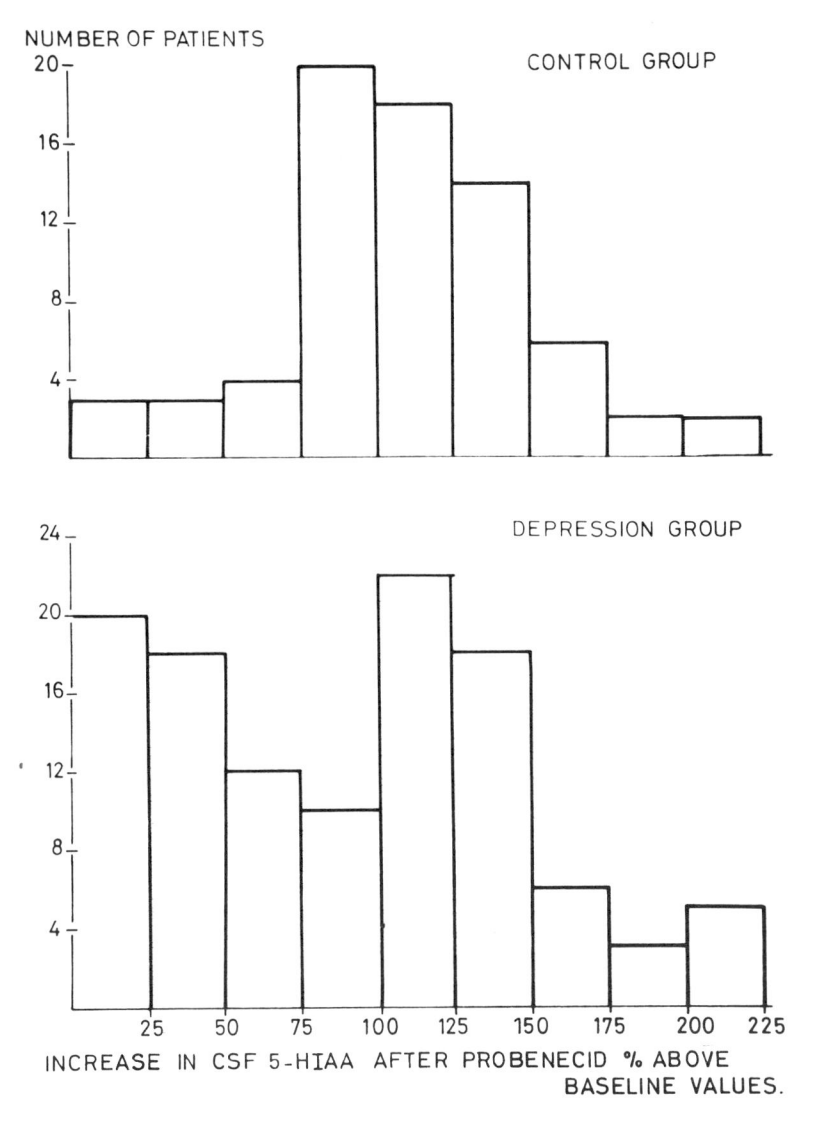

FIGURE 1. Increase of CSF 5-HIAA concentration after probenecid in patients suffering from melancholic major depression and in a nondepressed control group. The columns indicate the number of patients showing the increase in concentration given at the bottom of the column. (Reproduced from Reference 47 with permission from *Lancet.*)

Initially no psychopathological differences were demonstrated between depressed patients with and without lowered CSF 5-HIAA, apart from possibly higher anxiety ratings in the former group.[8] In 1976 Asberg et al. reported that low CSF 5-HIAA occurred preferentially in depressed patients who had attempted suicide before admission (FIGURE 3).[6] The correlation was strongest in the group that had made attempts with violent means (FIGURE 4).[39] Most studies, but not all,[37,57] confirmed the relationship between suicidal behavior and lowering of CSF 5-HIAA.[1,2,7,8,30,34,46,47] We confirmed the relation of low CSF 5-HIAA and attempted suicide, but found the correlation however to apply equally to violent and nonviolent attempters.[46,47] Van Praag measured postprobenecid 5-HIAA levels,[46,47] all others studied baseline values. In no study was the factor anxiety/distress analyzed separately as to its possible relation to lowered 5-HIAA levels.

Subsequent to the first report of Asberg et al.,[6] several groups claimed CSF 5-HIAA also to be lowered in patients admitted for suicide attempt, who after admission could not be diagnosed as being either depressed or psychotic (FIGURE 5).[7,11,12,34,39]

The correlation between low CSF 5-HIAA and suicidal behavior (particularly if attempts had been committed with violent means) both in depressed patients and in so-called nondepressed and nonpsychotic suicide attempters prompted the hypothesis

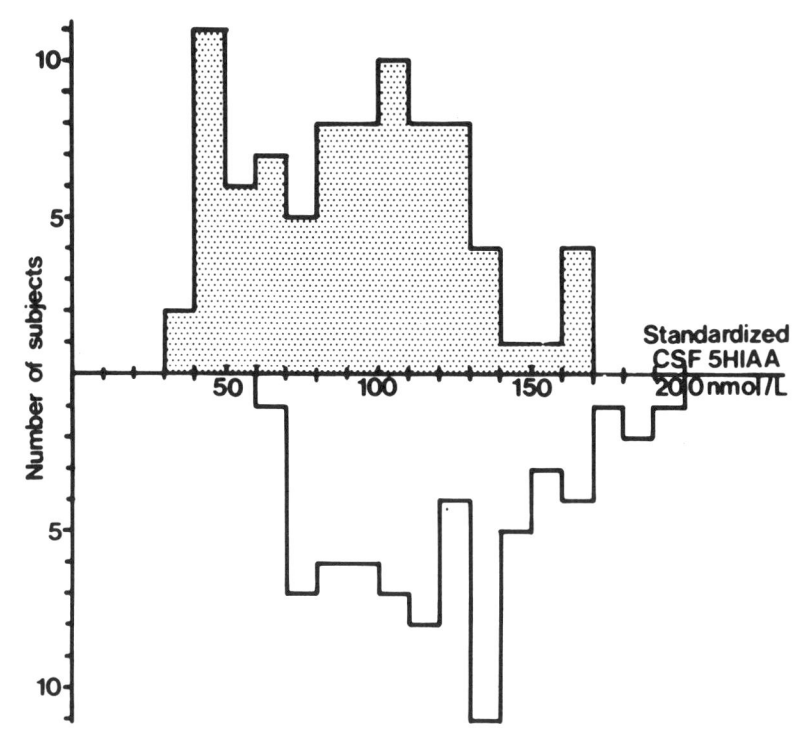

FIGURE 2. Frequency distributions of CSF 5-HIAA in patients with melancholia (upward) and healthy volunteer control subjects (downward). Because of the dependence of metabolite concentrations on sex, age, and body height of the subjects, the levels are not directly comparable between the two groups of subjects (controls are younger and taller than the patients and more often male). All values have therefore been standardized to common age (45 years), body weight (170 cm), and unit sex (female) by means of the multiple-regression equation. (Reproduced from Reference 5 with permission from *Acta Psychiatrica Scandinavica*.)

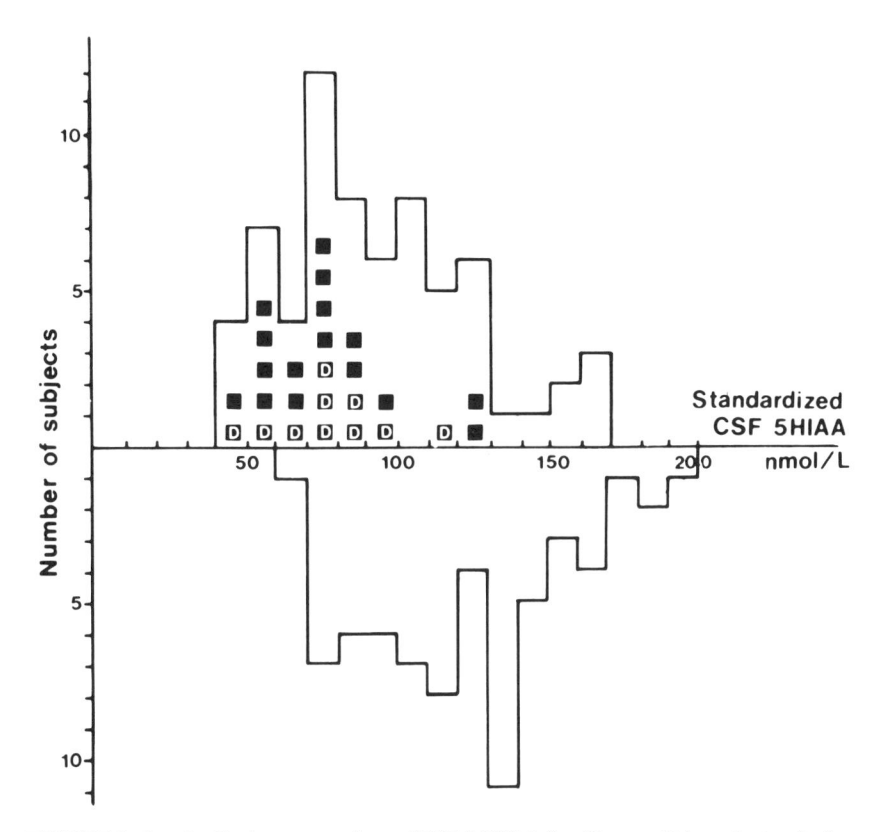

FIGURE 3. Standardized concentrations of CSF 5-HIAA (see FIGURE 2) in patients who have attempted suicide (upward) and healthy volunteer control subjects (downward). The squares indicate suicide attempts by a violent method (any method other than a drug overdose, taken by mouth, or a single wrist cut). D indicates a subject who subsequently died from suicide, in all cases but one within one year after the lumbar puncture. (Reproduced from Reference 5 with permission from *Acta Psychiatrica Scandinavica*.)

that lowered CSF 5-HIAA relates to disordered aggression rather than to disordered mood as had been assumed until then. Do the available data warrant the inference? They do not, we think, and our considerations will be discussed in the next section.

OBJECTIONS AGAINST LINKAGE OF LOW CSF 5-HIAA WITH (AUTO)AGGRESSION

Suicide Method and Type of Depression

The first objection we want to raise is that the incidence of suicide attempt with violent means is not the same in various depression types. Violent suicide attempt

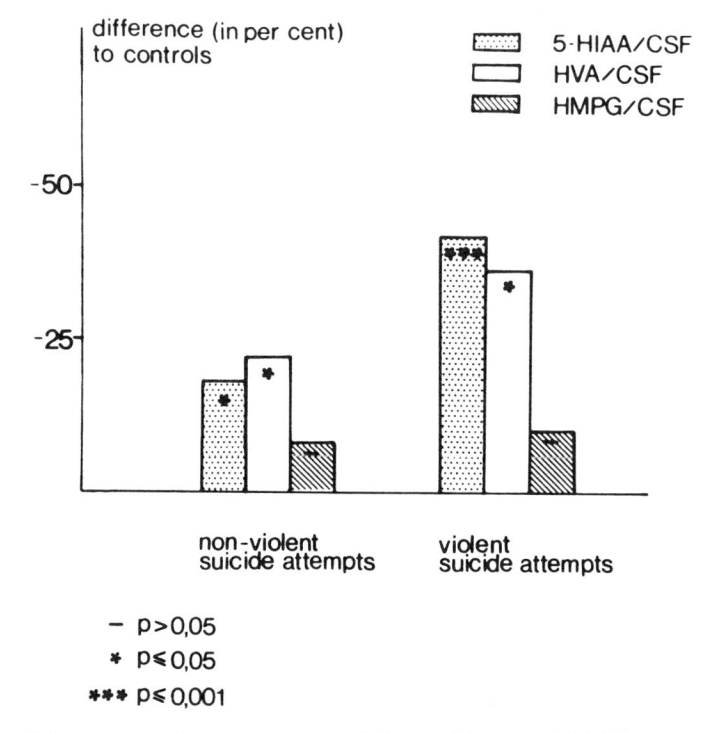

FIGURE 4. Differences in CSF monoamine levels (adjusted for age and height) between controls and violent and nonviolent suicide attempters. Symbols indicate significance levels of differences from mean of controls at following levels: minus sign, p > 0.05; asterisk, p ≤ 0.05; and three asterisks, p ≤ 0.001. 5-HIAA indicates 5-hydroxyindoleacetic acid; HVA, homovanillic acid; and MHPG, 3-methoxy-4-hydroxyphenyl glycol. (Reproduced from Reference 39 with permission from the *Archives of General Psychiatry*.)

occurs more frequently in major depression, melancholic type [*Diagnostic and Statistical Manual*, third edition (DSM III)], than in other forms of depression. Consequently it is impossible to decide whether low CSF 5-HIAA in violent suicide attempt relates to (auto)aggression or to that type of depression in which the risk of violent suicide attempt happens to be increased.

We based this conclusion on a study of suicide method in different types of depression.[55] Two groups of patients were compared. The first group consisted of 31 patients consecutively admitted to a psychiatric ward, in connection with a violent suicide attempt and a nonpsychotic depressive order. The second group consisted of 31 patients admitted during the same period, in connection with a nonviolent suicide attempt, likewise in the context of a (nonpsychotic) depressive disorder. These patients were matched in pairs for age and sex with those of the first group.

As usual in biological suicide research today, the classification of the suicide attempt as violent or nonviolent was based on the method used.[35] Drug overdose and superficial wrist cutting are classified as nonviolent, all other methods as violent. Psychopathological data were collected with a standard interview.[56] DSM III criteria were used to establish the diagnosis. Severity of depression was rated on a global five-point scale, independent of syndromal diagnosis.

When we compared the violent and nonviolent suicide group in terms of syndromal depression diagnosis, it was found that the diagnosis melancholic major depression had been made in 84% of cases in the violent group, and only in 43% of cases in the nonviolent group—a significant difference ($\chi^2 = 11.68$, $p < 0.001$) (TABLE 1).

The possibility exists that the increased frequency of melancholic depression in violent suicide attempters is due to greater severity of symptoms in melancholic depression; that, in other words, violent suicide attempt is related to depression severity rather than to depression type. To test this hypothesis we compared mean depression scores of patients with melancholic depression and patients with other types of depression. The severity level turned out to be the same (TABLE 2).

We concluded (1) that type of depressive syndrome is an important factor determining degree of violence manifested in suicidal behavior and (2) that it is impossible to decide whether the biological abnormalities found in depressed, violent suicide attempters relate to autoaggressive impulses or to the melancholic syndrome as such.

The Diagnosis Nondepressed Suicide Attempter

Our second objection is that the diagnosis nondepressive suicide attempter cannot be made after the attempt, but can only be based on presuicidal data. This statement

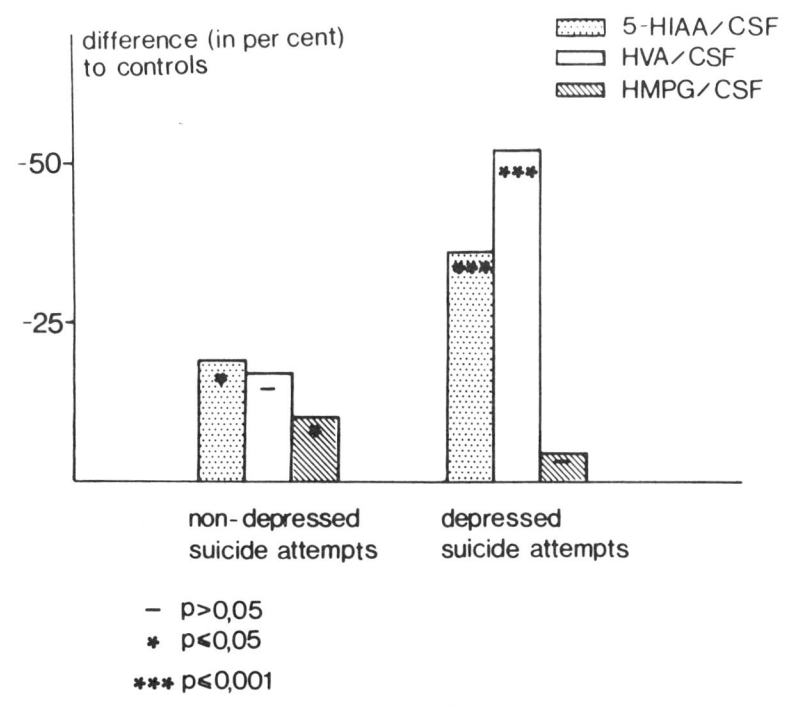

FIGURE 5. Differences in CSF monoamine levels (adjusted for age and height) between controls and depressed and nondepressed suicide attempters. Symbols and abbreviations are explained in FIGURE 4. (Reproduced from Reference 39 with permission from the *Archives of General Psychiatry*.)

TABLE 1. Syndromal Depression Diagnosis in 31 Depressed Patients Who Committed Violent Suicide Attempts and in 31 Depressed Patients Who Had Committed Nonviolent Suicide Attempts[a]

	Number	Diagnosis Major Depression (melancholic type)	Other Depression Types
Violent suicide attempt	31	26	5
Nonviolent suicide attempt	31	13	18

[a] Melancholic major depressions were found significantly more frequently in violent suicide attempters ($\chi^2 = 11.68$, $p < 0.001$). (Reproduced from Reference 55 with permission from *Psychiatry Research*.)

is based on two observations. First, in hospitalized suicide attempters, presuicidal depression is very common. Second, a substantial drop in depression rating occurs after the attempt as compared to the mood state prior to the attempt.

In the first study we explored the occurrence of depression in the two months prior to the suicide attempt in 100 consecutive suicide attempters admitted to a psychiatric unit. The diagnosis of depression prior to suicide attempt was based on self-reports of patients obtained with a standard interview. The diagnosis of presuicidal depression was made if the patients in the preceding two months had felt depressed continuously or frequently; if work performance, lust for life, and sleep quality had suffered considerably; and if the patient had felt to be in need of professional help: 82/100 of suicide attempters satisfied criteria for depression. In 24/82, melancholic depression was diagnosed; in the remaining 58, other depressive syndromes.[46,47]

We concluded that in a vast majority of admitted suicide attempters depression had occurred in the two months prior to the attempt.

In the second study we focused on mood state prior to and after the suicide attempt, and the question of possible systematic changes.[54] To this end we studied 25 suicide attempters within three to six days after admission to a psychiatric ward. The patients were interviewed by an independent physician in the presence of the treating physician. The interview focused on the mood condition prevailing (1) in the week

TABLE 2. Syndromal Depression Diagnosis and Global Severity of Depression in the Same Patients as in TABLE 1[a]

	Number	Mean Depression Rating	Standard Deviation
Major Depression (Melancholic type)	39	3.32	1.08
Other Forms of Depression	23	3.37	1.18

[a] Reproduced from Reference 55 with permission from *Psychiatry Research*.

prior to the attempt and (2) presently. On the basis of these data both physicians filled out the Hamilton Scale for Depression[21] — once related to the presuicidal, once related to the postsuicidal condition. In addition for each mood condition a global depression severity score was determined. Both raters made their assessment independently.

The patient was asked for a global depression score and to complete the Zung Depression Scale[65] likewise twice — once focusing on the week prior to the attempt, once describing the present condition.

Finally an important other, sharing life with the patient, was requested to give a global depression score related to the same periods of time.

As a control group we studied 50 patients consecutively admitted to the same inpatient service for various forms of nonpsychotic depression, but with no previous

TABLE 3. In a Group of 25 Suicide Attempters a Significant Drop in Depression Scores Occurred after Admission in Comparison with Those Scores in the Week Prior to the Attempt[a]

	Before $\bar{x}$	SD	After $\bar{x}$	SD	t
Global scores					
Independent physician	2.4	1.2	1.9	1.0	2.22[b]
Treating physician	2.4	1.1	1.7	0.9	2.63[b]
Patient	2.7	1.5	1.3	1.1	3.99[d]
Important others	2.0	1.4	1.3	0.8	2.38[b]
Hamilton Rating Scale					
Independent physician	18.6	6.6	15.6	5.2	2.17[b]
Treating physician	18.0	6.4	15.8	5.7	1.33
Zung Depression Scale	58.4	12.6	50.8	10.1	3.33[c]

[a] Reproduced from Reference 54 with permission from *Psychiatry Research*. SD is standard deviation.
[b] $p < 0.05$
[c] $p < 0.01$
[d] $p < 0.001$

suicide attempts. They were rated similarly as the suicide group, raters focusing on the week prior to and the week after admission respectively.

In the suicide group depression scores dropped significantly in the first week after admission. This was evident from every type of rating except one (TABLE 3). In the control group no systematic change of any of the measures was observed in the before/after comparisons, neither in the group with major depression (TABLE 4) nor in the group with other types of depression (TABLE 5).

We concluded that depression scores after suicide attempt tend to drop significantly, a confirmation of the assumed but never substantiated cathartic effect of suicide attempt.[17]

Our statement that the diagnosis nondepressed suicide attempter should be based on pre- rather than on postsuicidal data is based on this dual set of observations.

TABLE 4. Depression Ratings before and after Suicide Attempt in Control Patients Suffering from Major Depression ($n = 21$)[a]

	Before		After		
	$\bar{x}$	SD	$\bar{x}$	SD	t
Global score					
Independent physician	2.6	1.0	2.3	1.3	0.78
Treating physician	2.5	1.1	2.5	1.2	0.00
Patient	2.6	1.1	2.8	1.4	0.46
Important others	2.1	1.0	2.1	1.0	0.03
Hamilton Rating Scale					
Independent physician	21.1	4.4	19.8	4.9	1.36
Treating physician	20.4	4.0	19.2	4.4	1.18
Zung Depression Score	62.4	10.0	62.8	10.4	0.21

[a] Reproduced from Reference 54 with permission from *Psychiatry Research*. SD is standard deviation.

Suicide Method as an Index of Strength of Self-Destructive Impulses

Our third objection holds that suicide method is not a valid index of the strength of suicidal impulses and that for two reasons. First, suicide method pertains to seriousness of the *attempt,* defined as the probability of inflicting irreversible damage. It does not pertain to strength of the *intent* to die. It is conceivable that seriousness of attempt and seriousness of intent correlate highly, but up to now this has not been

TABLE 5. Depression Ratings before and after Suicide Attempt in Control Patients Suffering from Types of Depression Other than Major Depression ($n = 29$)[a]

	Before		After		
	$\bar{x}$	SD	$\bar{x}$	SD	t
Global score					
Independent physician	2.5	1.3	2.4	1.1	0.18
Treating physician	2.3	1.0	2.3	1.0	0.00
Patient	3.2	0.9	3.0	0.8	0.78
Important others	2.7	0.9	2.6	0.8	0.11
Hamilton Rating Scale					
Independent physician	19.7	3.9	19.2	3.8	0.82
Treating physician	19.5	3.5	19.7	3.9	0.34
Zung Depression Scale	56.1	9.2	53.6	8.4	1.72

[a] Reproduced from Reference 54 with permission from *Psychiatry Research*. SD is standard deviation.

demonstrated. Our group is presently engaged in a study of that kind. Secondly, seriousness of attempt is not only determined by risk factors, among which method is the most important one, but likewise by the chance of being rescued. Weisman and Worden constructed a quantitative method of measuring lethality of attempt expressed as a ratio of factors influencing risk and rescue.[60] High risk and low rescue chance result in the highest scores, low risk and high rescue chance in the lowest.

We computed risk/rescue scores in 44 patients admitted for suicide attempt. Twenty-three had used violent, the others nonviolent, methods. The violent group had slightly but not significantly higher risk/rescue scores than the nonviolent group (TABLE 6). In other words, violent method is not an adequate indicator of the seriousness of the attempt as measured with the Risk-Rescue Scale.

We concluded that suicide method is an imperfect indicator of the wish to die. Intent and attempt have to be assessed independently; and as far as attempt is concerned, its seriousness is a function of risk and rescue factors and not of the method that has been resorted to alone.

Based on the data discussed in this section, we feel justified to conclude that the data discussed here in the first section do not provide a solid base for the hypothesis that low CSF 5-HIAA is related to (auto)aggression. Other observations, however, do provide some such support. They will be discussed in the next section.

TABLE 6. Risk-Rescue Scores ($\pm$ Standard Deviation) and Suicide Method[a]

	Number	Risk-Rescue Score
Suicide attempt violent means	21	60.7 (± 12.7)
Suicide attempt nonviolent means	23	54.2 (± 15.3)

[a] Difference not significant ($t = 1.52$).

DATA SUPPORTING THE 5-HT HYPOTHESIS OF (AUTO)AGGRESSION

CSF 5-HIAA in Nondepressed, Psychotic Suicide Attempters

We compared postprobenecid CSF 5-HIAA levels in two groups of hospitalized schizophrenic patients without major affective symptoms and in a control group without psychiatric disturbances.[45] One group consisted of 10 schizophrenic patients who had attempted suicide because "voices" had ordered them to do so. The other group of 10 schizophrenic patients, matched with the first for age, sex, and symptomatology and likewise recently hospitalized, had never attempted suicide. In the first group, CSF 5-HIAA, though well within the normal range, was significantly lower than in the nonsuicidal group of schizophrenics and in the nonpsychiatric control group (FIGURE 6). Those who had scored high on the Risk-Rescue Scale[60] had the lowest 5-HIAA levels. Ninan *et al.*, studying schizophrenic patients, found a correlation between suicidal ideation and lowered CSF 5-HIAA.[32] The same group however found no correlation between CSF 5-HIAA and lifetime history of suicide attempts.[36]

Suicide, Hostility, and CSF 5-HIAA in Depression

Assuming that the regulation of aggressive impulses is "centralized" and taking into account the correlation in depressed patients between low CSF 5-HIAA and increased inward directed aggression, it seems reasonable to expect in low CSF 5-HIAA probands also augmented outward directed aggression.

A = Non-psychiatric control group
B = Schizophrenic without suicidal history
C = Schizophrenic with suicidal history
○ = Non-violent suicide
● = Violent suicide

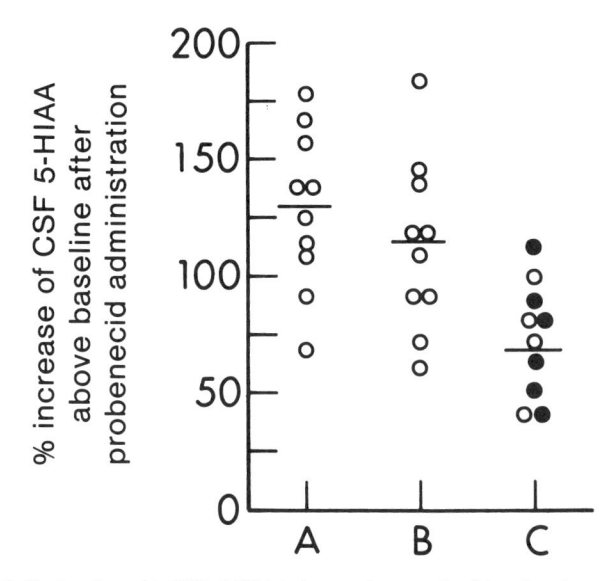

FIGURE 6. Postprobenecid CSF 5-HIAA in nondepressed schizophrenic patients with and without suicidal histories and in nonpsychiatrically disturbed controls. Mean CSF 5-HIAA in group c is lower than in the other two groups ($p < 0.05$, Fisher's exact test). (Reproduced from Reference 45 with permission from *Lancet.*)

TABLE 7. Low 5-HIAA Depressives Compared to Normal 5-HIAA Depressives Present[a]

1. More suicide attempts	$p < 0.01$
2. Greater number of contacts with police	$p < 0.05$
3. Increased arguments with	
• relatives	$p < 0.05$
• spouse	$p < 0.01$
• colleagues	$p < 0.05$
• friends	$p < 0.05$
4. More hostility at interview	$p < 0.05$
5. Impaired employment history (arguments)	$p < 0.05$

[a] Reproduced from Reference 43 with permission from the University of South Carolina.

In order to test this hypothesis, we compared two groups of 25 patients with major depression, melancholic type (DSM III), on several aggression measures.[43,44] The two groups were matched for age and sex but differed with respect to postprobenecid CSF 5-HIAA levels. In the patients of one group the level was normal, in the other it was decreased. In a psychopathological respect, the low 5-HIAA group differed from the other group in two ways (TABLE 6): (1) higher rate of suicide attempts and (2) higher hostility scores on a variety of measures (TABLE 7).

In the same vein, Brown et al. reported a trivariate relation between history of aggression, history of suicide, and low CSF 5-HIAA in patients with personality disorders.[11]

These data add a biological dimension to the observations of Weissman et al. demonstrating that the single most important factor distinguishing between patients admitted for depression and those admitted for attempted suicide is a higher degree of hostility in the suicidal patients.[61]

CSF 5-HIAA in Nondepressed Patients with Aggression Disorders

Several investigators studied CSF 5-HIAA in nondepressed patients with increased outward-directed aggression. These studies have been carried out in patients with several types of personality disorder[10-12] and in individuals who had committed violent crimes (TABLE 8).[25-27] Aggression was assessed with widely different means: from aggression scores on a personality inventory, to lifetime history of aggressive acts and measuring CSF 5-HIAA directly after a violent crime. Yet all studies reported a negative correlation between CSF 5-HIAA and outward directed aggression.

Two studies found evidence that it is not aggressive behavior per se but rather lack of impulse control that constitutes the behavioral correlate of deficient 5-HT metabolism.[26,27]

One should not overrate these data. In men the biology of aggression is hard to study. This behavioral state is preeminently influenced by environmental (social)

TABLE 8. Studies in Which CSF 5-HIAA and Aggression were Negatively Correlated

Study	Number Sex	Diagnosis	Measurement Aggression	Assay CSF 5-HIAA	Postprobenecid or Baseline 5-HIAA	Other MA Metabolites in CSF
Brown et al.[12] (1979)	26M	Personality disorder	• Checklist lifetime history aggressive acts	Fluorometrically	Baseline	HVA[b] unchanged MHPG[c] increased
Brown et al.[11] (1982)	12M	Borderline personality	• Checklist lifetime history aggressive acts • Buss-Durkee Inventory • MMPI[d]	Mass-fragmentography	Baseline	HVA unchanged MHPG unchanged
Bioulac et al.[10] (1980)	6M	xyy personality disorder	• Lifetime history of aggressive behavior	Fluorometrically	Postprobenecid	HVA unchanged MHPG not measured
Linnoila et al.[27] (1983)[a]	36M	Severe personality disorders	• 21 had killed; 15 had made attempts to kill. All were alcohol abusers.	Liquid chromatography	Baseline	HVA unchanged MHPG unchanged
Lidberg et al.[25] (1984)	2M 1F	Depression: 2 Acute psychotic episode: 1	• Killed one of their children and attempted suicide subsequently	Not stated	Baseline	Not mentioned
Lidberg et al.[26] (1985)	16M	Alcoholism: 10 Schizophrenia: 1 No further diagnoses mentioned.	• All had committed criminal homicide	Mass-fragmentography	Baseline	HVA unchanged MHPG unchanged

[a] Low CSF 5-HIAA in impulsive violent offenders as opposed to those who had premeditated their acts.
[b] Homovanillic acid, the main degradation product of dopamine.
[c] 3-Methoxy-4-hydroxyphenyl glycol, the main degradation product of noradrenaline in the CNS.
[d] Minnesota Multiphasic Personality Inventory.

factors for which it is difficult to control. It is often difficult to exclude that preceding drug and/or alcohol use has influenced the biological variables. In addition, disturbances in aggression regulation are generally short lasting, in contrast to pathological disturbances in mood regulation, and are therefore harder to study. Nevertheless, it would be inappropriate to ignore that no negative reports have so far been published, and that the animal literature provides a host of data implicating 5-HT in the regulation of (certain forms of) aggression.[40,41]

Self-Mutilation in the Lesch-Nyhan Syndrome

A possible case in point provides the Lesch-Nyhan syndrome, an inborn error of metabolism, characterized by deficiency of hypoxanthine-guanine phosphoribosyl transferase in male children and associated with severe neurological disturbances, mental retardation, and self-injurious behavior.[9] Some authors found CSF 5-HIAA in those patients to be lowered[15] and self-mutilative behavior ameliorated by administration of 5-hydroxytryptophan (5-HTP),[15,29,33] a 5-HT precursor readily transformed to 5-HT in the CNS. Others found 5-HTP to be ineffective.[3,16,59] Recent evidence suggest that the neuroleptic fluphenazine suppresses automutilative behavior in Lesch-Nyhan patients.[20] Together with the evidence that dopamine (DA) agonists induce self-mutilation in rats in whom DA receptors were rendered supersensitive,[14] these data suggest a role for DA in self-damaging behavior. 5-HT and DA pathology could be interrelated. 5-HT has a role in regulating DA release in the nigrostriatal pathway;[63] decrease in serotonergic activity leads to reduction of DA in the nigrostriatal pathway.[19] A DA deficit would render DA receptors supersensitive.

No studies of monoamine metabolism in other forms of self-mutilation have been published.

THERAPEUTIC IMPLICATIONS OF THE 5-HT HYPOTHESIS OF (AUTO)AGGRESSION

Assuming a causative relation to exist between diminished central 5-HT metabolism—as reflected in lowered CSF 5-HIAA—and disturbed regulation of (auto)aggression, one would expect compounds increasing central 5-HT availability to exert an ameliorating effect in (certain) aggression disorders. Compounds with such capacity are the so-called selective 5-HT reuptake inhibitors, the postsynaptic 5-HT agonists, and the 5-HT precursors tryptophan and 5-hydroxytryptophan (5-HTP). The latter, however, are not really selective, i.e., they exert an influence on central catecholamine metabolism as well.[52]

No studies focusing specifically and cross-diagnostically on the impact of 5-HT potentiating compounds on suicidal behavior have been published. Of possible significance in this context is the controlled observation that long-term administration of *l*-5-HTP (in combination with a peripheral decarboxylase inhibitor) reduces the relapse risk of depression in unipolar patients with high relapse frequency. This effect was most pronounced in patients with lowered postprobenecid CSF 5-HIAA as a trait characteristic.[51] The only controlled study on the effect of increased 5-HT availability on outward directed aggression is that of Morand et al.[31] They studied the effect of l-tryptophan, 4 g per day, on aggressive behavior in 12 schizophrenics and reported a beneficial effect. In a controlled study we are conducting presently in similar patients, the preliminary results are less promising.[58] Several studies have reported a beneficial effect of lithium on outward-directed aggression (e.g., Reference 24). This ion increases serotonergic "tone" in the brain, but since this effect is by no means selective, we do not know whether it is responsible for the reduction of aggression.

Clearly the issue of the therapeutic impact of increasing 5-HT availability in the brain in aggression disorders is wide open.

DEPRESSION, AGGRESSION, AND CENTRAL SEROTONIN, A POSSIBLE TRIVARIATE RELATIONSHIP

The data discussed in the third section, although preliminary in nature, do suggest a correlative relationship between low CSF 5-HIAA and disturbed aggression regulation. This increases the likelihood that lowered CSF 5-HIAA in suicidal patients is likewise related to disordered aggression regulation. The "5-HT hypothesis of aggression" does not per se contradict a relation between disturbed 5-HT metabolism and affective disorder. It is conceivable that disturbances in serotonergic regulation give rise to both mood and aggression disorders.[43] Several observations speak in favor of this assumption. Low CSF 5-HIAA has been found in depressed patients without suicidal history. In addition, CSF 5-HIAA was lowest in depressed patients who had made a violent attempt.[39] Finally, a trivariate relation has been found between suicide, outward-directed aggression, and low CSF 5-HIAA.[11,43,44] A common factor in the central regulation of mood and aggression would provide a biological explanation for (1) the psychoanalytic theory of aggressive impulses underlying depression and suicide,[18] (2) the empirical evidence for increased hostility and acts of aggression in suicide attempters;[22,43,44,61] and (3) the high incidence of suicide in murderers, amounting to more than 30% in some European countries.[62]

SUMMARY

Based on the relation found to exist between low CSF 5-HIAA and suicide attempt, in particular violent suicide attempt, both in depressed and in so-called nondepressed suicide attempters, the conclusion was drawn that decreased central 5-HT metabolism is related to (auto)aggression, rather than to depression. We challenged this conclusion and that for three reasons:

1. Violent suicide attempt accumulates in certain types of depression making it impossible to conclude whether the biological variable relates to (auto)aggression or to that type of depression as such.
2. Nondepressed suicide attempter is a diagnosis that should be based on presuicidal not on postsuicidal data, in order to avoid false-positive diagnoses.
3. Suicide method is not a reliable index of seriousness of the attempt. Risk/rescue ratio should be used instead.

Next the data are discussed that do support the hypothesis that diminished 5-HT metabolism in the brain is related to disregulation of aggression. Finally, the hypothesis is launched that both mood and aggression disorders are related to decreased 5-HT metabolism in the CNS. This would provide a biological explanation for the clinical observation that disorders in mood and in aggression often go hand in hand.

Biological research of psychiatric disorders gains in informative value as the psychopathological analysis of the phenomena one studies is more comprehensive. Biological suicide research is no exception to this rule.

REFERENCES

1. AGREN, H. 1983. Life at risk: markers of suicidality in depression. Psychiatr. Dev. 1: 87-103.
2. AGREN, H. 1980. Symptom patterns in unipolar and bipolar depression correlating with monoamine metabolites in the cerebrospinal fluid. Psychiatry Res. 3: 225-236.
3. ANDERSON, L. T., L. HERRMANN & J. DANCIS. 1976. The effect of *l*-5-hydroxytryptophan on self-mutilation in the Lesch-Nyhan disease: a negative report. Neuropadiatrie 7: 439-442.
4. APRISON, M. D., R. TAKAHASHI & K. TACHIKI. 1978. Hypersensitive serotonergic receptors involved in clinical depression. A theory. *In* Neuropharmacology and Behavior. B. Haber & M. H. Aprison, Eds. Plenum Press. New York, N.Y.
5. ASBERG, M., L. BERTILSSON, B. MARTENSSON, G-P. SCALIA-TOMBA, P. THOREN & L. TRASKMAN. 1984. CSF monoamine metabolites in melancholia. Acta Psychiatr. Scand. 69: 201-219.
6. ASBERG, M., L. TRASKMAN & P. THOREN. 1976. 5-HIAA in the cerebrospinal fluid: a biochemical suicide predictor? Arch. Gen. Psychiatry 33: 1193-1197.
7. BANKI, C. M. & M. ARATO. 1983. Amine metabolites and neuroendocrine responses related to depression and suicide. J. Affect. Disord. 5: 223-232.
8. BANKI, C. M., G. MOLNAR & M. VOJNIK. 1981. Cerebrospinal fluid amine metabolites, tryptophan and clinical parameters in depression: psychopathological symptoms. J. Affect. Disord. 3: 91-99.
9. BAUMEISTER, A. A. & G. D. FRYE. 1985. The biochemical basis of the behavioral disorder in the Lesch-Nyhan syndrome. Neurosci. Biobehav. Rev. 9: 169-178.
10. BIOULAC, B., M. BENEZICH, B. RENAUD, B. NOEL & D. ROCHE. 1980. Serotonergic functions in the 47, XYY syndrome. Biol. Psychiatry 15: 917-923.
11. BROWN, G. L., M. H. EBERT, P. F. GOYER, D. C. JIMERSON, W. J. KLEIN, W. E. BUNNEY & F. K. GOODWIN. 1982. Aggression, suicide and serotonin: relationships to CSF amine metabolites. Am. J. Psychiatry 139: 741-746.
12. BROWN, G. L., F. K. GOODWIN, J. C. BALLENGER, P. F. GOYER & L. F. MAJOR. 1979. Aggression in humans correlates with cerebrospinal fluid metabolites. Psychiatry Res. 1: 131-139.
13. BYERLEY, W. F. & S. C. RISCH. 1985. Depression and serotonin metabolism: rationale for neurotransmitter precursor treatment. J. Clin. Psychopharmacol. 5: 191-206.
14. CASAS-BRUGE, M., C. ALMENAR, I. M. GRAU & J. JANE. 1985. Dopaminergic receptor super-sensitivity in self-mutilatory behavior of Lesch-Nyhan disease. Lancet: 991-992.
15. CASTELLS, S., C. CHAKRABARTI, B. G. WINDSBERG, M. HURWIC, J. M. PEREL & W. L. NYHAN. 1979. Effects of *l*-5-hydroxytryptophan on monoamine and amino acids turnover in the Lesch-Nyhan syndrome. J. Autism Dev. Disord. 9: 95.
16. CIARNELLO, R., T. ANDERS, J. BARCHAS, P. BERGER & H. CANN. 1976. The use of 5-hydroxytryptophan in a child with Lesch-Nyhan syndrome. Child Psychiatry Hum. Dev. 7: 127-133.
17. FARBEROW, N. L. 1950. Personality patterns of suicidal mental hospital patients. Genet. Psychol. Monogr. 42: 3-79.

18. FREUD, S. 1956. Mourning and melancholia. *In* Collected papers. J. E. London, Ed. Hogarth Press. London, England.
19. FUENMAYOR, L. D. & M. BERMUDEZ. 1985. Effect of the cerebral tryptaminergic system on the turnover of dopamine in the striatum of the rat. J. Neurochem. **44:** 670-674.
20. GOLDSTEIN, M., L. T. ANDERSON, R. REUBEN & J. DANCIS. 1985. Self-mutilation in Lesch-Nyhan disease is caused by dopaminergic denervation. Lancet: 338-339.
21. HAMILTON, M. 1960. A rating scale for depression. J. Neurol. Neurosurg. Psychiatry **23:** 56-62.
22. HAWTON, K., J. ROBERTS & G. GOODWIN. 1985. The risk of child abuse among mothers who attempt suicide. Br. J. Psychiatry **146:** 486-489.
23. LAPIN, I. P. & G. F. OXENKRUG. 1969. Intensification of the central serotonergic process as a possible determinant of the thymoleptic effect. Lancet i: 132-136.
24. LENA, B. 1979. Lithium therapy in hyperaggressive behavior in adolescence. *In* Psychopharmacology of Aggression. M. Sandler, Ed.: 197-203. Raven Press. New York, N.Y.
25. LIDBERG, L., M. ASBERG & U. B. SUNDQUIST-STENSMAN. 1984. 5-Hydroxyindoleacetic acid in attempted suicides who have killed their children. Lancet ii: 928.
26. LIDBERG, L., J. R. TUCK, M. ASBERG, G. P. SCALIA-TOMBA & L. BERTILSSON. 1985. Homicide, suicide and CSF 5-HIAA. Acta Psychiatr. Scand. **71:** 230-236.
27. LINNOILA, M., M. VIRKHUNEN, M. SCHEININ, R. NUUTILA, R. RIMON & F. K. GOODWIN. 1983. Low cerebrospinal fluid 5-hydroxyindoleacetic acid concentration differentiates impulsive from non-impulsive violent behavior. Life Sci. **33:** 2609-2614.
28. MIGNOT, E., A. SERRANO, D. LAUDE, J-L. ELGHOZI, J. DEDEK & B. SCATTON. 1985. Measurement of 5-HIAA levels in ventricular CSF (by LCEC) and in striatum (by in vivo voltammetry) during pharmacological modifications of serotonin metabolism in the rat. J. Neural. Transm. **62:** 117-124.
29. MIZUNO, T. & Y. YUGARI. 1975. Prophylactic effect of *l*-5-hydroxytryptophan on self-mutilation in the Lesch-Nyhan syndrome. Neuropediatric **6:** 13.
30. MONTGOMERY, S. A. & D. MONTGOMERY. 1982. Pharmacological prevention of suicidal behavior. J. Affect. Disord. **4:** 291-298.
31. MORAND, C., S. N. YOUNG & F. R. ERVIN. 1983. Clinical response of aggressive schizophrenics to oral tryptophan. Biol. Psychiatry **18:** 575-578.
32. NINAN, P. T., D. P. VAN KAMMEN, M. SCHEININ, M. LINNOILA, W. E. BUNNEY & F. K. GOODWIN. 1984. CSF 5-hydroxyindoleacetic acid levels in suicidal schizophrenic patients. Am. J. Psychiatry **141:** 566-569.
33. NYHAN, W. L, H. G. JOHNSON, I. A. KAUFMAN & K. L. JONES. 1980. Serotonergic approaches to the modification of behavior in the Lesch-Nyhan syndrome. Appl. Res. Ment. Retard. **1:** 25-40.
34. ORELAND, L., A. WIDBERG, M. ASBERG, L. TRASKMAN, L. SJOSTRAND, P. THOREN, L. BERTILSSON & G. TYBRING. 1981. Platelet MAO activity and monoamine metabolites in cerebrospinal fluid in depressed and suicidal patients and in healthy controls. Psychiatry Res. **4:** 21-29.
35. PAYKEL, E. S. & E. RASSABY. 1978. Classification of suicide attempts by cluster analysis. Br. J. Psychiatry **133:** 45-52.
36. ROY, A., P. NINAN, A. MAZONSON, D. PICKAR, D. VAN KAMMEN, M. LINNOILA & S. M. PAUL. 1985. CSF monoamine metabolites in chronic schizophrenic patients who attempt suicide. Psychol. Med. **15:** 335-340.
37. ROY, P., R. M. POST, D. R. RUBINOW, M. LINNOILA, R. SAVARD & D. DAVIS. 1984. CSF 5-HIAA and personal and family history of suicide in affectively ill patients: a negative study. Psychiatry Res. **10:** 263-274.
38. TRASKMAN-BENDZ, L. 1983. CSF 5-HIAA and family history of psychiatric disorder. Am. J. Psychiatry **140:** 1257.
39. TRASKMAN, L., M. ASBERG, L. BERTILSSON & L. SJOSTRAND. 1981. Monoamine metabolites in CSF and suicidal behavior. Arch. Gen. Psychiatry **38:** 631-636.
40. VALZELLI, L. 1984. Reflections on experimental and human pathology of aggression. Prog. Neuropsychopharmacol. Biol. Psychiatry **8:** 311-325.
41. VALZELLI, L., Ed. 1981. Psychobiology of Aggression and Violence. Raven Press. New York, N.Y.

42. VAN PRAAG, H. M. Biochemical suicide research. Outcome and limitations. Biol. Psychiatry. (In press.)
43. VAN PRAAG, H. M. 1986. Affective disorders and aggression disorders. Evidence for a common biological mechanism. Suicide Life-Threat. Behav. **16:** 103-132.
44. VAN PRAAG, H. M. Brain serotonin and human (auto)aggression. *In* Perspectives in Psychopharmacology. J. D. Barchas, W. E. Bunney & A. R. Liss, Eds. (In press.)
45. VAN PRAAG, H. M. 1983. CSF 5-HIAA and suicide in non-depressed schizophrenics. Lancet. **i:** 977-978.
46. VAN PRAAG, H. M. 1982. Depression, suicide and the metabolism of serotonin in the brain. J. Affect. Disord. **4:** 275-290.
47. VAN PRAAG, H. M. 1982. Neurotransmitters and CNS disease: depression. Lancet **ii:** 1259-1264.
48. VAN PRAAG, H. M. 1977. Depression and Schizophrenia. A Contribution on their Chemical Pathologies. Spectrum Publications. New York, N.Y.
49. VAN PRAAG, H. M. 1977. Significance of biochemical parameters in the diagnosis, treatment and prevention of depressive disorders. Biol. Psychiatry **12:** 101-131.
50. VAN PRAAG, H. M. 1962. Monoamine oxidase inhibition as a therapeutic principle in depression. Thesis. Yanssen. Nymegen, Holland.
51. VAN PRAAG, H. M. & S. DE HAAN. 1980. Depression vulnerability and 5-hydroxytryptophan prophylaxis. Psychiatry Res. **3:** 75-83.
52. VAN PRAAG, H. M. & C. LEMUS. 1986. Uses of nutrients in treating psychiatric disease. *In* Nutrition and the Brain. R. J. Wurtman & J. J. Wurtman, Eds. **7:** 89-138. Raven Press. New York, N.Y.
53. VAN PRAAG, H. M., R. PLUTCHIK & H. CONTE. The serotonin hypothesis of (auto)-aggression: critical appraisal of the evidence. Ann. N.Y. Acad. Sci. (This volume.)
54. VAN PRAAG, H. M. & R. PLUTCHIK. 1985. An empirical study on the "cathartic effect" of attempted suicide. Psychiatry Res. **16:** 123-130.
55. VAN PRAAG, H. M. & R. PLUTCHIK. 1984. Depression-type and depression-severity in relation to risk of violent suicide attempt. Psychiatry Res. **12:** 333-338.
56. VAN PRAAG, H. M., A. M. ULEMAN & J. C. SPITZ. 1965. The vital syndrome interview. A structured standard interview for the recognition and registration of the vital depressive symptom complex. Psychiatr. Neurol. Neurochir. **68:** 329-346.
57. VESTERGAARD, P., T. SØRENSEN, E. HOPPE, O. J. RAFAELSEN, C. M. YATES & N. NICOLAOU. 1978. Biogenic amine metabolites in cerebrospinal fluid of patients with affective disorders. Acta Psychiatr. Scand. **58:** 88-96.
58. VOLAVKA, J., D. BRIZER, A. CONVIT, R. WOLNER, R. J. WURTMAN & H. M. VAN PRAAG. 1985. Tryptophan and aggression. Paper read at the IV World Congress of Biological Psychiatry, Philadelphia, Pennsylvania, September 9-11.
59. WATTS, R. W. E., E. SPELLACY, D. A. GIBBS, J. ALLSOP, R. O. MCKERAN & G. E. SLAVIN. 1982. Clinical post-mortem, biochemical and therapeutic observations on the Lesch-Nyhan syndrome with particular reference to the neurological manifestations. Q. J. Med. **201:** 43-78.
60. WEISMAN, A. D. & J. W. WORDEN. Risk/rescue rating in suicide assessment. Arch. Gen. Psychiatry **26:** 553-560.
61. WEISSMAN, J., K. FOX & J. L. KLERMAN. 1973. Hostility and depression associated with suicide attempts. Am. J. Psychiatry **130:** 450.
62. WEST, D. J., Ed. 1965. Murder followed by suicide. Heinemann. London, England.
63. WILLIAMS, J. & J. A. DAVIES. 1983. The involvement of 5-hydroxytryptamine in the release of dendritic dopamine from slices of rat substantia nigra. J. Pharm. Pharmacol. **35:** 734-737.
64. ZIS, A. P. & F. K. GOODWIN. 1982. The amine hypothesis. *In* Handbook of Affective Disorders. E. S. Paykel, Ed. The Guilford Press. New York, N.Y.
65. ZUNG, W. W. 1965. A self-rating depression scale. Arch. Gen. Psychiatry **12:** 63-70.

Serotonergic Function and Suicidal Behavior in Personality Disorders[a]

LIL TRÄSKMAN-BENDZ, MARIE ÅSBERG, AND DAISY SCHALLING

*Department of Psychiatry and Psychology
Karolinska Hospital and Institute
S-104 01, Stockholm, Sweden*

Many investigators have studied serotonergic function as reflected in concentrations of the serotonin metabolite 5-hydroxyindoleacetic acid (5-HIAA) in the cerebrospinal fluid (CSF) in patients suffering from various psychiatric and somatic illnesses,[1-11] and also in recovered depressed patients[12-14] and healthy volunteers.[15,16]

These studies suggest that serotonergic function is disturbed in subgroups of psychiatric patients. The results have not always been conclusive, which is probably due to the influence of confounding factors such as age, sex, body height, food intake, and diurnal and seasonal fluctuations (for an overview, see Reference 5). Low concentrations of CSF 5-HIAA have repeatedly been associated with suicidal behavior, and especially with serious suicide attempts and completed suicide regardless of the nature of the psychiatric disorder (for an overview, see Reference 17).

Low concentrations of CSF 5-HIAA have also been reported in healthy volunteers, and in depressed patients after recovery. A low CSF 5-HIAA, rather than being a sign of illness, may thus reflect personality traits associated with increased vulnerability for psychiatric illness and suicidal behavior.

A couple of studies indicate that this vulnerability may be genetically determined. Sedvall *et al.*, found an increased incidence of affective illness in families of low CSF 5-HIAA healthy volunteers.[15] Similarly, affective disorders were more common in families of depressed patients with low CSF 5-HIAA.[18]

PERSONALITY DISORDERS AND CSF 5-HIAA

There are several studies of serotonergic function in nondepressed, nonschizophrenic patients as shown in TABLE 1. In two consecutive studies, Brown *et al.* studied young military men who were diagnosed as personality disorders.[19,20] In the first study, the subjects were subgrouped into "more impulsive" and "less impulsive" personality disorders. Men classified according to the *Diagnostic and Statistical Manual,* second edition (DSM II) as "more impulsive" (antisocial, explosive, immature, and hysterical

---

[a] Research funded by the Swedish Medical Research Council (5454, 4545, 714/85).

personality disorders) had lower CSF 5-HIAA levels than those classified as "less impulsive" (passive-aggressive, passive-dependent, schizoid, obsessive-compulsive, or inadequate personality disorders). In their second study, the primary diagnostic category was borderline personality disorder (DSM III)[21] along with secondary diagnoses of explosive, immature, hysterical, and schizoid personality disorder (DSM III). In both investigations, there was a link between suicidal history and low CSF 5-HIAA.

Linnoila et al., who studied violent offenders,[22] subgrouped their subjects into "impulsive" offenders, who were diagnosed as intermittent explosive or antisocial personality disorders along with borderline personality disorder, and "nonimpulsive" offenders, who had paranoid or passive-aggressive personality disorders. The "impulsive" offenders had significantly lower CSF 5-HIAA concentrations than did the "nonimpulsive" offenders. "Impulsive" subjects with a history of suicide attempt had the lowest CSF 5-HIAA concentrations.

Banki and Arató classified their nondepressed, nonschizophrenic, and nonalcoholic patients as adjustment disorders, personality disorders, substance abuse, or somatization disorder.[23] The three patients who had used violent methods when attempting suicide had CSF 5-HIAA concentrations in the lower range.

In one of our earlier studies, 30 suicide attempters were examined, excluding patients with schizophrenia, substance abuse, and organic brain syndrome.[16] Eight were diagnosed as depressed, and 22 as nondepressed according to the Newcastle Inventory[24] (DSM III was not available in Sweden at that time). The patients were subgrouped into those who had made violent suicide attempts (such as hanging, drowning, several wrist cuts, or combinations of methods) and those who had made nonviolent attempts (drug overdoses, single wrist cuts). The nondepressed patients were diagnosed as anxiety disorder, minor depressive illness, manic-depressive illness in remission, and personality disorder (unspecified). Recently, the DSM III Axis II diagnostic system was applied in retrospect on these patients by scrutinizing their charts. The same procedure was applied to nondepressed patients in some other studies from our group. A reasonably satisfactory base for diagnosis was found in 26/28 patients (TABLE 2). Borderline personality disorder was the most common DSM III diagnostic category among the violent suicide attempters. CSF 5-HIAA concentrations below 80 nmol/L were found in 2 patients with antisocial, 2 with avoidant, and 1 with paranoid personality disorder.

In a follow-up study of 119 patients who had participated in our studies since 1970, we found that 7 patients had committed suicide. All of these had CSF 5-HIAA levels below the median.[16] Four of them were not diagnosed as depressed during the index illness period. In retrospect, among the nondepressed patients with completed suicides, 2 were classified as borderline personality disorder, 1 as paranoid, and 1 as histrionic personality disorder. These data support the assumption that disorders other than melancholia, schizophrenia, and substance abuse may be risk factors for suicide.

PERSONALITY MEASURES RELATED TO LOW CSF 5-HIAA AND SUICIDAL BEHAVIOR

The personality characteristics of low CSF 5-HIAA patients with suicidal behavior have been studied by means of projective psychological methods and personality inventories.

TABLE 1. Studies of Suicidal Patients with Diagnoses Other than Schizophrenia or Depression

Investigators	Number	Disorder	Finding
Brown et al., 1979[19]	24	Primary personality disorder (DSM II)	Low 5-HIAA/history of attempt
Träskman et al., 1981[16]	12	Personality disorder	Low 5-HIAA/violent suicide attempt
	7	Anxiety disorder	
	1	Manic-depressive in remission	
	2	Minor depressive illness	
Brown et al., 1982[20]	12	Borderline (DSM III)	Low 5-HIAA/history of attempt
Linnoila et al., 1983[22]	20	Intermittent explosive	Low 5-HIAA/history of attempt + explosive or antisocial personality
	7	Antisocial	
	9	Paranoid or passive-aggressive	
Banki & Arató, 1983[23]	12	Substance abuse	Low 5-HIAA/violent suicide attempt
		Somatization	
		Personality disorder	
		Adjustment disorders	

TABLE 2. DSM III Personality Disorder Diagnoses Given Retrospectively from Charts

Disorder	Number	Suicide Attempt Violent	Suicide Attempt Nonviolent	CSF 5-HIAA (nmol/L)[a]
Antisocial	2	1	1	27; 57
Avoidant	2	2	0	57; 76
Borderline	8	5	3	82 ± 31
Dependent	2	1	1	80; 109
Histrionic	6	1	5	96 ± 32
Paranoid	1	1	0	71
Passive-aggressive	1	0	1	104
Schizoid	4	1	3	92 ± 26
Nonclassifiable	2	1	1	95; 71
Total	28	13	15	

[a] Mean ± standard deviation.

In a study from our group, Rorschach protocols from psychiatric patients were rated blindly.[25] Patients with low 5-HIAA were compared with patients with high 5-HIAA, matched for sex, age, body height, and diagnosis. Low CSF 5-HIAA patients had significantly higher scores of anxiety level and lower scores of anxiety tolerance than did high 5-HIAA patients. From the Rorschach ratings, low CSF 5-HIAA patients also appeared more paranoid, and less able to handle conflict. Responses with aggressive content more often occurred in low 5-HIAA patients than in high 5-HIAA patients, and they had a hostile attitude during the examination.

Another projective test, the Thematic Apperception Test (TAT), was given in a follow-up study of 27 depressed and suicidal patients.[26] Patients with a history of attempted suicide had significantly higher hostility scores in TAT than did those who had not attempted suicide.

Schalling et al., have also investigated the relationship between personality inventory scales and CSF 5-HIAA in patient groups and healthy volunteers.[27] The Eysenck Personality Questionnaire (EPQ)[28] was used. It consists of three scales: extraversion, psychoticism, and neuroticism. Negative correlations were obtained between CSF 5-HIAA and EPQ psychoticism (i.e., nonconformity, aggressiveness) in nondepressed patients, suicide attempters, and healthy volunteers. In suicidal patients there was also a significantly negative correlation between CSF 5-HIAA and EPQ neuroticism (i.e., emotional instability) (TABLE 3).

TABLE 3. Correlations between CSF 5-HIAA and EPQ Scores[a]

	Suicide attempters ($n = 25$)	Volunteers ($n = 23$)
EPQ extraversion	NS	NS
EPQ psychoticism	—	—
EPQ neuroticism	—	NS

[a] Data from Schalling et al., 1985.[27] NS means not significant.

The Karolinska Scales of Personality (KSP), constructed by Schalling et al.,[29] were also applied. KSP consists of three groups of scales. Group I scales are impulsivity, sensation seeking (monotony avoidance), and socialization scales. All of these scales are associated with psychopathy, and they showed a consistent pattern in relation to CSF 5-HIAA in the patient groups: low CSF 5-HIAA was associated with high scores in monotony avoidance and impulsiveness, and low scores of socialization. The findings are in line with those reported by Brown and associates for the psychopathic deviate (Pd) scale of the Multiphasic Minnesota Personality Inventory (MMPI).[20]

The group II scales of the KSP deal with different aspects of anxiety and energy. Violent suicide attempters scored high on "somatic anxiety," i.e., panic attacks, autonomic symptoms, and a feeling of discomfort. A KSP scale associated with validity, a personality dimension from the Sjöbring personality model,[30] was also related to 5-HIAA in volunteers. Low 5-HIAA healthy volunteers rated themselves as energetic, efficient, assertive, and noninhibited according to this scale. Similarly, Banki and Arató, who studied female psychiatric patients, found a significant correlation between CSF 5-HIAA and a validity scale from the Marke-Nyman Temperament (MNT) inventory.[31]

In the group III scales of the KSP are included scales with items from the Buss Durkee Inventory (BDI)[32] of aggression. Scores from these scales were not significantly related to CSF 5-HIAA. Brown *et al.* also estimated aggressiveness from the BDI and found no association with CSF 5-HIAA,[20] whereas a history of aggressive behavior was related with low CSF 5-HIAA in their subjects.

CONCLUSION

Psychiatric patients with low CSF 5-HIAA appear to be more prone to suicidal behavior irrespective of diagnosis. In psychological tests and inventories these patients obtain high scores on aggression, hostility, anxiety, impulsivity, and monotony avoidance, and low scores in socialization. Similar characteristics are found in both borderline and antisocial personality disorders, as described in the DSM III.

REFERENCES

1. ÅSBERG, M., P. THORÉN, L. TRÄSKMAN, L. BERTILSSON & V. RINGBERGER. 1976. "Serotonin depression"—a biochemical subgroup within the affective disorders? Science **191:** 478-480.
2. MURPHY, D. L., I. C. CAMPBELL & J. L. COSTA. 1978. The brain serotonergic system in the affective disorders. Prog. Neuro-psychopharmacol. **2:** 1-31.
3. POST, R. M., J. C. BALLENGER & F. K. GOODWIN. 1980. Cerebrospinal fluid studies of neurotransmitter function in manic and depressive illness. *In* Neurobiology of Cerebrospinal Fluid I. J. H. Wood, Ed.: 685-717. Plenum Press. New York, N.Y.
4. VAN PRAAG, H. M. 1982. Depression, suicide and metabolism of serotonin in the brain. J. Affect. Disord. **4:** 275-290.
5. ÅSBERG, M., L. BERTILSSON, B. MÅRTENSSON, G.-P. SCALIA-TOMBA, P. THORÉN & L. TRÄSKMAN-BENDZ. 1984. CSF monoamine metabolites in melancholia. Acta Psychiatr. Scand. **69:** 201-219.
6. THORÉN, P., M. ÅSBERG, L. BERTILSSON, B. MELLSTRÖM, F. SJÖQVIST & L. TRÄSKMAN. 1980. Clomipramine treatment of obsessive compulsive disorder. II. Biochemical aspects. Arch. Gen. Psychiatry **37:** 1289-1294.
7. BALLENGER, J. C., F. K. GOODWIN, L. F. MAJOR & G. L. BROWN. 1979. Alcohol and central serotonin metabolism in man. Arch. Gen. Psychiatry **36:** 224-227.
8. BANKI, C. M. 1981. Factors influencing monoamine metabolites and tryptophan in patients with alcohol dependence. J. Neural Transm. **50:** 89-101.
9. NINAN, P. T., D. P. VAN KAMMEN, M. SCHEININ, M. LINNOILA, W. E. BUNNEY, JR. & F. K. GOODWIN. 1984. CSF 5-hydroxyindoleacetic acid in suicidal schizophrenic patients. Am. J. Psychiatry **141:** 566-569.
10. ANDERSEN, O., B. JOHANSSON & L. SVENNERHOLM. 1981. Monoamine metabolites in successive samples of spinal fluid—a comparison between healthy volunteers and patients with multiple sclerosis. Acta Neurol. Scand. **63:** 247-254.
11. HALLERT, C., J. ÅSTRÖM & G. SEDVALL. 1982. Psychic disturbances in adult coeliac diseases. III. Reduced central monoamine metabolites and signs of depression. Scand. J. Gastroenterol. **17:** 25-28.
12. COPPEN, A., A. J. PRANGE, JR., P. C. WHYBROW & R. NOGUERA. 1972. Abnormalities of indoleamines in affective disorders. Arch. Gen. Psychiatry **26:** 474-478.
13. VAN PRAAG, H. M. 1977. Significance of biochemical parameters in the diagnosis, treatment, and prevention of depressive disorders. Biol. Psychiatry **12:** 101-131.

14. TRÄSKMAN-BENDZ, L., M. ÅSBERG, L. BERTILSSON & P. THORÉN. 1984. CSF monoamine metabolites of depressed patients during illness and after recovery. Acta Psychiatr. Scand. **69:** 333-342.
15. SEDVALL, G., B. FYRÖ, B. GULLBERG, H. NYBÄCK, F.-A. WIESEL & B. WODE-HELGODT. 1980. Relationships in healthy volunteers between concentrations of monoamine metabolites in cerebrospinal fluid and family history of psychiatric morbidity. Br. J. Psychiatry **136:** 366-374.
16. TRÄSKMAN, L., M. ÅSBERG, L. BERTILSSON & L. SJÖSTRAND. 1981. Monoamine metabolites in CSF and suicidal behavior. Arch. Gen. Psychiatry **38:** 631-636.
17. ÅSBERG, M., P. NORDSTRÖM & L. TRÄSKMAN-BENDZ. 1986. Biological factors in suicide. *In* Suicide. A. Roy, Ed.: 47-71. Williams and Wilkins. Baltimore, Md.
18. VAN PRAAG, H. M. & S. DE HAAN. 1979. Central serotonin metabolism and the frequency of depression. Psychiatry Res. **1:** 219-224.
19. BROWN, G. L., F. K. GOODWIN, J. C. BALLENGER, P. F. GOYER & L. F. MAJOR. 1979. Aggression in humans correlates with cerebrospinal fluid amine metabolites. Psychiatry Res. **1:** 131-139.
20. BROWN, G. L., M. H. EBERT, P. F. GOYER, D. C. JIMERSON, W. J. KLEIN, W. E. BUNNEY & F. K. GOODWIN. 1982. Aggression, suicide, and serotonin: relationships to CSF amine metabolites. Am. J. Psychiatry **139:** 741-746.
21. American Psychiatric Association. 1980. Diagnostic and Statistical Manual of Mental Disorders. 3rd edit. Washington, D.C.
22. LINNOILA, M., M. VIRKKUNEN, M. SCHEININ, A. NUUTILA, R. RIMON & F. K. GOODWIN. 1983. Low cerebrospinal fluid 5-hydroxyindoleacetic acid concentration differentiates impulsive from nonimpulsive violent behavior. Life Sci. **33:** 2609-2614.
23. BANKI, C. M. & M. ARATÓ. 1983. Amine metabolites and neuroendocrine responses related to depression and suicide. J. Affect. Disord. **5:** 223-232.
24. GURNEY, C., J. ROTH, R. F. GARSIDE & A. KERR. 1972. Studies in the classification of affective disorder. Br. J. Psychiatry. **121:** 162-166.
25. RYDIN, E., D. SCHALLING & M. ÅSBERG. 1982. Rorschach ratings in depressed and suicidal patients with low levels of 5-hydroxyindoleacetic acid in cerebrospinal fluid. Psychiatry Res. **7:** 229-243.
26. SCHALLING, D., M. ÅSBERG, L. TRÄSKMAN-BENDZ, H. LUBLIN, V. RANTZÉN & E. RYDIN. Hostility, social support and suicidal behavior—a follow-up study of depressed patients. (Manuscript in preparation.)
27. SCHALLING, D., M. ÅSBERG & G. EDMAN. Personality and CSF monoamine metabolites. (Manuscript in preparation.)
28. EYSENCK, H. J. & S. B. G. EYSENCK. 1975. Manual of the Eysenck Personality Questionnaire. Hodder and Stoughton. London, England.
29. SCHALLING, D. & G. EDMAN, Eds. The Karolinska Scales of Personality (KSP). (Manual in preparation.)
30. SJÖBRING, H. 1973. Personality structure and development. A model and its application. Acta Psychiatr. Scand. (Suppl. 244).
31. BANKI, C. & M. ARATÓ. 1983. Relationship between cerebrospinal fluid amine metabolites, neuroendocrine findings and personality dimensions (Marke-Nyman scale factors) in psychiatric patients. Acta Psychiatr. Scand. **67:** 272-280.
32. BUSS, A. H. & A. DURKEE. 1957. An inventory for assessing different kinds of hostility. J. Consult. Psychol. **21:** 343-348.

Cerebrospinal Fluid Correlates of Suicide Attempts and Aggression

GERALD L. BROWN[a] AND FREDERICK K. GOODWIN[b]

[a]*Biological Psychiatry Branch*
Intramural Research Program
National Institute of Mental Health
Building 10, Room 3N212
NIH Clinical Center
Bethesda, Maryland 20892

[b]*Office of Scientific Director*
Intramural Research Program
National Institute of Mental Health
Building 10, Room 4N224
Bethesda, Maryland 20892

Human suicidal and aggressive behaviors have been studied extensively from sociopsychological perspectives. A stimulus for recent biochemical studies has been an interest in the relationship between suicide and aggression, a clinical relationship hypothesized by Freud.[1] The studies of Asberg et al.[2,3] and Brown et al.[4,5] have stimulated considerable further work on the suicide/aggression/impulsivity relationship from the point of view of central nervous system (CNS) biochemistry.

SELF-DESTRUCTIVE AND AGGRESSIVE BEHAVIOR IN ANIMALS

Animal models for suicidal behavior are problematic, whereas animal models for aggressive behavior have been widely reported.[6,7] Though cognitive and intentional mental processes can no doubt play an important role in suicidal behaviors, it would be an assumption necessarily to ascribe to them basic etiological roles. Distinguishing whether a behavior is self-destructive or "suicidal" in animals can be as difficult as making that distinction in humans. Jones writes, "While it is commonly assumed in human self-injury that thought initiates the act, the order may, in fact, be reversed, with thought being used to elaborate and transform, rather than to initiate ... the act."[8] He proposes that it is an "impulse to injure" that is induced by a stressful environment and that this impulse is transformed in its expression by the addition of cognitive and affective elements that shape the resulting behaviors. We might add to his views that the etiology of the "impulse" may be basically biological (with different individuals having differing propensities for such impulses) and that the "amount" of environmental stress that might induce such impulses could be different from time to time in the same individual. One might construct a model in which certain basic biological characteristics, such as the level of excitation-inhibition in areas of the CNS (influenced by internal and external biological stimuli) thought to interact with the laying down of short-term memory, the transformation of short-term memory to long-term memory, and the retrieval of the latter, all together form a system from which behavior originates.[9] Manifest behavior, then, e.g., suicide, would be influenced by both basic biological characteristics and predispositions (genetic or acquired) interacting with cognitive processes stimulated by environmental experience. Such a model could explain both the repeatedly impulsive individual (perhaps with a family history of the same) who manifests suicidal and/or aggressive/impulsive behavior triggered by seemingly mild to moderate environmental stress as an example of an individual with a "biological predisposition" toward such behaviors contrasted with the patriotic kamikaze pilot as an example of an individual who, at the very least, demonstrated a considerable cognitive contribution to suicidal behavior. (This model is not meant to imply that cognition is not related to biology, but simply that the biological contribution to "impulsive" behaviors and "cognitive" behaviors is probably different.) Human pathology could either affect the biological structure in which such processes (emotional, memory, and cognitive) are effected and/or provide another "external" stress decreasing the resiliency of the individual in coping with other stresses.

An advantage in looking at self-destructive behaviors in animals is that one might come to view possible evolutionary and genetic contributions to the "proneness" to suicide in humans that might otherwise be overlooked. Certain kinds of animal behaviors that often lead to their demise from causes other than a "disease" or accident have been carefully reviewed.[10] Among these general categories are altruistic behaviors, dispersal behaviors, stress-related behaviors, and laboratory models. Not all of these categories necessarily involve externally directed aggressive behaviors.

Altruistic behaviors may involve certain individuals, usually males, who might be viewed biologically as more expendable, e.g., "soldiering", in which the defense of the group, or certain members of a group, i.e., females and the young, leads to fighting and the likelihood of the male's death at some point. The kamikaze pilot above provided an example of cognitive contribution to self-destructive behavior; the "soldiering" of mountain gorillas in Rwanda, Uganda, and Zaire[11] involves similar behavior—is such behavior cognitive in apes? In human military operations, whether those who volunteer as point patrols may be the most aggressive or, possibly, "sensation seeking"[12] is not clear, but they are among the most likely to die if their volunteering persists. Some dispersal behaviors may reflect lack of survival by the more inadequate members of a species,[13] but an individual's "inadequacy" is partially the result of a lack of success in fighting or an avoidance of the same; thus such behaviors may relate to "passive" self-destruction as opposed to a more "aggressive" self-destruction. Confinement, in both animals and man, may lead to self-directed and other-directed destructive behaviors, i.e., the laboratory studies of rats by Calhoun[14] and the rageful and self-destructive behaviors found in human prisoners[15]—though this latter group is likely to be predisposed to externally directed aggressive behaviors. Each animal model has its relative advantages and disadvantages in making comparisons and contrasts to human self-destructive behavior, but the controlled laboratory model lends itself more to a possible understanding of biological bases and accompanying behavioral changes. Among such behaviors are "learned helplessness" in rats;[16–18] animals trained for "learned helplessness" have been found to have lower CNS serotonin (5-HT) release and lower 5-hydroxyindoleacetic acid (5-HIAA) levels in comparison with naive controls[19] and also to respond favorably to desipramine at the same time that hippocampal 5-HIAA is increased.[20] Another potentially self-destructive laboratory-induced behavior is that of the separation model in primates.[21,22]

Animals disadvantaged by those laboratory manipulations cited above would not long survive in a natural habitat, not unlike, perhaps, the relatively poor "survivability" of humans afflicted with significant psychopathology—especially without the "protective" elements of society, i.e., family and other care providers, institutions, etc. Suomi *et al.* have noted that "prolonged psychopathology is rarely observed among free-ranging animals other than man for a very elementary reason: Animals so afflicted are not apt to survive very long."[22] We have alluded to the protest-despair model in monkeys in earlier papers[4,5] as roughly analogous to the aggressive range (protest), sometimes followed by depressive affect (despair), that can be seen in humans; furthermore, the "despair" in such animals can often be therapeutically modified by those medications effective in the treatment of human depression.[23] Not only does this primate model have an analogy in the "anaclitic depression" (Spitz,[24] in infants) which can lead to death, but also infants who have experienced such social deprivation have been reported to show CNS changes related to the hypothalamic-pituitary axis and its regulation of hormones that influence glucose metabolism—these changes may or may not be entirely reversible with a restoration of the care-taker.[25] Perhaps of more interest is not the simple fact that such CNS changes have been reported but that, in order to pursue indications of a genetic contribution to suicidal behavior,[26,27] there would need to be further understanding of the relative vulnerability of different infants to such environmentally induced stresses. For example, a recent report linking adolescent suicide to perinatal respiratory distress and problem pregnancies[28] not only indicates the possibility of an interaction between biological and socioeconomic variables, but also raises questions as to whether a biological variable predisposing toward suicidal behavior was simply acquired, e.g., provoked by medical events, or whether certain individuals might be more genetically vulnerable to specific medically stressful conditions. That there has been a large increase in the number of adolescent suicides in the last 20 years (though the rate is disputed) might appear, superficially, to support the idea that some noxious change in the cultural or socioeconomic environment and/or some unique change in the psychology of adolescents has occurred. On the other hand, biological influences, especially those of a genetic nature, may be assumed to have occurred at a very slow rate. However, it is also possible that the kind of individual who would have been biologically vulnerable to suicide all along is now interacting with different nonbiological conditions in such a way as to result in a more lethal combination of determinants.

Certain neurotransmitters, i.e., 5-HT, gamma-aminobutyric acid (GABA), and dopamine (DA), largely inhibitory in the CNS, and norepinephrine (NE), largely excitatory in the CNS, as well as others, such as acetylcholine (AcH), have been associated with aggressive behaviors in animals.[28] Other biochemical compounds found in the CNS, i.e., the cyclic nucleotides, have also been sometimes associated with aggressive behaviors in animals.[30,31] Further, various pharmacological compounds that induce changes in the CNS, particularly in neurotransmission, have also been shown to alter aggressive behaviors in animals and humans.[32–34] Reviews of the animal literature have been provided by Eichelman[35] and Valzelli.[36]

Most laboratory-controlled animal studies focus on a highly controlled "state." Human studies that are associated with cerebrospinal fluid (CSF) neurotransmitter metabolites—i.e., 5-HIAA, a major metabolite of 5-HT; 3-methoxy-4-hydroxyphenylglycol (MHPG), a major metabolite of NE; and homovanillic acid (HVA), a major metabolite of DA—and aggressive behavior have largely focused on "trait," though those studies that have distinguished "violent" vs. "nonviolent" suicide attempts are not so easily categorized with regard to "state" or "trait," since, in most of these studies, longitudinal behavioral history is not reported. As both suicide[37] and aggression[38] are best predicted by a history of similar behavior, one might wonder if those individuals who make a "violent" suicidal attempt have not generally been more repetitively impulsive in previous other behaviors. That suicide not associated with violence has not been so consistently associated with decreased CSF 5-HIAA as that associated with violence might indicate that aggression/impulsivity is a more basic and primitive response than depression and suicide (45-85% of suicides are associated with depression as a syndrome or symptom).[39]

Another important difference between animal and human studies is the greater memory capacity in humans. A human, for example, may show less aroused, aggressive, and sometimes self-destructive behavior when exposed to a novel environment than is often the case for animals.[40] Possibly, with a greater store of memory and a greater cognitive capacity to search and utilize such a store, the human is more likely to be able to make some association between the new environment and past experience to ameliorate the adjustment process. In any case, muricidal behavior in rats with decreased CNS 5-HT is attenuated by prior exposure to mice.[41] How likely a proneness to act on "impulse" is influenced by prior experience is surely variable in humans and, perhaps, in animals as well. The animal data certainly would be consistent with the notion that, in general, CNS biochemistry may be more related to patterns of behavior than to psychiatric diagnoses, as has been discussed in an earlier review.[42]

In large part because of such animal data, we initiated one study in 1979[4] and reported a replication in 1982.[5] The independent studies were a joint effort between the National Naval Medical Center and the National Institute of Mental Health, both in Bethesda, Maryland, involving inpatient, active-duty military men of normal intelligence; the first study was comprised of 26 subjects and the second 12 (more subjects were not available for the second study). Their physical characteristics, be-

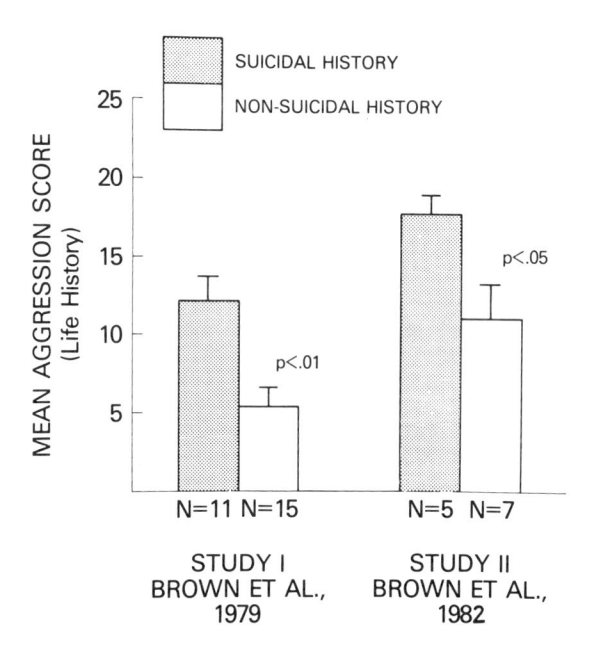

FIGURE 1. Suicidal history and aggression.

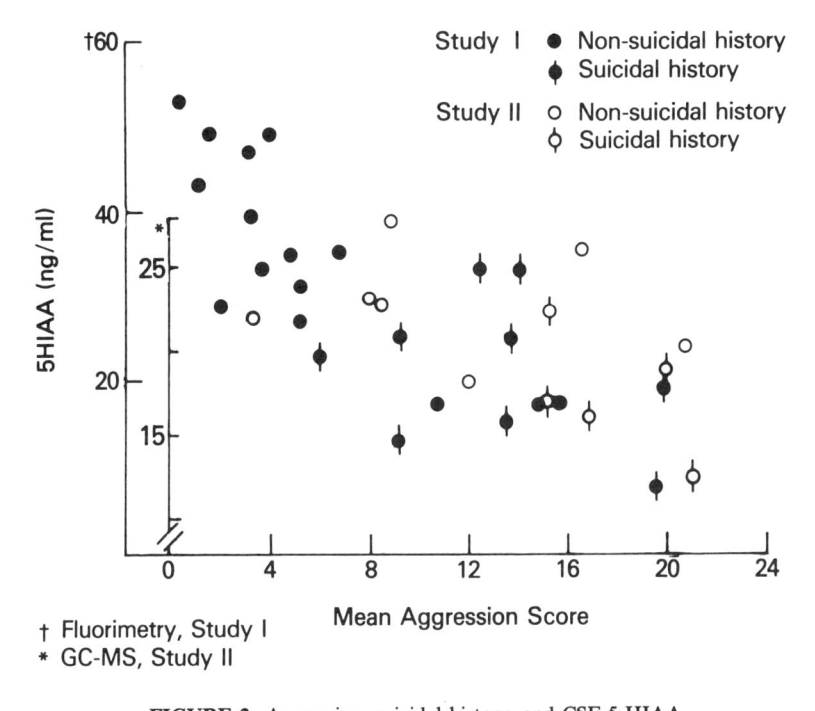

FIGURE 2. Aggression, suicidal history, and CSF 5-HIAA

havior histories, clinical symptomatology, and psychiatric diagnoses (primarily personality disorders) are described elsewhere in detail.[4,5] Exclusion criteria, methods to increase the likelihood of drug history veracity, clinical material available for evaluating each patient, the psychological and psychometric instruments used, biological procedures and assays, and statistical methods have also been reported elsewhere.[4,5,9,42-45]

In both studies, CSF 5-HIAA was negatively correlated with a history of aggressive behavior ($r = -0.78$; $n = 24$; $p < 0.01$ and $r = -0.53$; $n = 12$; $p < 0.08$, both two-tailed t-tests, respectively). In the second study, CSF 5-HIAA was negatively correlated with the psychopathic deviate (PD) scale of the Minnesota Multiphasic Personality Inventory (MMPI) ($r = 0.77$; $n = 12$; $p < 0.004$). Further, in both studies, life histories characterized by higher levels of aggression were associated with a history of suicidal behavior (FIGURE 1) and both patterns were associated with decreased CSF 5-HIAA. The trivariate relationship between a history of aggressive behavior, a history of suicidal behavior, and CSF 5-HIAA is readily apparent (FIGURE 2). Though CSF MHPG was correlated with a history of aggressive behavior in the first study, this finding was not replicated in a somewhat different diagnostic group in the second study. No relationship between aggression, suicide, and CSF HVA was found in either study.

Aggression history correlated significantly with Buss-Durkee Inventory (BDI) scores for total aggression, behavioral aggression, and hostility and with the PD scale of the MMPI as well. The PD scale score did not correlate significantly with the BDI scores for total aggression or behavioral aggression but did with the score for hostility.

LITERATURE REVIEW

Though suicide for many years had largely been attributed to sociopsychological variables, two human *in vivo* studies by Bunney et al.,[46,47] predating those of Asberg et al.[2,3] and Brown et al.,[4,5] did indicate a possible increased urinary steroid metabolite excretion in depressed patients who had made a suicidal attempt. Several follow-up studies provided conflicting results.[48-53] In three studies, plasma cortisol appears to correlate with suicidal behavior;[54-56] a single study of CSF cortisol[57] found no relationship with suicidal behavior. Earlier (1957-1976) autopsy studies of completed suicides,[58-63] usually in patients who were primarily depressed, indicated that either 5-HT or 5-HIAA was decreased in five of the six studies; other neurotransmitters (NE and DA) or their metabolites showed either inconsistent results or none at all. More recent autopsy studies of suicides report some changes in CNS neurotransmitter receptors with regard to 5-HT,[64-69] but more conflicting results with regard to AcH[65] and other receptors.[69]

Since the initial clinical and biological studies linking suicide[2,3] and aggression,[4,5] there have been five additional studies published relating aggressive/impulsive behavior, suicidal behavior, and CSF 5-HIAA (see TABLE 1).[70-74] CSF MHPG and HVA have yielded inconsistent results. Those of Bioulac et al. from France reported decreased CSF 5-HIAA turnover (via the probenecid method) in 47, XYY institution-

TABLE 1. Aggressive/Impulsive Behavior, Suicidal Behavior, and CSF 5-HIAA[a]

		CSF 5-HIAA	
Study	Diagnosis	Aggressive/ Impulsive Behavior	Suicidal Behavior
1. Brown et al., 1979	Personality disorders (military)	↓	↓
2. Bioulac et al., 1978, 80	Personality disorders XYY (prisoners)	↓[b]	?
3. Brown et al., 1982	Borderline disorders (military)	↓	↓
4. Linnoila et al., 1983	Personality disorders (prisoners)	↓	↓
5. Lidberg et al., 1984	Murderers of own children (forensic)	↓[c]	↓
6. Lidberg et al., 1985	Murderers—depression anxiety, personality disorders (forensic)	↓[c,d]	↓

[a] One of 4 studies in which CSF HVA was examined found it lower in more aggressive subjects; 1 of 3 studies in which CSF MHPG was examined found it higher in more aggressive subjects ↓ = decrease; ? = not reported (see study for details). Branchey et al., 1984 (alcoholics)—↓ plasma tryptophan/neutral amino acids in more aggressive subjects.

[b] Postprobenecid.

[c] Not necessarily a history of aggressivity/impulsivity.

[d] Only if victims were sexual partners and subjects were not alcoholics.

TABLE 2. Violent and Nonviolent Suicidal Behavior and CSF 5-HIAA[a]

		CSF 5-HIAA	
Study	Diagnosis	Violent Suicide	Nonviolent Suicide
1. Asberg et al., 1976 (2)	Unipolar depression	↓↓	NS
2. Oreland et al. 1981; Traskman et al., 1981	Depression and controls (anxiety; personality disorders)	↓↓	↓
3. van Praag, 1982	Depression	↓↓	↓
4. van Praag, 1983	Schizophrenia	↓↓	↓
5. Roy-Byrne et al., 1983	Unipolar depression Bipolar depression	NS[b] NS	NS NS
6. Banki et al., 1983 (2), 1984	Depression, schizophrenia, alcoholism, adjustment disorder	↓	NS
7. Roy et al., 1985	Schizophrenia	NS	NS

[a] One of three studies in which CSF HVA was examined found it lower in violent attempts; CSF MHPG was examined in two studies and was lower in neither. ↓ = decrease; ↓↓ = greater decrease; NS = nonsignificant change (see study for details).

[b] Nonsignificantly lower in unipolar depressives.

alized criminals[70,71]—though the history of aggression was not quantified in these reports, descriptions of aggressive behaviors were provided. Linnoila et al. studied incarcerated murderers in Finland;[72] of further interest, it was noted that those personality disorder diagnoses associated particularly with impulsivity, i.e., antisocial and explosive, had the lowest levels of CSF 5-HIAA. These more specific clinical findings replicated the earlier work of Brown et al.[4,43,44] Lower CSF 5-HIAA was also associated with a history of suicidal behavior in the Finnish group. Lidberg et al. in Sweden have published reports of three suicidal individuals who killed their own children; all three individuals had quite low levels of CSF 5-HIAA. Lidberg et al. have more recently reported a larger group of murderers in whom suicide was related to lower CSF;[74] however, only those who murdered sexual partners (and were not alcoholics) had lower levels of CSF 5-HIAA contrasted to nonemotional or nonviolent murderers, e.g., a murderer who had killed a number of patients in a nursing home because of a belief in euthanasia. All of these studies taken together tend to lend credence to the idea that some form of impulsivity, disinhibition, or dyscontrol is the behavioral variable linked to CSF 5-HIAA and not antisocial acts in and of themselves.

Following the initial Asberg reports, nine studies have assessed the relationship between CSF 5-HIAA and violent vs. nonviolent suicidal behavior (TABLE 2).[75-83] CSF MHPG and HVA have yielded inconsistent results. Five of seven groups of patients with lower CSF 5-HIAA also had a history of violent suicidal attempt, whereas four of seven groups had lower (but less so) CSF 5-HIAA if they had had a history of suicidal behavior by nonviolent means. Two studies showed no relationship between low CSF 5-HIAA in those with histories of violent or nonviolent suicidal attempts.[79-83] In general, the distinction between violent and nonviolent suicide has been using guns, knives, and/or hanging for the former and minor cuts and overdoses for the latter. Among studies in TABLE 1, the diagnoses are primarily personality disorders; whereas among those in TABLE 2, the diagnoses are primarily major affective disorders and schizophrenia.

Another nine studies (TABLE 3)[84-92] have also reported observations of suicidal behavior and CSF 5-HIAA, MHPG, and HVA in which the aggressivity or violent nature of the suicide was not reported, nor was any life history of the subject's aggressivity/impulsivity. In these studies, seven of nine have reported a lower level of CSF 5-HIAA and suicidal behavior. Again, among these studies, CSF MHPG and HVA have yielded inconsistent results. These studies have primarily been comprised of major affective disorders. The subjects in all previously cited CSF 5-HIAA-suicide-aggression studies have been either European or American, but one study in this last group reports decreased CSF 5-HIAA in depressive Indian patients with a history of suicidal behavior (though no biochemical findings were related specifically to subtypes of depression).[90] A more recent study from Spain, not tabulated, further corroborates a significant negative correlation between suicidal/self-aggressive behavior and CSF 5-HIAA in unipolar depressives; aggressivity within fifteen days prior to lumbar puncture did not correlate with CSF 5-HIAA.[93] The fact that a similar behavioral-biochemical association has been found from such diverse social, cultural, and national backgrounds could be some evidence for a biological contribution in some suicidal/aggressive behaviors that is more basic than environmental and/or social variables.

TABLE 3. Suicidal Behavior and CSF Amine Metabolites

Study	Diagnosis	5-HIAA	HVA	MHPG
1. Vestergard et al., 1978	Unipolar depression Bipolar depression	NS	—	—
2. Agren, 1980	Unipolar depression Bipolar depression	↓ NS	NS NS	↓ NS
3. Leckman et al., 1981	Affective and schizophrenic psychoses	↓[b]	NS	NS
4. Banki et al., 1981	Major depression	↓	NS	—
5. Montgomery et al., 1982	Depression and personality disorder	↓	↓	—
6. Agren, 1983	Unipolar depression Bipolar depression	↓ NS	NS NS	↓ NS
7. Palaniappan et al., 1983	Depression	↓	↓	NS
8. Ninan et al., 1984	Schizophrenia	↓	—	—
9. Berrettini et al., 1985	Euthymic bipolar depression	NS	NS	—

[a] ↓ = decrease; NS = nonsignificant change; — = not measured (see study for details).
[b] Suicidal ideation.

TABLE 4. Relationship of Aggressivity/Impulsivity, Suicide, and CSF 5-HIAA

	No. of Studies Identifying Suicidal Behavior	No. of Studies Identifying Other Aggressive/ Impulsive Behavior	CSF 5-HIAA Decrease
Diagnoses			
Aggressive personality disorder	6	6	6/6 (100%)
Unipolar depression	12	0	10/12 (83%)
Schizophrenia	4	0	3/4 (75%)
Alcoholics	2	2	1/2 (50%)
Bipolar depression	6	0	0/6 (0%)
Suicide Method			
Violent	7	0	5/7 (71%)
Nonviolent	7	0	3/7 (43%)

Of particular interest is that a relationship between suicidal behavior and CSF 5-HIAA has not been observed in any of five studies in TABLES 2 and 3 in which the diagnoses were bipolar affective illness.

Though relatively little has been published that pertains to the behavioral interactions of suicide, aggression/impulsivity, and 5-HIAA in alcoholics, several studies are of interest. Two early studies have shown no difference between alcoholics and nonalcoholic controls during an abstinent state with regard to CSF 5HVA;[94,95] however, the latter group of investigators later showed that CSF 5-HIAA decreased with the interval of time between acute intoxication and a period of "drying out."[96] Branchey et al. (see TABLE 1) have shown the plasma tryptophan (TP)/neutral amino acid (NAA) ratio to be lower in alcoholics, particularly those with a history of suicidal and aggressive/impulsive behaviors.[97] The TP/NAA ratio[98,99] is important in that it is directly related to the amount of TP, the dietary precursor of 5-HT, that is transported across the blood-brain barrier for the synthesis of 5-HT in the CNS. Furthermore, these alcoholics showed a statistically significant relationship between suicidal behavior and aggressive behavior much as that reported in the two studies by Brown et al.[4,5] Of further interest, the murderers reported by Lidberg et al., who were also alcoholics, tended to have normal levels of CSF 5-HIAA.[73] Though more studies need to be done in alcoholics, the studies thus far reported suggest the hypothesis that some alcoholics may be subject to excessive drinking as an attempt to treat themselves for depressive, aggressive, and suicidal affects.

Though the studies reviewed above would generally support the notion that CNS biochemistry may be more related to patterns of behavior than to psychiatric diagnoses,[42] and further, such a concept would be more consistent with the animal data cited above, a now obvious problem is the data from those subjects with bipolar illness (see TABLE 4). The data from bipolar illness are nonsupportive of the suicide/CSF 5-HIAA association; whereas, the data are generally supportive of that association in aggressive personality disorders, unipolar illness, schizophrenia, and, equivocally, alcoholism. Yet, the incidence of suicide is quite high in manic-depressive illness[100] and alcoholism.[101] Possibly, CSF 5-HIAA is less strongly linked to suicidal behavior than it is to aggressive behavior, since none of the studies reporting bipopolar illness have included any assessment of repetitive aggressive, impulsive behaviors. Are manic-depressives generally aggressive/impulsive during euthymic intervals? Further, are there predispositions to suicidal behaviors in bipolar illness other than the possible suicide/CSF 5-HIAA link observed in other disorders? With regard to alcoholism, the hypothesis that drinking might be a form of self-medication to elevate CNS 5-HT levels (as indirectly suggested by CSF 5-HIAA studies) was proposed above. Similarly, lithium, the most prevalent treatment for bipolar illness, elevates CSF 5-HIAA;[92,102,103] importantly, studies involving bipolars have been variable with regard to histories of suicidal and aggressive/impulsive behaviors as well as medication status. Carbamazepine, a more recent treatment for manic-depressive illness, has also been reported to reduce aggressive/impulsive behaviors,[33] possibly by having an influence on peripheral TP.[104]

The central question appears to be a necessary, but not sufficient, role for 5-HT in both suicidal and aggressive behaviors. In that sense, an affect of aggressive rage may be critical for the development of depression and, in some instances, suicide; thus, aggression being a more primitive affective response to the environment than depression. Such a construct appears consistent with the fact that aggression is found at all ages in all species (and probably in all individuals),[105] but clinically significant depression and suicide are not. Furthermore, since a small number of "normal" subjects, i.e., those that do not report a history of either suicidal or aggressive/impulsive behaviors, have also been shown to have a lower CSF 5-HIAA than other normals, one would question whether the former group might be different in some ways other than CSF 5-HIAA. For example, normals show a significant negative correlation between a measure of sensation seeking[12] and CSF NE.[106] If so, what kind of "compensating" mechanisms—biological, psychological, or social—might be coming into play? Perhaps of equal interest, are there individuals with histories of suicidal and/or aggressive/impulsive behaviors who have high levels of CSF 5-HIAA?

Since considerable new data have been added to the literature in recent years regarding the possible biological contributions to suicidal and aggressive/impulsive behavior, it would now appear an important period to reassess some of the nonbiological questions that might be further studied. For example, if a certain propensity for self-destructive behavior exists in certain individuals "waiting for the right kind of environmental stress," what new clinical studies might be done to assess the families and childhood of such individuals, since biological data seem to suggest the strong possibility of a trait, just as earlier studies have indicated the strong possibility of a genetic contribution to both suicidal behavior[26] and aggressive, antisocial behavior.[107,108] Brown et al. have recently reported that the level of self-reported childhood problems (particularly conduct problems and those associated with "minimal brain dysfunction") were significantly negatively related to the levels of CSF 5-HIAA found in young adult males.[45] Stoff et al. also recently reported a decrease in platelet [³H]imipramine binding (thought to be a periphral marker of 5-HT activity) in boys with aggressive, conduct disorders vs. pediatric controls.[109] Both studies would tend to buttress the argument that CSF 5-HIAA is related to human aggressive/impulsive behavior as a trait variable.

In summary, there have now been a substantial number of scientific reports indicating that CNS 5-HT may be altered in suicidal and aggressive/impulsive behaviors in humans, largely consistent with the animal data, and these reports constitute one of the most highly replicated finding in biological psychiatry. That CNS 5-HT has been associated with animal aggression prior to its hypothesized relationship to suicidal behavior in humans might suggest that some suicidal behavior may be a special kind of self-destructive behavior in humans, though perhaps not absolutely unique to humans.

REFERENCES

1. FREUD, S. 1953. Mourning and melancholia. *In* Standard Edition of the Complete Psychological Works of Sigmund Freud. J. Strachey, A. Strachey & A. Tyson, Eds.: 237-260. Hogarth Press. London, England.
2. ASBERG, M., P. THOREN & L. TRASKMAN. 1976. Science **191**: 478-480.
3. ASBERG, M., L. TRASKMAN & P. THOREN. 1976. Arch. Gen. Psychiatry **33**: 1193-1197.
4. BROWN, G. L., F. K. GOODWIN, J. C. BALLENGER, P. F. GOYER & L. F. MAJOR. 1979. Psychiatry Res. **1**: 131-139.
5. BROWN, G. L., M. H. EBERT, P. F. GOYER, D. C. JIMERSON, W. J. KLEIN, W. E. BUNNEY, JR. & F. K. GOODWIN. 1982. Am. J. Psychiatry **139**: 741-746.
6. MOYER, K. E. 1968. Commun. Behav. Biol. Part A **2**: 65-87.
7. REIS, O. J. 1974. Res. Publ. Assoc. Res. Nerv. Ment. Dis. **52**: 119-148.
8. JONES, I. H. 1982. Perspect. Biol. Med. **26**: 137.
9. BROWN, G. L. & F. K. GOODWIN. 1984. Aggression, adolescence and psychobiology. *In* The Aggressive Adolescent: Clinical Perspectives. C. Keith, Ed.: 63-95. The Free Press, MacMillan Inc. New York, N.Y.
10. CRAWLEY, J. N., M. E. SUTTON & D. PICKAR. 1985. Animal models of self-destructive behavior and suicide. *In* Symposium on Self-Destructive Behavior. Psychiatr. Clin. North Am. **8**: 299-310.
11. FOSSEY, D. 1972. Living with mountain gorillas. *In* The Marvels of Animal Behavior. P. R. Marder, Ed.: 208. National Geographic Society. Washington, D.C.
12. ZUCKERMAN, M. 1983. *In* Biological Bases of Sensation Seeking, Impulsivity, and Anxiety. M. Zuckerman, Ed.: 37-76. Lawrence Erlbaum Associates. Hillside, N.J.
13. CARL, E. A. 1971. Ecology **52**: 395.
14. CALHOUN, J. B. 1962. Sci. Am. **206**: 139.
15. BACH-Y-RITA, G. & A. VERO. 1974. Am. J. Psychiatry **131**: 1015.
16. MAIER, S. F. & M. E. SELIGMAN. 1976. J. Exp. Psychol. **1**: 3.
17. OVERMIER, J. B. & M. D. SELIGMAN. 1976. J. Comp. Physiol. Psychol. **63**: 23.
18. SHERMAN, A. D., *et al.* 1982. Pharm. Biochem. Behav. **16**: 449.
19. PETTY, F. & A. D. SHERMAN. 1983. Pharm. Biochem. Behav. **18**: 649-650.
20. PETTY, F. & A. D. SHERMAN. 1980. Life Sci. **26**: 1447-1452.
21. HARLOW, H. F. & M. K. HARLOW. 1959. Sci. Am. **200**: 68-74.
22. SUOMI, S. J., H. F. HARLOW & W. T. MCKINNEY. 1972. Am. J. Psychiatry **128**: 927.
23. MCKINNEY, W. T., E. C. MORAN & G. W. KRAEMER. 1984. Separation in nonhuman primates as a model for human depression: neurobiological implications. *In* Neurobiology of Mood Disorders. R. M. Post & J. C. Ballenger, Eds. **1**: 393-406. Williams & Wilkins. Baltimore, Md.
24. SPITZ, R. A. & K. M. WOLF. 1946. Anaclitic depression: an inquiry into the genesis of psychiatric conditions in early childhood. II. *In* Psychoanalytic Study of the Child. P. Greenacre *et al.*, Eds. **2**: 313-339. International Universities Press. New York, N.Y.
25. POWELL, G. F., J. A. BRASEL, S. RAITI & R. M. BLIZZARD. 1967. N. Engl. J. Med. **276**: 1279.
26. KETY, S. S. 1979. Sci. Am. **241**: 202-214.
27. SCHULSINGER, F., S. S. KETY, D. ROSENTHAL & P. H. WENDER. 1979. A family study of suicide. *In* Origin, Prevention and Treatment of Affective Disorders. M. Schou & E. Stromgren, Eds.: 277-287. Academic Press. London, England.
28. SALK, L., L. P. LIPSITT, W. Q. STURNER, B. M. REILLY & R. H. LEVAT. 1985. Lancet: 624-627.
29. WEST, L. J. 1977. Psychopharmacol. Bull. **13**: 14-25.
30. ORENBERG, E. K., J. RENSON, G. R. ELIOTT, J. D. BARCHAS & S. KESSLER. 1975. Commun. Psychopharmacol. **1**: 99-107.
31. ANGEL, C., D. C. DELUCA & O. D. MURPHREE. 1976. Biol. Psychiatry **11**: 743-753.
32. SHEARD, M. 1971. Nature **230**: 113-114.
33. LUCHINS, D. J. 1983. Lancet i: 766.
34. LEVENTHAL, B. L. 1984. The neuropharmacology of violent and aggressive behavior. *In* The Aggressive Adolescent: Clinical Perspectives. C. R. Keith, Ed.: 299-358. The Free Press, MacMillan Inc. New York, N.Y.

35. EICHELMAN, B. 1979. Role of biogenic amines in aggressive behavior. *In* Psychopharmacology of Aggression. M. Sandler, Ed.: 61-93. Raven Press. New York, N.Y.
36. VALZELLI, L. 1981. Psychobiology of Aggression and Violence. Raven Press. New York, N.Y.
37. POKORNY, A. D. 1983. Arch. Gen. Psychiatry **40:** 249-257.
38. ROBINS, L. N. 1978. Psychol. Med. **8:** 611-622.
39. BESKOW, J. 1979. Acta Psychiatr. Scand. (Suppl.) **277:** 85-88.
40. CHRISTMAS, A. J. & D. R. MAXWELL. 1970. Neuropharmacology **9:** 17-29.
41. MARKS, P., M. O'BRIEN & G. PAXINOS. 1977. Brain Res. **135:** 383-388.
42. BROWN, G. L., F. K. GOODWIN & W. E. BUNNEY, JR. 1982. Human aggression and suicide: their relationship to neuropsychiatric diagnoses and serotonin metabolism. Adv. Biochem. Psychopharmacol. **34:** 287-307.
43. BROWN, G. L., J. C. BALLENGER, M. D. MINICHIELLO & F. K. GOODWIN. 1979. Human aggression and its relationship to cerebrospinal fluid 5-hydroxyindoleacetic acid, 3-methoxy-4-hydroxyphenylglycol and homovanillic acid. *In* Psychopharmacology of Aggression. M. Sandler, Ed.: 131-148. Raven Press. New York, N.Y.
44. BROWN, G. L. & F. K. GOODWIN. 1984. Clin. Neuropharmacol. **7:** 756-757.
45. BROWN, G. L., W. J. KLINE, P. F. GOYER, M. D. MINICHIELLO, M. J. P. KREUSI & F. K. GOODWIN. 1986. Relationship of childhood characteristics to cerebrospinal fluid 5-hydroxyindoleacetic acid in aggressive adults. *In* Biological Psychiatry, 1985. C. Shagass, R. C. Josiassen, W. H. Bridger, K. J. Weiss, D. Stoff & G. M. Simpson, Eds. **7:** 177-179. Elsevier. New York, N.Y.
46. BUNNEY, W. E., JR. & J. A. FAWCETT. 1965. Arch. Gen. Psychiatry **13:** 232-239.
47. BUNNEY, W. E., JR., J. A. FAWCETT, J. M. DAVIS & S. GIFFORD. 1969. Arch. Gen. Psychiatry **21:** 138-150.
48. LEVY, B. & E. HANSEN. 1969. Arch. Gen. Psychiatry **20:** 415-418.
49. KRIEGER, G. 1970. Dis. Nerv. System **31:** 478-482.
50. FINK, E. B. & W. L. CARPENTER. 1976. Dis. Nerv. System **37:** 341-343.
51. ROCKWELL, D. A., C. M. WINGET, L. S. ROSENBLATT, E. A. HIGGINS & N. W. HETHERINGTON. 1978. J. Nerv. Ment. Dis. **166:** 851-858.
52. OSTROFF, R., E. GILLER, K. BONESE, E. EBERSOLE, L. HARKNESS & J. MASON. 1982. Am. J. Psychiatry **139:** 1323-1325.
53. PRASAD, A. J. 1985. Neuropsychobiology **13:** 157-159.
54. PLATMAN, J. R., R. PLUTCHIK & B. WEINSTEIN. 1971. J. Psychiatr. Res. **8:** 127-137.
55. KRIEGER, G. 1974. Dis. Nerv. System **35:** 237-240.
56. MELTZER, H. Y., R. PERLINE, B. J. TRICOU, M. LOWRY & A. ROBERTSON. 1984. Arch. Gen. Psychiatry **41:** 379-390.
57. TRASKMAN, L., G. TYBRING, M. ASBERG, L. BERTILSSON, O. LANTTO & D. SCHALLING. 1980. Arch. Gen. Psychiatry **37:** 761-767.
58. SHAW, D. M., F. E. CAMPS & E. G. ECCLESTON. 1967. Br. J. Psychiatry **113:** 1407-1411.
59. BOURNE, H. R., W. E. BUNNEY, JR., R. W. COLBURN, J. M. DAVIS, J. N. DAVIS, D. M. SHAW & A. COPPEN. 1968. Lancet **2:** 805-808.
60. PARE, C. M. B., D. P. H. YEUNG, K. PRICE & R. S. STACEY. 1969. Lancet **2:** 133-135.
61. LLOYD, K. G., I. J. FARLEY, J. H. N. DECK & O. HORNYKIEWICZ. 1974. Serotonin and 5-hydroxyindoleacetic acid in discrete areas of the brainstem of suicide victims and control patients. *In* Serotonin: New Vistas. E. Costa, G. L. Gessa & M. Sandler, Eds.: 387-397. Raven Press. New York, N.Y.
62. BESKOW, J., C. G. GOTTFRIES, B. E. ROOS & B. WINBLAD. 1976. Acta Psychiatr. Scand. **53:** 7-20.
63. COCHRAN, E., E. ROBINS & S. GROTE. 1976. Biol. Psychiatry **11:** 283-294.
64. STANLEY, M., J. VIRGILIO & S. GERSHON. 1982. Science **216:** 1337-1339.
65. MEYERSON, L. R., L. P. WENNOGLE, M. S. ABEL, J. COUPET, A. S. LIPPA, C. E. RAU & B. BEER. 1982. **17:** 159-163.
66. STANLEY, M. & J. J. MANN. 1983. Lancet **i:** 214-216.
67. PERRY, E. K., E. F. MARSHALL, G. BLESSED, B. E. TOMLINSON & R. H. PERRY. 1983. Br. J. Psychiatry **142:** 188-192.
68. STANLEY, M. & J. J. MANN. 1984. Lancet **i:** 349.

69. CROW, T. J., A. J. CROSS, S. J. COOPER, J. F. W. DEAKIN, I. N. FERRIER, J. A. JOHNSON, M. H. JOSEPH, F. OWEN, M. POULTER, R. LOFTHOUSE. J. A. N. CORSELLIS, D. R. CHAMBERS, G. BLESSED, E. K. PERRY, R. H. PERRY & B. E. TOMLINSON. 1984. Neuropharmacology 23: 1561-1569.
70. BIOULAC, B., M. BENEZECH, B. RENAUD, D. ROCHE & B. NOEL. 1978. Neuropsychopharmacology 4: 366-370.
71. BIOULAC, B., M. BENEZECH, B. RENAUD, B. NOEL & D. ROCHE. 1980. Biol. Psychiatry 15: 917-923.
72. LINNOILA, M., M. VIRKKUNEN, M. SCHEININ, A. NUUTILA, R. RIMON & F. K. GOODWIN. 1983. Life Sci. 33: 2609-2614.
73. LIDBERG, L., M. ASBERG & U. B. SUNQUIST-STENSMAN. 1984. Lancet ii: 928.
74. LIDBERG, L., J. R. TUCK, M. ASBERG, G. P. SCALIA-TOMBA & L. BERTILSSON. 1985. Acta Psychiatr. Scand. 71: 230-236.
75. ORELAND, L., A. WEIBERG, M. ASBERG, L. TRASKMAN, L. SJOSTRAND, P. THOREN, L. BERTILSSON & G. TYBRING. 1981. Psychiatry Res. 4: 21-29.
76. TRASKMAN, L., M. ASBERG, L. BERTILSSON & L. SJOSTRAND. 1981. Arch. Gen. Psychiatry 38: 631-636.
77. VAN PRAAG, H. M. 1982. J. Affect. Disord. 4: 275-290.
78. VAN PRAAG, H. M. 1983. Lancet ii: 977-978.
79. ROY-BYRNE, P., R. M. POST, D. R. RUBINOW, M. LINNOILA, R. SAVARD & D. DAVIS. 1983. Psychiatry Res. 10: 263-274.
80. BANKI, C. M. & M. ARATO. 1983. J. Affect. Disord. 5: 223-232.
81. BANKI, C. M. & M. ARATO. 1983. Psychiatry Res. 10: 253-261.
82. BANKI, C. M., M. ARATO, Z. PAPP & M. KURCZ. 1984. J. Affect. Disord. 6: 341-350.
83. ROY, A., P. NINAN, A. MAZONSON, D. PICKAR, D. VAN KAMMEN, M. LINNOILA & S. M. PAUL. 1985. Psychol. Med. 15: 335-340.
84. VESTERGAARD, P., T. SORENSEN, E. HOPPE, O. J. RAFAELSON, C. M. YATES & N. NICOLAOU. 1978. Acta Psychiatr. Scand. 58: 88-96.
85. AGREN, H. 1980. Psychiatry Res. 3: 225-236.
86. LECKMAN, J. F., D. S. CHARNEY, C. R. NELSON, G. R. HENINGER & M. B. BOWERS, JR. 1981. CSF tryptophan, 5HIAA and HVA in 132 psychiatric patients categorized by diagnosis and clinical state. In Recent Advances in Neuropsychopharmacology. B. Angrist, G. D. Burrows, M. Lader, D. Lingjaerde, G. Sedvall & D. Wheatley, Eds.: 289-297. Pergamon Press. New York, N.Y.
87. BANKI, C. M., G. MOLNAR & M. VOJNIK. 1981. J. Affect. Disord. 3: 91-99.
88. MONTGOMERY, S. A. & D. B. MONTGOMERY. 1982. J. Affect. Disord. 4: 291-298.
89. AGREN, H. 1983. Psychiatr. Dev. 1: 87-104.
90. PALANIAPPAN, V., V. RAMACHANDRAN & D. SOMASUNDARAM. 1983. Indian J. Psychiatry 25: 286-292.
91. NINAN, P. T., D. P. VAN KAMMEN, M. SCHEININ, M. LINNOILA, W. E. BUNNEY, JR. & F. K. GOODWIN. 1984. Am. J. Psychiatry 141: 566-569.
92. BERRETTINI, W. H., J. I. NURNBERGER, JR., M. SCHEININ, T. SEPPALA, M. LINNOILA, W. NARROW, S. SIMMONS-ALLING & E. S. GERSHON. 1985. Biol. Psychiatry 20: 257-269.
93. LÓPEZ-IBOR, J. J., JR., J. SAIZ-RUIZ & J. C. PÉREZ DE LOS COBOS. 1985 Neuropsychobiology 14: 67-74.
94. TAKAHASKI, S., H. YAMANE, H. KONDO & N. TANI. 1974. Folia Psychiatr. Neurol. Jpn. 28: 347-354.
95. MAJOR, L. F., J. C. BALLENGER, F. K. GOODWIN & G. L. BROWN. 1977. Biol. Psychiatry 12: 635-642.
96. BALLENGER, J. C., F. K. GOODWIN, L. F. MAJOR & G. L. BROWN. 1979. Arch. Gen. Psychiatry 36: 224-227.
97. BRANCHEY, L., M. BRANCHEY, S. SHAW & C. S. LIEBER. 1984. Psychiatry Res. 12: 219-226.
98. OLENDORF, W. H. & J. SZABO. 1976. Am. J. Physiol. 230: 94-98.
99. GESSA, G. L., G. BIGGLIO, F. FADDA, C. V. CORSINI & A. TAGLIAMONTE. 1974. J. Neurochem. 22: 869-870.

100. JAMISON, K. R. 1986. *In* Manic-Depressive Illness. F. K. Goodwin & K. R. Jamison, Eds. Oxford Press. New York, N.Y. (In press.)
101. ROY, A. & M. LINNOILA. 1986. Suicide and alcoholism. Suicide Life-Threat. Behav. (In press.)
102. BOWERS, M. B., JR., G. R. HENINGER, & F. A. GERBODE. 1969. Int. J. Neuropharmacol. **8:** 255-262.
103. FYRO, B., U. PETTERSON & G. SEDVALL. 1975. Psychopharmacologia. **44:** 99-103.
104. PRATT, J., P. JENNER, A. L. JOHNSON, S. D. SHOWON & E. H. REYNOLDS. 1984. J. Neurol. Neurosurg. Psychiatry **47:** 1131-1133.
105. ARNOLD, L., R. FLEMING & B. A. BELL. 1979. Can. J. Psychiatry **24:** 762-766.
106. BALLENGER, J. C., R. M. POST, D. C. JIMERSON, C. R. LAKE, D. L. MURPHY, M. ZUCKERMAN & C. CRONIN. 1984. Personality Indiv. Dif.: 1-11.
107. HUTCHINGS, B. & S. A. MEDNICK. 1975. Registered criminality in the adoptive and biological parents of registered male criminal adoptecs. *In* Genetic Research in Psychiatry. R. R. Fieve, D. Rosenthal & H. Brill, Eds.: 105-116. The Johns Hopkins University Press. Baltimore, Md.
108. MEDNICK, S. A. & B. HUTCHINGS. 1978. J. Am. Acad. Child Psychiatry **17:** 209-223.
109. STOFF, D. M., L. POLLOCK & W. H. BRIDGER. 1986. Platelet imipramine binding sites correlate with aggression in adolescents. *In* Biological Psychiatry, 1985. C. Shagass, R. C. Josiassen, W. H. Bridger, K. J. Weiss, D. Stoff & G. M. Simpson, Eds. **7:** 180-182. Elsevier. New York, N.Y.

Suicide and Aggression in Schizophrenia

Neurobiologic Correlates

DAVID PICKAR, ALEC ROY, ALAN BREIER,
ALLEN DORAN, OWEN WOLKOWITZ,
JEAN COLISON, AND HANS AGREN[a]

*Section on Clinical Studies
Clinical Neuroscience Branch
National Institute of Mental Health
Building 10, Room 4N214
9000 Rockville Pike
Bethesda, Maryland 20892*

Whereas affective illness is the most prevalent psychiatric diagnosis associated with attempted and completed suicide,[1] suicide risk in schizophrenic patients is high and its management important to the long-term care of the schizophrenic patient. In a retrospective analysis of 127 *Diagnostic and Statistical Manual,* third edition (DSM III) diagnosed schizophrenic patients consecutively admitted to our National Institute of Mental Health research ward, Roy *et al.* reported a 55% incidence of life history of attempted suicide,[2] a figure that, though high for schizophrenia overall, reflects the prevalence of suicide attempts in chronically ill schizophrenic patients. These authors also reported significantly higher incidences of depressive symptomatology, sufficient in severity to meet DSM III criteria for major depression episode, and higher numbers of previous hospital admissions in suicide attempters in comparison to nonattempters. Taken together, clinical data suggest that young schizophrenic patients, particularly male, suffering from a severe, chronic illness with intermittent depressive symptoms are at greatest risk of suicide attempt.[3] Although suicide attempts are often made when patients are treated with neuroleptic medications, specific neuroleptics appear not to be directly related to enhanced suicide risk.[4,5]

In contrast to suicidal behavior, aggressive and hostile behaviors are more common among schizophrenic than depressed patients,[6] particularly when violent suicide attempts are excluded. While aggression is neither restricted to nor necessarily more frequent in schizophrenic than selected other groups such as criminal populations, drug abusers, or certain personality disorders, aggressive behaviors in schizophrenic patients are not infrequent in inpatient settings and represent a particular challenge to clinical management. In a recent prospective study using factor analysis methodology, Yesavage reported that the best predictor of aggressive or violent acts among inpatient schizophrenics was low neuroleptic serum levels, although severity of symptomatology and history of prior violence were also significant predictors.[7]

---

[a] Section on Clinical Pharmacology, Laboratory of Clinical Science, NIMH.

Studies attempting to identify the biologic substrates underlying suicidal behavior have suggested an association between suicidality and (1) hyperactivity of the hypothalamic-pituitary-adrenal axis[8-10] and (2) diminished central nervous system (CNS) serotonin metabolism as reflected by low levels of cerebrospinal fluid (CSF) 5-hydroxyindoleacetic acid (5-HIAA).[11-13] Of these factors, disordered serotonin metabolism has received the greatest attention with some data suggesting that low levels of CSF 5-HIAA may represent a trait marker for suicidal and aggressive behavior across diagnostic categories.[13-17] Although most studies have focused on depressed or mixed patient groups, van Praag et al.[16] and Ninan et al.[17] have reported lower levels of CSF 5-HIAA in schizophrenic patients with histories of violent attempted suicide.

We have previously reported levels of CSF 5-HIAA, homovanillic acid (HVA), and 3-methoxy-4-hydroxyphenylglycol (MHPG) in a group of 54 DSM III diagnosed schizophrenic patients, 27 (50%) with histories of suicide attempt.[18] Analysis, including consideration of violent and nonviolent attempts and covariance for height and age, revealed no significant relationship between the CSF amine metabolite levels and suicide histories. In this current study we have examined a new cohort of 28 schizophrenic patients, focusing on life histories of suicide attempts and measures of aggressive behavior when free from neuroleptics in comparison to levels of CSF amine metabolites, response to the dexamethasone suppression test (DST), and measures of ventricular size by computerized tomography (CT) scan.

METHODS

Subjects

Twenty-eight consecutively admitted DSM-III[19] diagnosed schizophrenic inpatients of the NIMH 4-East research ward of the National Institutes of Health Clinical Center (14 male, 14 female) granted informed written consent to participate in these studies of neurochemical correlates of illness and behavior. These patients are representative of relatively young [mean ± standard error of the mean (SEM) age: 28 ± 2 years], chronically ill schizophrenic patients. Patients with histories of seriously violent, criminal, or persistent suicidal behaviors were excluded from admission and study. All patients were free from medical and neurological illnesses. Double-blind medications were begun within two weeks of hospital admission; patients who were treated with neuroleptics prior to admission were first placed on clinically determined doses of fluphenazine. After at least three weeks on a stabilized fluphenazine regimen, placebo was substituted. Behavioral ratings throughout were performed blind to medication status.

Behavioral Variables

Past history of suicide attempt was determined for each patient on the basis of detailed record review. Number of suicide attempts ranged from 0-6; for data analysis the presence or absence of a history of any suicide attempt was used.

Physician ratings of the Brief Psychiatric Rating Scale (BPRS)[20] items "hostility" and "uncooperativeness" provided a reflection of aggression-related behaviors. The effect of double-blind neuroleptic treatment on these BPRS items was studied in a representative subgroup of 19 patients. Ratings made during the week of lumbar puncture were used for comparisons with levels of CSF monoamine metabolites. The use of the following two clinical interventions to manage aggressive behaviors were also recorded: (1) seclusion room restriction and (2) sedative wet sheet pack (SWSP) restraint. The need for these restrictions was determined clinically by the ward staff.

Neurobiologic Measures

Lumbar punctures (LP) were performed in 25 patients after at least three weeks of placebo (mean ± SEM drug-free days: 29 ± 4); the remaining 3 patients were free from neuroleptic treatment for greater than six months at the time of study. All patients followed a low monoamine, alcohol-free, and caffeine-restricted diet beginning on admission to the ward. LPs were performed between 8:30 and 9:00 with the patients in the lateral decubitus position following an overnight fast and bed-rest restriction. The first 10 ml of CSF was collected as a pool and placed on ice at the bedside, subsequently aliquoted, and then frozen at $-80°C$ until time of assay. CSF was assayed using high-pressure liquid chromatography with electrochemical detection for levels of 5-HIAA, HVA, and MHPG.[21] CSF levels were not corrected for age or height.

The DST was performed in 24 of the patients after at least two weeks on placebo medication. Blood for cortisol determinations was drawn at 4:00 PM on the day prior to an 11:00 PM dose of dexamethasone (1 mg) and again at 4:00 PM and 11:00 PM on the following day. Cortisol determinations were performed using a radioimmunoassay (Diagnostic Products Corporation). A maximum postdexamethasone cortisol value of 5 $\mu g\%$ or greater identified dexamethasone "nonsuppressors."

All patients underwent CT scans without contrast on a GE-8800 machine, at 15 to the canthomeatal line, with 1-cm cuts as part of their clinical examination within one month of admission. Ventricular brain ratio (VBR) was calculated planimetrically at the slice with the largest ventricles, and the width of the third ventricle was measured using a magnifying rule with divisions of 0.2 mm as previously described.[22]

Statistical Analysis

Behavioral measures were dichotomized so that levels of CSF amine metabolites, VBR, and third ventricular width in patients with and without suicide attempt histories, with and without the need for seclusion and SWSP were compared by t-test. Patients who received a score of 4-7 on BPRS items were considered as having a high degree of "hostility" and "uncooperativeness," whereas those receiving ratings of 0-3 were considered to have a low degree of these symptoms; these distinctions were based on rating scores reflecting distinct behaviors. t-Test comparison was made for the neurobiologic variables corresponding to the high and low symptom group profiles. DST results were analyzed by comparing the incidence of suppression/nonsuppression for the dichotomized clinical variables by Fisher Exact Test. All probabilities reported are two-tailed.

RESULTS

History of Suicide Attempt

Thirteen of the 28 (46%) patients studied had past histories of suicide attempt. No significant differences between levels of CSF 5-HIAA, HVA, and MHPG between groups were observed (FIGURE 1). Similarly, neither VBR nor third ventricular width differed between patients with and without suicide histories. Two of 12 patients without and 3 of 12 patients with a past history of suicide attempts showed nonsuppression (NS) to dexamethasone administration.

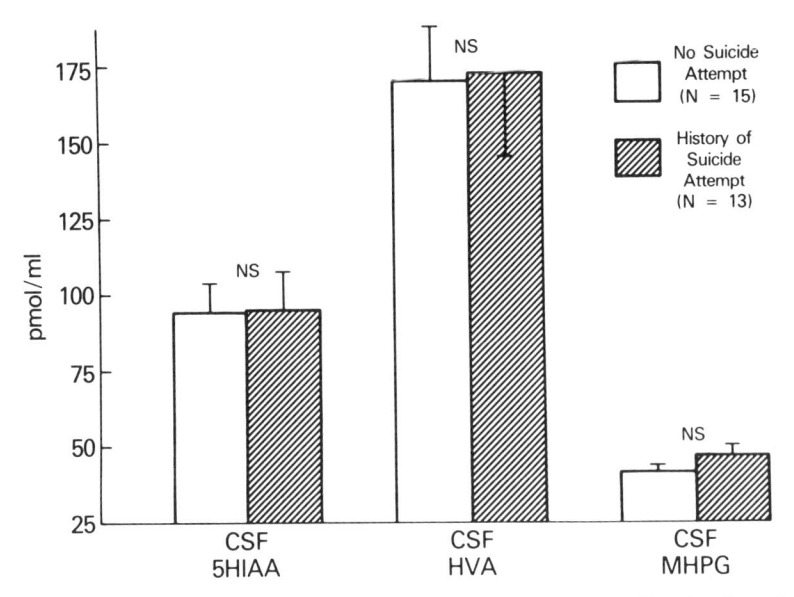

FIGURE 1. Levels of CSF 5-HIAA, HVA, and MHPG in drug-free schizophrenic patients with and without lifetime histories of suicide attempt.

Measures of Aggression

Neuroleptic treatment was associated with significant decreases in BPRS "hostility" and "uncooperativeness" ratings (FIGURE 2). When drug-free ratings were examined in the overall patient group, 7 of 28 patients were characterized by high uncooperativeness and 17 of 28 by high hostility. FIGURES 3 and 4 show levels of CSF metabolites in high and low rating groups. Lower levels of CSF 5-HIAA were observed in patients with higher hostility ($p = 0.10$) and uncooperativeness ratings ($p = 0.04$). Lower levels of CSF HVA were also found in patients with higher levels of these ratings, although near significance was achieved only for ratings of uncooperativeness ($p = 0.07$). No significant differences in CSF MHPG were observed between groups. In

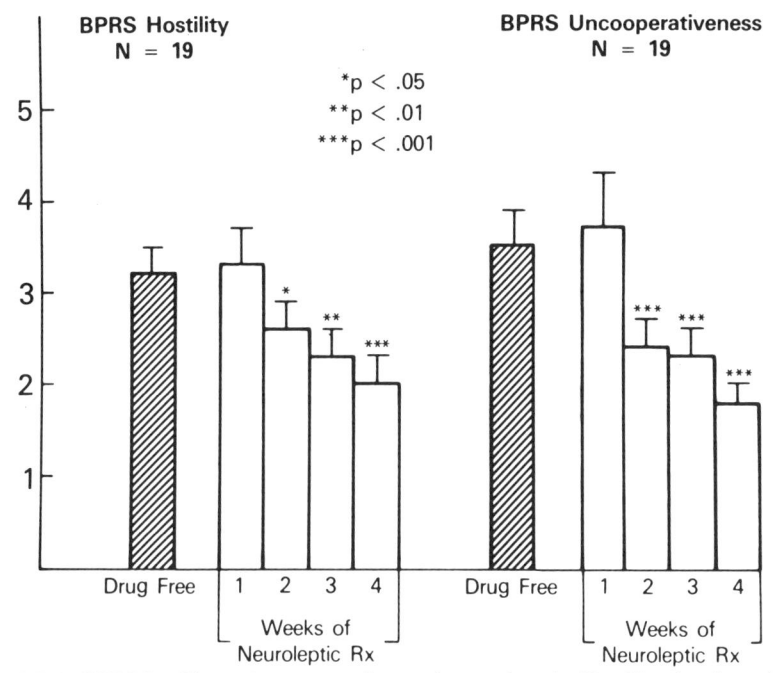

FIGURE 2. BPRS hostility and uncooperativeness item ratings in 19 schizophrenic patients undergoing double-blind fluphenazine administration (mean ± SEM daily dose: 30.3 ± 5 mg/day). Patients were drug-free for at least four weeks prior to the initiation of fluphenazine.

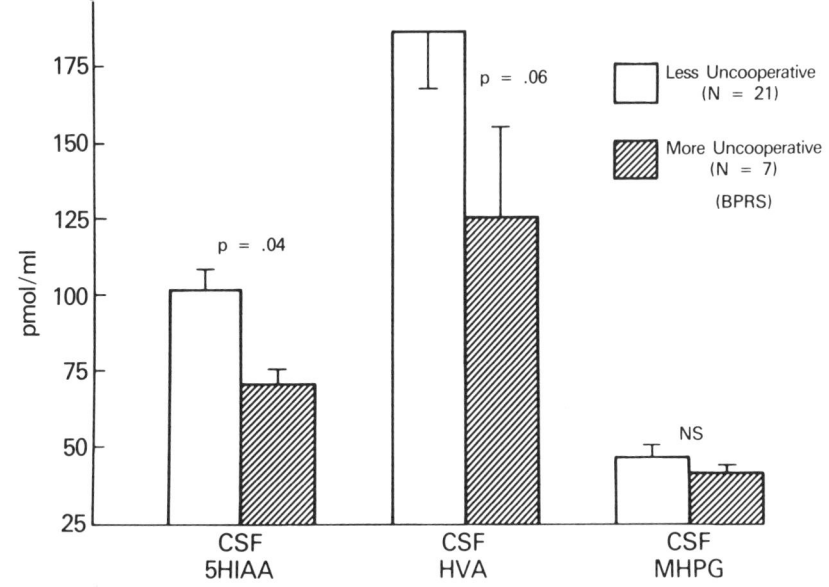

FIGURE 3. Levels of CSF 5-HIAA, HVA, and MHPG in drug-free schizophrenic patients with "more" and "less" uncooperativeness by BPRS ratings.

CT scan analysis, larger third ventricular width was found in patients with lower hostility ratings (mean ± SEM: 1.27 ± 0.1 vs. 0.95 ± 0.37 mm, p = 0.04); no significant differences between groups were found in VBRs. No significant or near significant differences were found with regard to DST suppression/nonsuppression distinction and the BPRS items.

The incidence of both seclusion room and SWSP was 7 of 28 patients (21%), although there was not complete overlap in patients. No significant differences between patients requiring and those not requiring behavioral restriction was observed for levels of CSF monoamine metabolites or for CT measures. A trend for a higher incidence

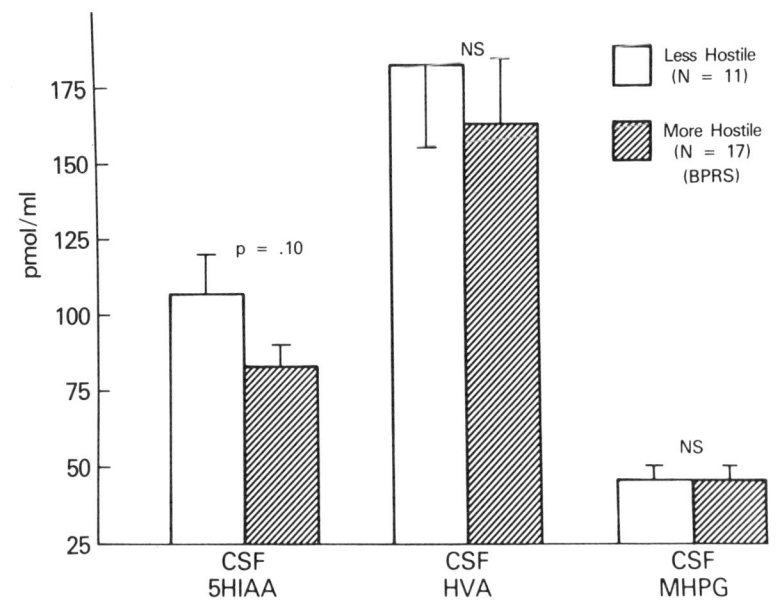

FIGURE 4. Levels of CSF 5-HIAA, HVA, and MHPG in drug-free schizophrenic patients with "more" and "less" hostility by BPRS ratings.

of DST nonsuppression was found among patients requiring seclusion (3 of 6 vs. 2 of 16, respectively, p = 0.07).

COMMENT

Consistent with our previous report,[18] we observed no significant differences in levels of CSF 5-HIAA, HVA, and MHPG between schizophrenic patients with and without a history of suicide attempt. Further, response to the DST and ventricular size by CT scan were nonpredictive of positive past histories of suicide attempt. It is of interest that 2 of the 28 patients studied committed suicide, in both cases by shooting, within two years of hospital discharge. Both were male and both experienced clinically significant depressive symptoms during their hospitalization. Neither, however, was a nonsuppressor on the DST. Levels of CSF HVA in these patients were 154 and 120 pmol/ml and levels of CSF 5-HIAA were 80 and 79 pmol/ml, in each case below the mean levels of suicide attempters (FIGURE 1) and below the total schizophrenic group means: 171 ± 15 (SEM) pmol/ml for CSF HVA and 94 ± 7 (SEM) pmol/ml for CSF 5-HIAA. In this regard, some support for an association between violent suicide attempt and low levels of CSF 5-HIAA in schizophrenic patients is found in our data.

The effectiveness of neuroleptic treatment in reducing aggression was demonstrated by our double-blind fluphenazine study using BPRS items "hostility" and "uncooperativeness" as reflectors of aggressive behaviors. Similarly, our experience indicates that the need for seclusion or SWSP is markedly lower in neuroleptic-treated than in drug-free schizophrenic patients. As we have previously shown that a neuroleptic-induced time-dependent decrease in dopamine turnover, as reflected by levels of plasma HVA, is related to the antipsychotic effects of neuroleptics,[23,24] it may be supposed that aggressive behaviors, when found in the context of overt psychosis, are diminished by decreasing dopamine activity.

Higher drug-free ratings of hostility and uncooperativeness each showed some relation to lower levels of CSF 5-HIAA and CSF HVA. The CSF 5-HIAA finding is consistent with reported aggression/5-HIAA relationships.[13,15] The lack of relationship between seclusion room and SWSP interventions and levels of CSF amine metabolites should caution the interpretation of this finding, however, since these behavioral interventions are used in the most seriously symptomatic and aggressive patients. As the total group of schizophrenic patients had significantly higher levels of 5-HIAA in comparison to age-matched controls (data not shown), illness-related factors may have diminished an association between decreased serotonin metabolism and aggressive behaviors. The trend towards lower levels of CSF HVA in the more uncooperative patients seems to be in disagreement with the postulate that decreased dopamine function in schizophrenia reduces aggressive behavior. Differential neuroleptic responsiveness of specific CNS brain dopamine systems (e.g., mesolimbic vs. mesocortical)[25] coupled with their differential contribution to levels of CSF HVA may prove to be related to this apparent discrepancy.

The DST and CT data revealed little association with the behavioral measures studied. The trend for a higher incidence of DST nonsuppression in patients requiring seclusion is of interest and may indicate a stress response in these severely ill patients; our experience in larger numbers of schizophrenic patients has indicated that DST nonsuppression is not particularly associated with depressive symptoms. The finding of low hostility ratings in patients with larger third ventricular width is compatible with some data suggesting that morphologic brain changes in schizophrenic patients are associated with more "negative" or muted positive symptoms.[26] The lack of CT relation to suicide history differs from previous reports[27,28] but is in agreement with data from larger series of our patients.

SUMMARY

In this study of schizophrenic patients, we were unable to find an association between past history of suicide attempt and levels of CSF amine metabolites, response to DST, and ventricular size by CT scan, neurobiologic variables each of which have been reported to be associated with attempted suicide in some patient groups. Our data, however, demonstrate the marked responsiveness of measures of aggressive behavior to neuroleptic treatment, suggesting a dopaminergic involvement in these behaviors when observed in the presence of overt psychotic symptoms. Some support for an association between decreased CNS serotonin function and aggressive behavior was found in drug-free schizophrenics, although difficulty in separating illness from trait factors is an important confounding variable. The need for clinical interventions required to treat severely disturbed and aggressive behavior in the schizophrenic patients studied could not be predicted by any of the neurobiologic variables.

REFERENCES

1. ROY, A. 1985. Suicide in psychiatric patients. Psychiatr. Clin. North Am. **8:** 227-241.
2. ROY, A., A. MAZONSON & D. PICKAR. 1984. Br. J. Psychiatry **144:** 303-306.
3. DRAKE, R. E., C. GATES, A. WHITAKER & P. G. COTTON. 1985. Compr. Psychiatry **26:** 90-100.
4. ROY, A. 1982. Br. J. Psychiatry **41:** 171-177.
5. HOGAN, T. P. & A. G. AWAD. 1983. Can. J. Psychiatry **28:** 277-281.
6. SHADER, R. I., A. H. JACKSON, J. S. HARMATZ & P. S. APPLEBAUM. 1977. Dis. Nerv. Syst. **38:** 13-16.
7. YESAVAGE, J. A. 1984. J. Psychiatry Res. **3:** 225-231.
8. BUNNEY, W. E., JR. & J. A. FAWCETT. 1965. Arch. Gen. Psychiatry **33:** 201-215.
9. TARGUM, S., R. ROSEN & A. CAPODANNO. 1983. Am. J. Psychiatry **140:** 877-879.
10. BANKI, C., M. ARATO, A. PAPP & M. KURCZ. 1984. J. Affect. Disord. **6:** 341-350.
11. ASBERG, M., L. TRASKMAN & P. THOREN. 1976. Arch. Gen. Psychiatry **33:** 1193-1197.
12. VAN PRAAG, H. 1982. J. Affect. Disord. **4:** 275-290.
13. BROWN, G., M. EBERT, P. GOYER, D. JIMERSON, W. KLEIN, W. E. BUNNEY, JR. & F. K. GOODWIN. 1982. Am. J. Psychiatry **139:** 741-746.
14. BROWN, G., F. K. GOODWIN, J. BALLENGER, P. GOYER & L. E. MAJOR. 1979. Psychiatry Res. **1:** 131-139.
15. LINNOILA, M., M. VIRKKUNEN, M. SCHEININ, A. NUUTILA, R. RIMON & F. K. GOODWIN. 1983. Life Sci. **33:** 2609-2614.
16. VAN PRAAG, H. 1983. Lancet ii: 977-978.
17. NINAN, P., D. VAN KAMMEN, M. SCHEININ, M. LINNOILA & W. E. BUNNEY, JR. 1984. Am. J. Psychiatry **141:** 566-569.
18. ROY, A., P. NINAN, A. MAZONSON, D. PICKAR, D. VAN KAMMEN, M. LINNOILA & S. M. PAUL. 1985. Psychol. Med. **15:** 335-340.
19. 1980. Diagnostic and Statistical Manual. 3rd edit. American Psychiatric Association. Washington, D.C.
20. OVERALL, J. E. & D. E. GORHAM. 1961. Psychol. Rep. **10:** 799-812.
21. SCHEININ, M., W. CHANBG, K. KIRK & M. LINNOILA. 1983. Ann. Clin. Biochem. **131:** 246-253.
22. BORONOW, J., D. PICKAR, P. J. NINAN, A. ROY, D. HOMMER, M. LINNOILA & S. M. PAUL. 1985. Arch. Gen. Psychiatry **42:** 266-271.
23. PICKAR, D., R. LABARCA, M. LINNOILA, A. ROY, D. HOMMER, D. EVERETT & S. M. PAUL. 1984. Science **225:** 457-459.
24. PICKAR, D., R. LABARCA, A. DORAN, O. WOLKOWITZ, A. ROY, A. BREIER, M. LINNOILA & S. M. PAUL. 1986. Arch. Gen. Psychiatry **43:** 669-676.
25. PICKAR, D. 1986. Neuroleptics, dopamine and schizophrenia. Psychiatr. Clin. North Am. **9(1):** 35-48.
26. ANDREASEN, N. C., S. A. OLSEN, J. DENVERT & M. R. SMITH. 1982. Am. J. Psychiatry **139:** 297-312.
27. LEVY, A. B., N. KURTZ & A. S. KLING. 1984. Am. J. Psychiatry **141:** 438-439.
28. NASRALLAH, H. A., M. MCCALLEY-WHITTERS & S. CHAPMAN. 1984. Am. J. Psychiatry **141:** 919.

Cerebrospinal Fluid Studies of Bipolar Patients with and without a History of Suicide Attempts

WADE H. BERRETTINI, JOHN I. NURNBERGER, JR.,
WILLIAM NARROW, SUSAN SIMMONS-ALLING,
AND ELLIOT S. GERSHON

Clinical Neurogenetics Branch
Intramural Research Program
National Institute of Mental Health
Building 10, Room 3N218
Bethesda, Maryland 20892

INTRODUCTION

In the past decade a number of studies have reported abnormalities of serotonin metabolism in individuals with a history of suicide attempts or other violent acts.[1-10] A number of investigators have reported that cerebrospinal fluid (CSF) 5-hydroxyindole acetic acid (5-HIAA) is lower in those individuals with a history of suicide attempts. Low CSF 5-HIAA was found more often in those individuals with a history of violent attempts. These studies initially were focused on individuals who attempted suicide during an episode of depression.[1-5] Subsequently, low CSF 5-HIAA was found in suicide attempters with diagnoses of personality disorders[6] and schizophrenia.[7,8]

Further, postmortem studies of successful suicides have shown decreased ^{3}H-imipramine binding, another finding compatible with altered serotonin metabolism in suicide.[9,10] These postmortem studies include individuals who probably had major depressive disorders, schizophrenia, alcoholism, and personality disorders.

Given the reports suggestive of altered serotonin function in suicide across several diagnostic boundaries, one hypothesis is that low CSF 5-HIAA may be a biologic marker for impulsive violent behavior, directed toward the self or others. Clearly, this hypothesis is problematic for the study of suicide, because some suicide attempts are repeated violent impulsive events, while others are solitary carefully premeditated acts.

One confounding variable is altered serotonin metabolism in the particular diagnostic category. For example, numerous studies have reported low CSF 5-HIAA (for review see Reference 11) and low platelet ^{3}H-imipramine binding in major depressive disorder.[12-14] These abnormalities are not found in schizophrenia.[15,16] Another confounding variable is drug effect. Individuals may be treated with medicines, such as lithium[17] and tricyclic antidepressants,[18] which may alter CSF 5-HIAA.

To avoid these two confounding variables, we chose to study unmedicated bipolar patients who had been recovered from their most recent episode of illness for at least three months. Study of recovered bipolar individuals (with and without a history of suicide attempts) may avoid confusion of state-dependent, illness-specific abnormalities (such as low platelet ³H-imipramine binding in actively depressed subjects)[12] with possible markers for suicide attempts. Thus we studied CSF biochemistry in unmedicated euthymic bipolar patients (with and without a history of suicide attempts) and normal volunteers.

METHODS

Thirty normal volunteers and 15 unmedicated euthymic bipolar patients (6 of whom had made a suicide attempt at some point in their illnesses) underwent a lumbar

TABLE 1. CSF Studies of Euthymic Bipolar Patients

Substance	Method	Reference
5-HIAA	HPLC/EC detection	17
Homovanillic acid (HVA)	HPLC/EC detection	17
Dihydroxy-phenylacetic acid (DOPAC)	HPLC/EC detection	17
Norepinephrine (NE)	HPLC/EC detection	17
3-Methoxy-4-hydroxyphenylglycol (MHPG)	HPLC/EC detection	17
Dopamine sulfate (DPS)	HPLC/EC detection	17
Gamma-aminobutyric acid (GABA)	HPLC/fluorometric detection	19
Beta-lipotropin (B-LPH)	Radioimmunoassay	20
Beta-endorphin (BE)	Radioimmunoassay	20
Alpha-melanocyte stimulating hormone (α-MSH)	Radioimmunoassay	20
Adrenocorticotropin (ACTH)	Radioimmunoassay	20
N-terminal fragment of proopiomelanocortin (N-POMC)	Radioimmunoassay	20
Corticotropin releasing factor (CRF)	Radioimmunoassay	21
Neurotensin	Radioimmunoassay	21
Somatostatin (SRIF)	Radioimmunoassay	21
Vasoactive intestinal peptide (VIP)	Radioimmunoassay	21
Vasopressin	Radioimmunoassay	21
Substance P	Radioimmunoassay	22
Neuropeptide Y (NPY)	Radioimmunoassay	unpublished data
Atrial natriuretic factor (ANF)	Radioimmunoassay	unpublished data
Calcitonin	Radioimmunoassay	unpublished data
Calmodulin	Radioimmunoassay	unpublished data

puncture as previously described.[17] Additionally, 25 patients underwent a lumbar puncture after a minimum of three weeks on lithium, as the sole drug therapy (with the exception of several individuals who were taking levothyroxine for lithium-induced hypothyroidism).

CSF monoamines and their metabolites, gamma-aminobutyric acid (GABA), and 15 neuropeptides were measured in CSF aliquots from these patients (see TABLE 1).

Of the six individuals who had attempted suicide, three were drug overdoses, all resulting in hospitalization. One individual attempted asphyxiation by sitting in her enclosed garage with her car motor running. Another patient attempted to hang himself. Lastly, one patient attempted suicide by inflicting a knife wound. All patients were depressed at the time of attempt. For five of these six, this was the only attempt. One individual took a drug overdose three times.

All 25 bipolar patients admitted to suicidal thoughts during depression. Approximately half of these made plans but never acted on those plans.

RESULTS

None of the substances measured differentiated the bipolar patients, with or without a history of suicide attempts, from the normal volunteers (TABLE 2). There were

TABLE 2. Levels of CSF Biochemicals in Euthymic Bipolar Patients and Controls[a]

Substance	Control value ($n = 30$)	Euthymic Bipolars: History of Suicide Attempt Positive ($n = 6$)	Negative ($n = 20$)
5-HIAA (pmol/ml)	72.3 ± 21.3	105 ± 49	98 ± 31
HVA (pmol/ml)	176 ± 57	176 ± 94	204 ± 87
DOPAC (pmol/ml)	2.77 ± 1.26	1.80 ± 0.74	2.81 ± 0.91
MHPG (pmol/ml)	44.7 ± 7.6	42.7 ± 6.1	51.9 ± 27.0
NE (pmol/ml)	0.40 ± 0.19	0.46 ± 0.23	0.52 ± 0.29
DPS (pmol/ml)	3.4 ± 2.0	2.4 ± 0.9	4.2 ± 2.0
GABA (pmol/ml)	127 ± 44	113 ± 46	135 ± 23
B-LPH (pg/ml)	73.1 ± 20.1	61.8 ± 8.3	82.9 ± 23.9
BE (pg/ml)	40.2 ± 6.9	41.3 ± 12.6	37.0 ± 5.8
α-MSH (pg/ml)	22.1 ± 2.6	21.5 ± 4.7	22.2 ± 1.9
ACTH (pg/ml)	22.8 ± 5.8	24.3 ± 5.8	20.7 ± 5.7
N-POMC (pg/ml)	436 ± 184	561 ± 266	372 ± 169
CRF (pg/ml)	33.0 ± 11.9	28.2 ± 21.3	30.2 ± 11.3
Calmodulin (pg/ml)	29.5 ± 15.9	21.7 ± 18.6	28.4 ± 20.4
Neurotensin (pg/ml)	65.2 ± 6.8	65.8 ± 11.9	65.0 ± 5.6
Calcitonin (pg/ml)	77.6 ± 17.2	79.1 ± 14.2	77.3 ± 17.2
Substance P (pg/ml)	17.1 ± 5.6	16.5 ± 2.8	14.9 ± 2.1
SRIF (pg/ml)	32.5 ± 15.8	26.3 ± 19.3	33.7 ± 14.8
VIP (pg/ml)	18.0 ± 7.4	17.6 ± 7.3	15.2 ± 5.7
Vasopressin (pg/ml)	4.0 ± 1.0	5.0 ± 1.2	4.5 ± 0.9
NPY (pg/ml)	103 ± 21	96 ± 36	101 ± 24
ANF (pg/ml)	15.1 ± 2.9	22.0 ± 3.9	15.4 ± 5.7

[a] Values are mean ± standard deviation.

trends ($0.01 < p < 0.05$) for lithium to increase 5-HIAA and decrease vasoactive intestinal peptide.

DISCUSSION

The results of this study are in agreement with those of Roy-Byrne et al.,[19] and Asberg et al. (personal communication), in that low CSF 5-HIAA does not appear to be associated with suicide attempts in *bipolar* patients, as is the case among unipolar patients. However, the sample size reported here is small ($n = 6$) and a type II error is certainly possible.

It seems more likely that low CSF 5-HIAA is a marker for individuals predisposed to repeatedly violent impulsive behavior. Our patients (and those of Roy-Byrne *et al.*) may have been selected for the absence of such repeatedly violent behavior. In general, repeated violent behavior is an exclusion criterion for the outpatient clinic from which our subjects were selected. Similar exclusion criteria exist for the inpatient unit from which Roy-Byrne *et al.* selected their subjects. Thus, the populations for these two studies may have excluded those individuals most likely to have low CSF 5-HIAA.

From the existing literature, it seems that low CSF 5-HIAA is most likely to be found in impulsive repeatedly violent subjects, regardless of their psychiatric diagnosis. The often impulsive behavior of overtly psychotic individuals may be an exception.

REFERENCES

1. ASBERG, M., L. TRASKMAN & P. THOREN. 1976. 5-HIAA in the cerebrospinal fluid: a biochemical suicide predictor. Arch. Gen. Psychiatry 33: 93-97.
2. AGREN, H. 1980. Symptom patterns in unipolar and bipolar depression correlating with monoamine metabolites in the cerebrospinal fluid. II. Suicide. Psychiatry Res. 3: 225-236.
3. VAN PRAAG, H. 1982. Depression, suicide and metabolism of serotonin in the brain. J. Affect. Disord. 4: 275-290.
4. TRASKMAN, L., M. ASBERG, L. BERTILSSON & L. SJOSTRAND. 1981. Monoamine metabolites in CSF and suicidal behavior. Arch. Gen. Psychiatry 38: 631-636.
5. BANKI, C., M. ARATO, Z. PAPP & M. KURCZ. 1984. Biochemical markers in suicidal patients: investigations with cerebrospinal fluid amine metabolites and neuroendocrine tests. J. Affect. Disord. 6: 341-350.
6. BROWN, G., F. K. GOODWIN, J. BALLENGER, P. GOYER & L. MAJOR. 1979. Aggressions in humans correlates with cerebrospinal fluid amine metabolites. Psychiatry Res. 1: 131-139.
7. NINAN, P., D. VAN KAMMEN, M. SCHEININ, M. LINNOILA, W. E. BUNNEY & F. K. GOODWIN. 1984. Cerebrospinal fluid 5-HIAA in suicidal schizophrenic patients. Am. J. Psychiatry 141: 566-569.
8. VAN PRAAG, H. 1983. CSF 5-HIAA and suicide in non-depressed schizophrenics. Lancet ii: 977-978.
9. PAUL, S. M., M. REHAVI, P. SKOLNICK & F. K. GOODWIN. 1984. *In* Neurobiology of Mood Disorders. R. M. Post & J. C. Ballenger, Eds.: 846-853. Williams and Wilkins, Baltimore, Md.
10. STANLEY, M., J. VIRGILIO & S. GERSHON. 1982. Tritiated imipramine binding sites are depressed in frontal cortex of suicides. Science 216: 1337-1339.
11. JIMERSON, D. C. & W. H. BERRETTINI. 1984. *In* Pathochemical Markers in Major Psychoses H. Beckmann & P. Riederer, Eds. 129-143. Springer Verlag. Berlin, FRG.
12. SURANYI-CADOTTE, B. E., P. L. WOOD, N. P. V. NAIR & G. SCHWARTZ. 1982. Normalization of platelet ^{3}H-imipramine binding in depressed patients during remission. Eur. J. Pharmacol. 85: 357-358.
13. BRILEY, M. S., S. Z. LANGER & R. RAISMAN. 1980. Tritiated imipramine binding sites are decreased in platelets of untreated depressed patients. Science 209: 303-305.
14. PAUL, S. M., M. REHAVI, P. SKOLNICK, J. C. BALLENGER & F. K. GOODWIN. 1981. Depressed patients have decreased binding of tritiated imipramine to the platelet serotonin "transporter." Arch. Gen. Psychiatry 38: 1315-1318.
15. WOOD, P. L., B. E. SURANYI-CADOTTE, N. P. V. NAIR, F. LAFAILLE & G. SCHWARTZ. 1983. Lack of association between ^{3}H-imipramine binding sites and uptake of serotonin in control, depressed and schizophrenic patients. Neuropharmacology 22: 1211-1214.

16. BERGER, P. A., K. F. FAULL, J. KILKOWSKI, P. J. ANDERSON, H. KRAEMER, K. L. DAVIS & J. D. BARCHAS. 1980. CSF monoamine metabolites in depression and schizophrenia. Am. J. Psychiatry 137: 174-180.
17. BERRETTINI, W. H., J. I. NURNBERGER, JR., M. LINNOILA, W. NARROW, M. SCHEININ, T. SEPPALA, S. SIMMONS-ALLING & E. S. GERSHON. 1985. CSF and plasma monoamines and their metabolites in euthymic bipolar patients. Biol. Psychiatry 20: 257-275.
18. POTTER, W. Z., M. SCHEININ, R. N. GOLDEN, M. V. RUDORFER, R. W. COWDRY, H. M. CALIL, R. J. ROSS & M. LINNOILA. Selective antidepressants lack specificity on norepinephrine and serotonin metabolites in CSF. Arc. Gen. Psychiatry. (In press.)
19. BERRETTINI, W. H., J. I. NURNBERGER, JR., T. A. HARE, S. SIMMONS-ALLING, E. S. GERSHON & R. M. POST. 1983. Reduced plasma and CSF GABA in affective illness: effect of lithium carbonate. Biol. Psychiatry 18: 185-194.
20. BERRETTINI, W. H., J. I. NURNBERGER, JR., N. G. SEIDAH, G. P. CHROUSOS, J. S. D. CHAN, P. W. GOLD, S. SIMMONS-ALLING, L. R. GOLDIN, M. CHRETIEIN & E. S. GERSHON. 1986. Pro-opiomelanocortin-related peptides in CSF: a study of manic-depressive disorder. Psychiatry Res. 16: 287-302.
21. BERRETTINI, W. H., J. I. NURNBERGER, JR., P. W. GOLD, R. L. ZERBE, G. P. CHROUSOS, T. TOMAI, S. SIMMONS-ALLING & E. S. GERSHON. CSF neuropeptides in euthymic bipolar patients and controls. Br. J. Psychiatry. (In press.)
22. BERRETTINI, W. H., D. R. RUBINOW, J. I. NURNBERGER, JR., S. SIMMONS-ALLING, R. M. POST & E. S. GERSHON. 1985. CSF substance P immunoreactivity in affective disorders. Biol. Psychiatry 20: 965-970.

Indices of Serotonin and Glucose Metabolism in Violent Offenders, Arsonists, and Alcoholics

ALEC ROY, MATTI VIRKKUNEN,[a] SALLY GUTHRIE,
AND MARKKU LINNOILA

National Institute of Alcohol Abuse and Alcoholism
9000 Rockville Pike
Building 10, Room 3B-19
Bethesda, Maryland 20892

In recent years, there have been several reports of studies on central monoamine metabolites in patients exhibiting suicidal behaviors. The first such report was by Asberg et al., who found a bimodal distribution of levels of the serotonin metabolite 5-hydroxyindoleacetic acid (5-HIAA) in the lumbar cerebrospinal fluid (CSF) of 68 depressed patients.[1] Significantly more of the depressed patients in the low CSF 5-HIAA mode had attempted suicide in comparison with those in the high mode, leading to the proposal that low CSF 5-HIAA levels may be associated with suicidal behaviors. Since then other studies in personality disordered,[2,3] schizophrenic,[4,5] and depressed patients[6,7] have also reported an association between low levels of CSF 5-HIAA and aggressive and suicidal behaviors, though there have also been some negative reports.[8-10]

It is of note that low CSF 5-HIAA levels have been particularly associated with violent suicide attempts. In fact, in an early study, Traskman et al. reported that CSF 5-HIAA levels were significantly lower only among those patients who had made a violent suicide attempt (hanging, drowning, shooting, gassing, several deep cuts), and that levels were not reduced among those who had made a nonviolent suicide attempt (overdosage).[11] More recently Banki et al. also found that among 141 female psychiatric patients suffering from depression, schizophrenia, alcoholism, or adjustment disorder, levels of CSF 5-HIAA were significantly lower in the violent suicide attempters in all four diagnostic categories.[12]

VIOLENT OFFENDERS

Initial studies of CSF 5-HIAA levels and aggressive behaviors were reported by Brown et al.[2,3] The relationship of low CSF 5-HIAA levels to impulsive violent behavior has been further explored by Linnoila et al.[13] They examined CSF 5-HIAA levels among 36 male murderers and attempted murderers undergoing an intensive one to two month forensic psychiatry evaluation. Twenty-seven of these individuals formed

[a] Department of Forensic Psychiatry, University of Helsinki, Helsinki, Finland.

a group of impulsive offenders, 20 were assessed as having an intermittent explosive disorder, and 7 an antisocial personality disorder. All these subjects also met *Diagnostic and Statistical Manual,* 3rd edition (DSM III) criteria for alcohol abuse and borderline personality disorder. The 9 violent offenders, who had premeditated their crimes, formed the nonimpulsive group and were individuals assessed as having paranoid or passive-aggressive personality disorders. The authors found that CSF 5-HIAA levels were significantly lower among the group of impulsive violent offenders than among the nonimpulsive violent offenders (FIGURE 1). Also, the 17 offenders (14 impulsive

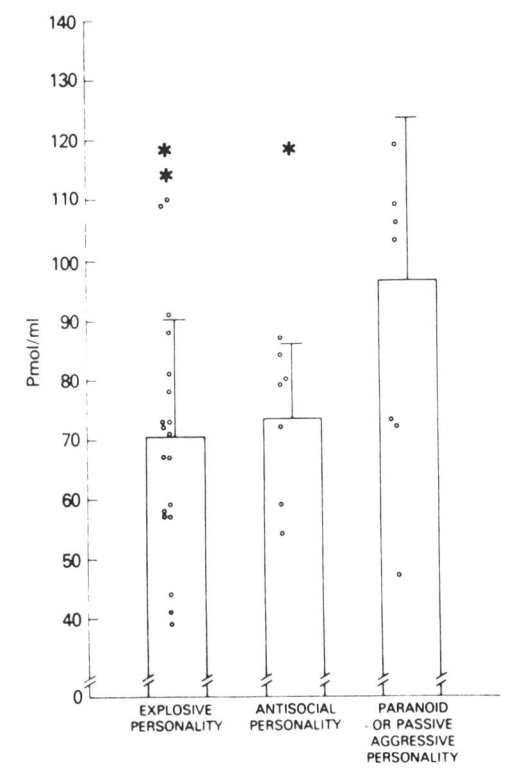

FIGURE 1. CSF 5-HIAA concentration in three diagnostic subgroups of violent offenders. I = impulsive and II = nonimpulsive offenders. Anova p < 0.01 between the groups. ** = p < 0.01, * = < 0.05 Students t-test, two-tailed, between the nonimpulsive and the two subgroups of impulsive offenders.

and 3 nonimpulsive) who had committed more than one violent crime had CSF 5-HIAA levels significantly lower than those found among offenders who had committed only one violent crime (mean 67.9 ± 12.1 vs. 87.1 ± 23.7 nM, p < 0.02). Furthermore, the impulsive offenders who at some time had attempted suicide were found to have significantly lower CSF 5-HIAA levels than did violent offenders who had never attempted suicide (mean 67.4 ± 19.7 vs. 91.2 ± 22.0 nM, p < 0.01).

Because of these findings the authors suggested that low CSF 5-HIAA levels may be associated with a tendency toward impulsive violent behavior which may manifest itself either as violence toward others or as attempts at suicide. They also suggested that in previous studies of depressed patients the presence of subgroups of depressed impulsive suicide attempters with low CSF 5-HIAA levels may have been obscured by low CSF 5-HIAA levels produced in other patients by withdrawal from their antidepressant medication. If this is correct they believe that the association between impulsive suicide attempts and low CSF 5-HIAA levels may, in fact, be stronger than previously claimed.

The authors cautioned that the implications of their study are limited at the present time as the number of subjects was relatively small and consisted of offenders who had exhibited extreme forms of impulsive violent behavior. However, they speculated that there may be individuals who have a defect in their central serotonin metabolism who, at an early age, start to abuse alcohol and later manifest impulsive violent behavior toward themselves and others. Furthermore, they suggested that experimental prospective prophylactic studies with serotonergic drugs should be considered, particularly for impulsive individuals who also have a family history of impulsive behavior.

ARSONISTS

In a later study Virkkunen et al. performed lumbar punctures on 20 male arsonists also undergoing intensive evaluation at the Forensic Psychiatry Department at the Helsinki University Central Hospital.[14] They matched the arsonists for age, height, and sex with a subgroup of the previously studied violent offenders and also compared them with 10 normal controls studied at the National Institutes of Health in Maryland. CSF 5-HIAA levels were significantly lower among the arsonists than the other two groups. CSF levels of the noreprinephrine metabolite 3-methoxy-4-hydroxyphenylglycol (MHPG) were also significantly lower among the arsonists. When patients who had made past violent suicide attempts were excluded from the groups, the arsonists again showed significantly lower CSF 5-HIAA and CSF MHPG levels than the other two groups (TABLE 1).

All of the arsonists also met DSM III criteria for borderline personality disorder and many of them had exhibited occasional explosive behavior, usually after consuming alcohol. Only one of the 20 arsonists met DSM III criteria for a major depressive episode. Thus, Virkkunen et al. argued that these results also suggest that low brain serotonin turnover, as indicated by low CSF 5-HIAA levels, may be associated with violent behavior through a primary effect on poor impulse control.

They also noted that among the arsonists the motive of revenge was not significantly associated with low CSF 5-HIAA levels and that the arsonists did not consider themselves to be aggressive. Similarly, Asberg et al. observed that low CSF 5-HIAA levels were not associated with self-reported aggressive feelings[15] but that elevated scores on the impulsiveness scale of the Karolinska Scales of Personality correlated negatively with CSF 5-HIAA levels.[16]

Urinary Free Cortisol

Serotonin plays an excitatory role in the regulation of the release of corticotropin releasing hormone (CRH) from the hypothalamus.[17] CRF is carried via the portal

TABLE 1. Cerebrospinal Fluid Levels Comparing Arsonists, Violent Offenders, and Normal Controls[a]

		Arsonists Group A	Violent Offenders Group B	Normal Controls Group C	df	F	p	Post Hoc	t-Test
All cases									
5-HIAA	Adjusted means	48.52	68.05	90.00	3,39	9.244	<0.001	A/B = < 0.002 B/C = < 0.001	A/C = p < 0.001
	SD	18.19	18.19	29.00					
MHPG	Adjusted means	17.34	28.90	42.30	3,39	6.487	<0.001	A/B = p < 0.001	A/C = p < 0.001 B/C = p < 0.001
	SD	6.12	6.12	8.50					
HVA	Adjusted means	223.9	216.6	206.0	3,39	3.482	NS		
	SD	86.63	86.63	64.00					
Groups excluding cases who had made a violent suicide attempt									
5-HIAA	Adjusted means	46.38	69.56	90.00	3,29	7.633	<0.001	A/B = p < 0.005 B/C = p < 0.042	A/C = p < 0.001
	SD	17.37	17.37	29.00					
MHPG	Adjusted means	17.28	28.18	42.30	3,29	39.96	<0.001	A/B = p < 0.001	A/C = p < 0.001 B/C = p < 0.001
	SD	5.79	5.79	8.50					
HVA	Adjusted means	216.1	213.1	206.0	3,29	3.199	NS		
	SD	92.32	92.32	64.00					

[a] Analyses of variance were performed. SD is standard deviation. NS is not significant. HVA is homovanillic acid. Reproduced from Reference 14 with permission from *Archives of General Psychiatry*.

system to the anterior pituitary where it stimulates the secretion of adrenocorticotropic hormone (ACTH) into the blood.[17] Thus, Virkkunen also compared the various groups of these male offenders with each other and with male controls for their excretion of urinary free cortisol.[18] Habitually violent offenders with an antisocial personality disorder had a significantly lower excretion rate of urinary free cortisol than did all the other groups of offenders or controls (TABLE 2).

Furthermore, offenders who had shown poor attention in school, truancy, or who had an undersocialized aggressive conduct disorder had significantly lower excretion rates of urinary free cortisol than did offenders who had not shown these characteristics during their adolescence (TABLE 3).

Reactive Hypoglycemic Tendency

In a series of studies Virkkunen has also investigated glucose metabolism among these violent and impulsive offenders.[19-23] Approximately half of these subjects had also exhibited suicidal behavior. The purpose of the first study was to determine whether results on the glucose tolerance test (GTT) differed between offenders who had an antisocial personality and habitually committed acts of violence, usually under the influence of alcohol, when compared with offenders who had intermittent explosive disorder and the same kind of habitual violent tendency. A consecutive series of 68 habitually violent offenders were investigated. Of these, 37 had an antisocial personality and 31 an intermittent explosive disorder. Blood glucose levels fell below the basal level to a nadir of 2.4 ± 0.5 mmol/l in the antisocial personality group and to 2.3 ± 0.4 mmol/l in the intermittent explosive disorder group. The blood glucose nadir for the psychiatric personnel controls was 3.1 ± 0.5 mmol/l, which was significantly higher than that found in both of the violent offender groups ($p < 0.001$). Also, the duration of hypoglycemia was greatest in the antisocial personality disorder group (195.4 ± 44.4 minutes) and shortest in the intermittent explosive disorder group (125.8 ± 48.3 minutes); the value for the controls was intermediate (165.0 ± 39.1 minutes) (TABLE 4).

Reactive hypoglycemic levels were related to two factors in the violent groups: (1) disturbances of memory about the violent and impulsive acts; and (2) the opinion of the offender's relatives that he was quarrelsome and aggressive under the influence of alcohol. A long duration of hypoglycemia correlated with a low verbal IQ, the presence of tattoos and slashing scars, and behavioral and sleeping problems (TABLE 5). There were also significant correlations between a long duration of hypoglycemia and truancy, stealing, crimes against property, having multiple sentences, and having a father who was violent under the influence of alcohol (TABLE 6).

In the second study the GTTs of 59 arsonists were studied. Twenty-seven of them (45.8%) had a glucose nadir under 3.0 mmol/l. In comparison to 39 adult males, of approximately the same age and weight, who had a GTT only 5 subjects had such low values (17%)—a significant difference compared with the arsonists ($p < 0.01$). The fires of "hypoglycemic" arsonists were usually very dramatic, and, in some cases, the arsonists had also intended to burn themselves, although the motives were very chaotic and conflicting. They seemed to be "confused" when they set the fires, and the crimes had been preceded by alcohol abuse. Sometimes the arson was immediately regretted and the arsonist himself alerted the fire department or tried to get the fire under control, supporting the hypothesis that there had been some short-lived "confusion."

TABLE 2. Urinary (24 hour) Free Cortisol Excretion in Male Offenders and Controls[a]

	Group A (n = 34)	Group B (n = 39)	Group C (n = 17)	Group D (n = 10)	Group E (n = 15)	Group F (n = 20)
Age (years)	28.5 ± 7.4	28.1 ± 5.8	29.2 ± 10.7	27.3 ± 4.5	30.4 ± 5.9	30.2 ± 9.7
Total IQ (WAIS)	93.9 ± 13.0	106.1 ± 14.6	104.4 ± 20.8	96.2 ± 16.1	NA	106.7 ± 18.6
Urine volume (ml/24 hours)	1580 ± 353	1797 ± 581	1600 ± 463	1556 ± 489	1754 ± 510	1619 ± 997
Urinary cortisol (μg/24 hours)	36.2 ± 11.7[b]	73.1 ± 25.0	71.2 ± 32.6	78.8 ± 23.3	74.2 ± 22.3	69.5 ± 27.9

[a] Means ± SD. Group A = antisocial personality with habitually violent tendency (DSM III 312.34). Group B = habitually violent offenders with intermittent explosive disorder (DSM III 312.34). Group C = other violent offenders (DSM III 301.84 + 301.00). Group D = residivous arsonists (DSM III 312:33). Group E = psychiatric male personnel controls. Group F = antisocial personality without the habitually violent tendency (DSM 301.70). NA = not available. F = 9.43; df = 5, 129; p < 0.01. Reproduced from Reference 18 with permission from *Acta Psychiatrica Scandinavica*.

[b] Group A had lower urinary cortisol levels than each of the other groups (p < 0.01).

Insulin Secretion during the Glucose Tolerance Test

In the first of these studies, free insulin secretion during the GTT was examined in 23 young violent offenders with antisocial personality. Those with and without an undersocialized aggressive conduct disorder in adolescence were compared. Insulin secretion during the GTT was greater in those who had an early undersocialized aggressive conduct disorder. There were significant differences in the 30, 60, 90, and 120 minute values (TABLE 7). The glucose values, however, did not differ among the groups. Mean individual peak values in insulin secretion were significantly higher among subjects with an early onset of alcohol abuse (TABLE 8). Also, subjects who had experienced attention problems into late adolescence had higher peak insulin values than subjects who did not (TABLE 8). Day-night rhythm disturbances, sleeping difficulties, and increasing behavioral problems observed during the evaluation were more characteristic of subjects who developed high insulin peak values.

TABLE 3. Urinary (μg/24 hours) Free Cortisol Excretion, Behavioral Aspects in Adolescence, and Background Factors in 73 Habitually Violent Male Offenders[a]

	Present	Not Present	t-Test
Marks for attention only fair (5 or 6 in 10-grade system) at the end of school in late adolescence (n = 27)	40.1 ± 19.3	67.6 ± 32.4	3.91[b]
Truancy (n = 41)	44.2 ± 22.4	71.0 ± 37.2	3.81[b]
Undersocialized aggressive conduct disorder (n = 31)	36.2 ± 15.2	70.5 + 34.2	5.21[b]
Violent suicide attempt or attempts (n = 23)	49.9 ± 34.6	58.7 ± 31.3	1.08
Violent suicides among first-degree relatives (n = 9)	57.1 ± 37.1	55.8 ± 32.1	0.11
Father violent under influence of alcohol (n = 50)	55.0 ± 34.6	57.9 + 27.9	0.34

[a] Means ± SD. Reproduced from Reference 18 with permission from *Acta Psychiatrica Scandinavica*.
[b] $p < 0.001$ (two-tailed t-test).

In the second study, free insulin secretion during the GTT was examined in all the violent and impulsive offenders among both the antisocial personality disorder and intermittent explosive disorder groups. Because of differences between the groups for basal values of glucose, only Δ glucose and Δ insulin values (values = basal values) were compared. The Δ mean 60-minute glucose values showed a significantly more rapid decline among offenders with explosive disorder than among those with antisocial personality disorder. The Δ 180-minute value also demonstrated a significantly more severe reactive hypoglycemia in both groups of offenders compared to controls. In the Δ 300-minute value, there was a significantly more rapid return to normal blood glucose levels from reactive hypoglycemia among explosive disorder offenders. Differences in Δ insulin values were seen within 15 minutes due to enhanced insulin secretion among offenders with explosive disorder. Also, in that group Δ insulin secretion ended more rapidly than in the other groups (TABLE 9).

These GTT and insulin secretion results are of particular interest, as in rats lesions of the suprachiasmactic nucleus altered not only the circadian rhythm of sleep and feeding behavior, but also the glucagon responses to intracranial injection of 2-deoxy-

TABLE 4. Glucose Tolerance Test Results in Groups of Habitually Violent Male Offenders and Male Controls[a]

	Habitually Violent Offenders with Antisocial Personality ($n = 37$) (A)	Habitually Violent Offenders with Intermittent Explosive Disorder ($n = 31$) (B)	Psychiatric Personnel Controls ($n = 20$) (C)	A/B	A/C	B/C
Age (years)	30.9 ± 9.3	29.3 ± 8.1	28.7 ± 3.6	NS	NS	NS
Weight (kilograms)	72.8 ± 8.7	70.0 ± 8.1	69.3 ± 7.3	NS	NS	NS
Basal level of glucose (mmol/l)	3.9 ± 0.4	3.6 ± 0.4	4.0 ± 0.5	<0.01	NS	<0.01
Hyperglycemic level (mmol/l)	6.8 ± 1.6	6.6 ± 1.8	6.2 ± 1.7	NS	NS	NS
Blood glucose nadir (mmol/l)	2.4 ± 0.5	2.3 ± 0.4	3.1 ± 0.5	NS	<0.001	<0.001
Difference between hyper- and hypoglycemic levels (mmol/l)	4.5 ± 0.2	4.4 ± 0.2	3.2 ± 0.1	NS	<0.01	<0.05
Duration of hypoglycemic phase (minutes)	195.4 ± 44.4	125.8 ± 48.3	165.0 ± 39.1	<0.001	<0.05	<0.001

[a] Means ± SD. Student's t-test (two-tailed) was used. Reproduced from Reference 19 with permission from *Neuropsychobiology*.

TABLE 5. Background Factors, Reactive Hypoglycemic Levels, and Duration of Hypoglycemia among 68 Habitually Violent Male Offenders[a]

	Person Quarrelsome and Aggressive under Influence of Alcohol (n = 58)			Loss of Memory about Violent Acts (n = 52)		
	yes	no	p	yes	no	p
Reactive hypoglycemia level (mmol/l)	2.3 ± 0.4	2.9 ± 0.3	<0.001	2.3 ± 0.4	2.7 ± 0.4	<0.001
Duration of hypoglycemic phase (minutes)	195.5 ± 44.6	158.2 ± 58.2	NS	165.0 ± 58.8	159.4 ± 55.1	NS

	Verbal IQ Less than Performance IQ (n = 31)			Kahn Value under 80 (n = 38)		
	yes	no	p	yes	no	p
Reactive hypoglycemia level (mmol/l)	2.4 ± 0.5	2.3 ± 0.4	NS	2.3 ± 0.5	2.4 ± 0.4	NS
Duration of hypoglycemic phase (minutes)	182.3 ± 61.1	148.1 ± 50.2	<0.05	178.2 ± 52.0	141.2 ± 63.0	<0.05

	Tatoos (n = 31)			Slashing Scars (n = 17)		
	yes	no	p	yes	no	p
Reactive hypoglycemia level (mmol/l)	2.4 ± 0.5	2.3 ± 0.4	NS	2.5 ± 0.5	2.3 ± 0.5	NS
Duration of hypoglycemic phase (minutes)	181.4 ± 58.0	148.8 ± 53.7	<0.05	192.9 ± 49.1	153.9 ± 57.4	<0.05

	Behavioral Problems and Sleeping Difficulties during Admission (n = 17)		
	yes	no	p
Reactive hypoglycemia level (mmol/l)	2.3 ± 0.5	2.4 ± 0.5	NS
Duration of hypoglycemic phase (minutes)	185.6 ± 49.7	149.3 ± 58.5	<0.01

[a] Means ± SD. Reproduced from Reference 19 with permission from *Neuropsychobiology*.

TABLE 6. Background Factors, Reactive Hypoglycemic Levels, and Duration of Hypoglycemia among 68 Habitually Violent Male Offenders[a]

	Father Violent under the Influence of Alcohol ($n = 39$)			Father's Criminality ($n = 13$)		
	yes	no	p	yes	no	p
Reactive hypoglycemia level (mmol/l)	2.3 ± 0.5	2.4 ± 0.4	NS	2.1 ± 0.4	2.4 ± 0.4	<0.05
Duration of hypoglycemic phase (minutes)	178.7 ± 53.1	129.3 ± 56.9	<0.01	174.2 ± 58.9	161.2 ± 57.6	NS

	Father Absent (Deaths or Separations) in Puberty ($n = 22$)			Truancy ($n = 37$)		
	yes	no	p	yes	no	p
Reactive hypoglycemia level (mmol/l)	2.5 ± 0.5	2.3 ± 0.5	<0.05	2.4 ± 0.5	2.3 ± 0.4	NS
Duration of hypoglycemic phase (minutes)	175.0 ± 51.8	158.3 ± 60.0	NS	188.9 ± 45.0	133.5 ± 57.0	<0.001

	Stealing Including Theft at Home in Childhood ($n = 29$)			Crimes against Property ($n = 46$)		
	yes	no	p	yes	no	p
Reactive hypoglycemia level (mmol/l)	2.4 ± 0.5	2.3 ± 0.5	NS	2.4 ± 0.5	2.3 ± 0.4	NS
Duration of hypoglycemic phase (minutes)	180.2 ± 53.8	150.6 ± 57.5	<0.05	175.7 ± 56.5	138.6 ± 52.8	<0.05

	More than Two Sentences for Crimes of Any Kind ($n = 38$)		
	yes	no	p
Reactive hypoglycemia level (mmol/l)	2.4 ± 0.5	2.3 ± 0.5	NS
Duration of hypoglycemic phase (minutes)	182.4 ± 51.9	140.0 ± 56.6	<0.01

[a] Means ± SD. Reproduced from Reference 19 with permission from *Neuropsychobiology*.

TABLE 7. Insulin Secretion during a 4 Hour Glucose Tolerance Test Comparing Male Subjects with Antisocial Personality, with and without Undersocialized Aggressive Conduct Disorder, and Controls[a]

	Antisocial Personality Disorder with Undersocialized Agressive Conduct Disorder ($n = 16$) (A)	Antisocial Personality Disorder without Undersocialized Aggressive Conduct Disorder ($n = 17$) (B)	Psychiatric Personnel Controls ($n = 10$) (C)	A/B	A/C	B/C
Age (years)	20.6 ± 3.7	25.3 ± 4.5	23.0 ± 4.9	NS	NS	NS
Weight (kilograms)	69.9 ± 12.5	71.3 ± 8.3	70.6 ± 7.6	NS	NS	NS
Glucose values (mmol/l)						
0 hour	4.2 ± 0.4	4.1 ± 0.4	4.4 ± 0.5	NS	NS	NS
15 minutes	5.9 ± 1.0	5.7 ± 0.9	6.1 ± 0.8	NS	NS	NS
30 minutes	7.4 ± 1.5	6.4 ± 1.2	7.4 ± 1.6	NS	NS	NS
60 minutes	7.1 ± 1.9	4.9 ± 1.1	6.3 ± 2.2	<0.05	NS	NS
90 minutes	5.6 ± 1.8	4.7 ± 1.3	5.7 ± 1.8	NS	NS	NS
120 minutes	4.7 ± 1.5	4.2 ± 1.1	5.0 ± 1.6	NS	NS	NS
180 minutes	3.5 ± 0.7	3.4 ± 0.4	4.1 ± 0.9	NS	NS	NS
240 minutes	3.7 ± 0.5	3.8 ± 0.3	4.0 ± 0.7	NS	NS	NS
Blood glucose nadir	3.0 ± 0.5	3.1 ± 0.5	3.5 ± 0.5	NS	NS	NS
Insulin values (mU/l)						
0 hour	8.6 ± 3.6	4.6 ± 2.6	6.5 ± 4.2	<0.05	NS	NS
15 minutes	36.1 ± 17.2	24.0 ± 12.5	23.4 ± 14.7	NS	NS	NS
30 minutes	54.8 ± 21.5	36.8 ± 10.5	36.2 ± 23.4	<0.05	<0.05	NS
60 minutes	60.2 ± 23.5	22.4 ± 7.8	29.2 ± 23.7	<0.001	<0.01	NS
90 minutes	49.6 ± 17.9	21.5 ± 10.9	24.9 ± 11.9	<0.01	<0.001	NS
120 minutes	32.6 ± 17.1	10.0 ± 5.9	21.4 ± 11.7	<0.01	NS	<0.05
180 minutes	10.4 ± 3.7	3.7 ± 1.7	9.3 ± 8.9	<0.01	NS	NS
Mean of the individual peak values	68.3 ± 20.7	38.0 ± 9.9	45.7 ± 21.9	<0.001	<0.05	NS

[a] Means + SD. Reproduced from Reference 21 with permission from the *British Journal of Psychiatry*.

D-glucose making the rats more vulnerable to hypoglycemia.[24] The suprachiasmactic nucleus, which is thought to be the major pacemaker of many circadian rhythms, has a major serotonergic input. Thus, one might speculate that low brain serotonin levels in impulsive violent offenders and alcoholics might in addition to impulsivity produce the insomnia and changes in feeding and glucose metabolism that are reported in these groups, through a dysfunction of a suprachiasmatic regulatory mechanism.

ALCOHOLICS

In 1977, Miles reviewed 15 follow-up studies reporting mortality among alcoholics.[25] He estimated that 15% of alcoholics died by committing suicide. He also

TABLE 8. Mean of Individual Peak Values of Insulin Secretion (mU/l) during Glucose Tolerance Test in Relation to Aspects of Adolescence and Early Adulthood among Subjects with Antisocial Personality ($n = 23$)[a]

	Present	Not Present	t-Test[b]
In adolescence			
Physically aggressive behavior ($n = 18$)	64.9 ± 21.9	38.0 ± 11.1	0.05
Bullying ($n = 10$)	61.2 ± 21.5	57.5 ± 24.6	NS
Stealing outside the home ($n = 18$)	63.2 ± 22.9	40.6 ± 10.1	0.05
Repeative abusive language ($n = 11$)	69.4 ± 16.4	49.6 ± 24.5	0.05
Chronic lying ($n = 18$)	64.2 ± 22.9	40.6 ± 10.1	0.05
Alcohol abuse started between 12-14 years ($n = 15$)	69.6 ± 20.6	39.5 ± 11.1	0.01
Marks for attention only fair (5 or 6 in 10 grade system) in first year of school ($n = 9$)	71.5 ± 18.2	51.1 ± 22.5	0.05
Marks for attention only fair at end of school in late adolescence ($n = 11$)	72.8 ± 21.7	48.6 ± 16.1	0.01
Observations and findings in the department			
Sleeping difficulties ($n = 14$)	71.2 ± 20.1	40.2 ± 11.1	0.001
Behavioral problems ($n = 11$)	72.7 ± 18.5	46.6 ± 19.5	0.01
Minor EEG changes ($n = 7$)	75.5 ± 23.3	51.9 ± 19.2	0.05

[a] Means ± SD. Reproduced from Reference 21 with permission from the *British Journal of Psychiatry*.
[b] Student's t-test (two-tailed) was used.

estimated that the suicide rate for alcoholics is approximately 270 per 100,000 per year and that in the United States there are between 6900 and 13,000 alcoholic suicides each year.

Also, there have been five carefully carried out general population studies, which have retrospectively assigned psychiatric diagnoses to suicide victims. The percent of alcoholic suicides in these five studies ranges from 15 to 26.9.[26] The total number of suicide victims is 748, of whom 158 were determined to be alcoholic—21.1% (TABLE 10).

It is estimated that between 0.5% and 1% of the general population die by committing suicide.[32] It is also estimated that up to 5% of the general population are

TABLE 9. Glucose Tolerance Test and Insulin Secretion among Habitually Violent Offenders and Controls[a]

	Group A[b]	Group B[c]	Group C[d]	F Value	F Significance	A/B	A/C	B/C
Age (years)	25.4 ± 6.5	25.5 ± 8.9	27.2 ± 8.7	0.24	NS			
Weight (kilograms)	71.1 ± 8.9	72.1 ± 14.7	73.1 ± 7.4	2.46	0.097			
RBW% (relative body weight)	92.1 ± 9.2	90.7 ± 18.2	93.4 ± 8.4	7.91	0.001			
Δ Glucose values (mmol/l)								
15 minutes	1.8 ± 0.6	1.6 ± 1.0	1.8 ± 0.7	1.12	0.335	NS	NS	NS
30 minutes	2.2 ± 1.1	3.2 ± 1.7	2.9 ± 1.4	1.22	0.305	NS	NS	NS
60 minutes	0.7 ± 1.5	3.3 ± 2.1	2.2 ± 2.0	5.75	0.006	<0.05	NS	NS
90 minutes	0.6 ± 1.5	1.5 ± 2.3	1.3 ± 1.8	2.05	0.142	NS	NS	NS
120 minutes	−0.1 ± 1.1	0.4 ± 1.2	0.6 ± 1.6	7.41	0.002	NS	NS	NS
180 minutes	−0.9 ± 0.6	−1.0 ± 0.7	0.1 ± 1.2			NS	<0.05	<0.05
240 minutes	−0.3 ± 0.3	−0.5 ± 0.3	−0.4 ± 0.3			NS	NS	NS
300 minutes	0.1 ± 0.3	−0.3 ± 0.3	−0.1 ± 0.4			<0.05	NS	NS
Δ Blood glucose nadir (mmol/l)	−1.4 ± 0.6	−1.4 ± 0.3	−0.9 ± 0.5	4.34	0.019	NS	<0.05	NS
Δ Insulin values (mU/l)								
15 minutes	43.8 ± 33.3	24.1 ± 15.4	20.5 ± 13.5	4.36	0.019	NS	<0.05	NS
30 minutes	62.1 ± 47.2	44.6 ± 21.5	31.8 ± 20.3	3.07	0.057	NS	NS	NS
60 minutes	48.1 ± 48.8	54.3 ± 24.7	26.3 ± 23.0	2.10	0.135	NS	NS	NS
90 minutes	30.9 ± 28.8	41.8 ± 21.5	20.7 ± 10.7	2.76	0.075	NS	NS	NS
120 minutes	18.6 ± 25.8	27.9 ± 21.5	19.1 ± 15.7	0.79	0.462	NS	<0.05	NS
180 minutes	−1.5 ± 5.0	2.5 ± 5.7	4.0 ± 7.7	3.58	0.036	NS	NS	NS
Δ Insulin peak value (mU/l)	66.3 ± −46.6	60.0 ± 22.7	41.9 ± 19.3	1.98	0.151	NS	NS	NS

[a] Mean ± SD. Group A[b] = habitually violent offenders with intermittent explosive disorder. Group B[c] = antisocial personality with habitually violent tendency. Group C[d] = psychiatric male personnel controls. Reproduced from Reference 22 with permission from *Aggressive Behavior*.

TABLE 10. Alcoholism among Suicide Victims in Studies on Suicide in the General Population

Author	Place	Number of Suicides	Number and Percent of Suicides with a Primary Diagnosis of Alcoholism
Robins et al., 1959[27]	St. Louis	134	31 (23.1%)
Dorpat and Ripley, 1960[28]	Seattle	108	29 (26.9%)
Barraclough et al., 1974[29]	Portsmouth	100	15 (15%)
Beskow, 1979[30]	Stockholm	271	60 (22.1%)
Chynoweth et al., 1980[31]	Brisbane	135	23 (17.0%)
Total		748	158 (21.1%)

alcoholics.[33] As the mean percent of deaths from suicide among the follow-up studies of alcoholics was 15 and a mean 21.1% of the suicide victims in the five general population studies were alcoholic, it appears that the suicide rate is substantially raised among alcoholics.

Previous Suicide Attempt

A previous suicide attempt is generally considered to be the best long-range indicator that an individual has an increased risk of eventually committing suicide.[34] Studies of completed suicides reveal that among those who commit suicide, 25% to 50% have made a previous suicide attempt.[35] The four studies reporting the number of alcoholic suicides who have made a previous suicide attempt report a total of 104 alcoholic suicides, of whom 38 (36.5%) had made a previous suicide attempt (TABLE 11). Thus, a sizable proportion of alcoholic suicide victims have exhibited prior suicidal behavior.

Sex

More men than women are found among alcoholic suicides. The ratio of men to women is about 5 to 1. In all 11 studies that reported the sex distribution there was

TABLE 11. Previous Suicide Attempt among Alcoholic Suicides

	Number Alcoholic Suicides	Number and Percent Who Had Made a Previous Suicide Attempt
Robins et al., 1959[27]	31	6 (19.4%)
Ritson, 1968[36]	8	7 (87.5%)
Barraclough et al., 1974[29]	15	10 (66%)
Murphy et al., 1979[37]	50	15 (30%)
Total	104	38 (35.5%)

a clear overrepresentation of men among the suicide victims (TABLE 12). Among the total number of 311 suicide victims in these 11 studies, 84.9% were men. This male preponderance reflects both that suicide is found more among men than women[32] and that alcoholism is found more among men than women by a ratio of 5 to 1.[44]

Also, it is noteworthy that there are many differences between men and women alcoholics. These differences include the family history of psychiatric disorder, developmental history, drinking behavior, gender-related effects of ethanol, and patterns of alcohol misuse.[45,46] Relevant to the issue of impulsivity, Schuckit and Morrissey have argued that some of these sex differences are partially due to the relative rates of different subtypes of secondary alcoholism in the two sexes[47] — in particular, that the major secondary alcoholic subtype among men is the sociopathic alcoholic subtype, which makes up about 25% of all of male alcoholism, while among women alcoholics the major secondary alcoholic subtype is the affective disorder subtype, which makes up about 30% of all of female alcoholism. In Swedish adoption studies, Cloninger et al.[48] and Bohman et al.[49] have reported evidence for two types of genetic influence on alcoholism in men and women. Other adoption studies have also suggested a genetic

TABLE 12. Sex Distribution among Alcoholic Suicides

	Men	Women
Robins et al., 1959[27]	27	4
Kessel and Grossman, 1961[38]	13	0
Tashiro and Lipscomb, 1964[39]	6	0
Ritson, 1968[36]	6	2
Gillis, 1969[40]	10	1
Virkkunen, 1971[41]	43	7
Schmidt and deLint, 1972[42]	47	4
Nicholls et al., 1974[43]	39	7
Barraclough et al., 1974[29]	12	3
Murphy et al., 1979[37]	43	7
Chynoweth et al., 1980[31]	18	12
Total	264	47

factor in antisocial personality disorder and that alcohol abuse can be regarded in some men to be a consequence of antisocial personality.[50,51]

Cerebrospinal Fluid Monoamine Metabolite Studies

There is considerable evidence from animal studies that alcohol causes significant alterations in central indoleamine and catecholamine turnover.[52-58] There are also animal studies demonstrating that serotonin plays a role in the regulation of aggression.[59] Thus it is of interest that in recent years there have been several CSF monoamine metabolite studies among alcoholics. Takahashi et al. found no significant difference for CSF 5-HIAA levels between alcoholics studied one week after alcohol withdrawal and controls.[60] However, when the alcoholics were divided into subgroups it was only the subgroup with delirium tremens and other florid withdrawal symptoms who had significantly lower CSF 5-HIAA levels than controls. Repeat lumbar punctures in this subgroup four weeks later showed that the CSF 5-HIAA levels remained low. Takahashi et al. speculated that an abnormality of brain serotonin metabolism might be a factor causing the psychiatric symptoms, including suicidal ideation, that are commonly found among alcoholics.[60]

Later, Ballenger et al. studied CSF monoamine metabolite levels in alcoholic patients, firstly within 48 hours of admission when being detoxified and secondly after four weeks of abstinence.[61] CSF 5-HIAA levels were significantly lower during the abstinent phase than in the postintoxication phase, or when compared to levels found in personality disordered controls. Also Banki, working in Hungary, performed lumbar punctures on 36 female alcoholic patients and found a significant negative correlation between the number of days abstinent and CSF 5-HIAA levels.[62]

The interpretation of these findings suggested by Ballenger et al. was that alcoholics may have preexisting low brain serotonin levels that are transiently raised by alcohol consumption, which in turn eventually leads to further depletion of brain serotonin levels. They speculated that a pattern may become established where the alcoholic drinks repeatedly in order to pharmacologically modify a serotonin deficiency in the brain. Ballenger et al. reviewed the animal studies that demonstrated that alcohol does, in fact, release serotonin in the brain and noted that genetic strains of rats that prefer alcohol to water have low brain serotonin levels.

In another alcohol-related CSF study, Rosenthal et al. examined the CSF monoamine metabolite data obtained from 69 depressed patients.[63] Depressed patients with a positive family history of alcoholism had significantly lower CSF levels of both 5-HIAA and of the norepinephrine metabolite 3-methoxy-4-hydroxyphenylglycol than those without a family history of alcoholism. Lidberg et al. found, however, that alcoholic murderers had significantly higher CSF 5-HIAA levels than did nonalcoholic murderers.[64]

Postmortem studies examining serotonin metabolite levels and receptors in the brains of suicide victims have also provided evidence suggesting a relationship between decreased brain serotonin metabolism and suicidal behavior.[65] Studying brains from alcoholic suicide victims, Gotfries et al. measured the activity of monoamine oxidase (MAO)[66]—an enzyme involved in serotonin metabolism. They compared 8 alcoholic suicide victims with 20 normal controls and found significantly decreased MAO activity among the alcoholic suicide victims in all 13 parts of the brain that they studied. Cochran et al., however, found no significant differences for levels of 5-hydroxytryptamine (5-HT, serotonin) in any of 33 brain areas when they compared 6 alcoholic suicides with 6 depressed suicide victims and 6 normal controls.[67] Further postmortem studies among alcoholic suicide victims are needed.

CONCLUSION

Scientific literature on violent behavior, suicide, and alcoholism has one common biochemical theme: a deficient serotonin metabolism indicated by a low CSF 5-HIAA concentration. As reviewed above, the literature is not unanimous but a number of reports implicate a deficiency of the serotonin system to be associated with these disorders. Our own research has provided evidence for a relatively specific association between a low CSF 5-HIAA concentration and poor impulse control in humans. Furthermore, hypoglycemia during the oral glucose tolerance test and insomnia are very common among the individuals with poor impulse control and low CSF 5-HIAA concentration. Recent animal research has implicated the suprachiasmatic nucleus, which has a dense serotonergic innervation, to play an important role in controlling both circadian rhythms and glucose metabolism. We interpret the insomnia of the individuals with poor impulse control as an indicator of a circadian rhythm disturbance and point out that insomnia is a very common complaint of alcoholics as well. The hypoglycemic tendency during the oral glucose test provides direct evidence of a disturbed glucose metabolism in a majority of individuals with a poor impulse control. Thus, we postulate that a functional serotonergic deficit is conducive of poor impulse control and circadian rhythm and glucose metabolism disturbances, and that these disturbances increase the incidence of violent outbursts, suicide attempts, and alcohol abuse.

REFERENCES

1. ASBERG, M., L. TRASKMAN & P. THOREN. 1976. 5-HIAA in the cerebrospinal fluid: a biochemical suicide predictor. Arch. Gen. Psychiatry 33: 93-97.
2. BROWN, G., M. EBERT, P. GOYER, D. JIMERSON, W. KLEIN, W. BUNNEY & F. K. GOODWIN. 1982. Aggression, suicide, and serotonin. Am. J. Psychiatry 139: 741-746.
3. BROWN, G., F. K. GOODWIN, J. BALLENGER, P. GOYER & L. MAJOR. 1979. Aggression in humans correlates with cerebrospinal fluid amine metabolites. Psychiatry Res. 1: 131-139.
4. NINAN, P., D. VAN KAMMEN, M. SCHEININ, M. LINNOILA, W. E. BUNNEY & F. K. GOODWIN. 1984. Cerebrospinal fluid 5-HIAA in suicidal schizophrenic patients. Am. J. Psychiatry 141: 566-569.
5. VAN PRAAG, H. 1983. CSF 5-HIAA and suicide in non-depressed schizophrenics. Lancet 2: 977-978.
6. AGREN, H. 1980. Symptom patterns in unipolar and biopolar depression correlating with monoamine metabolites in the cerebrospinal fluid. II. Suicide. Psychiatry Res. 3: 225-236.
7. VAN PRAAG, H. 1982. Depression, suicide and metabolism of serotonin in the brain. J. Affect. Disord. 4: 275-290.
8. ROY-BYRNE, P., R. POST, D. R. RUBINOW, M. LINNOILA, R. SAVARD & D. DAVIS. 1983. CSF 5-HIAA and personal and family history of suicide in affectively ill patients: a negative study. Psychiatry Res. 10: 263-274.
9. ROY, A., H. AGREN, D. PICKAR, M. LINNOILA, A. DORAN, N. CUTLER & S. M. PAUL. Reduced cerebrospinal fluid homovanillic acid and lower ratio of homovanillic acid to 5-hydroxyindoleacetic acid in depressed patients: relationship to suicidal behavior and dexamethasone nonsuppression. Am. J. Psychiatry. (In press.)
10. ROY, A., P. NINAN, D. PICKAR, D. VAN KAMMEN, M. LINNOILA & S. PAUL. 1985. CSF monoamine metabolites in chronic schizophrenic patients who attempt suicide. Psychol. Med. 15: 335-340.
11. TRASKMAN, L., M. ASBERG, L. BERTILSSON & L. SJOSTRAND. 1981. Monoamine metabolites in CSF and suicidal behavior. Arch. Gen. Psychiatry 38: 631-636.
12. BANKI, C., M. ARATO, Z. PAPP & M. KURCZ. 1984. Biochemical markers in suicidal patients: investigations with cerebrospinal fluid amine metabolites and neuroendocrine tests. J. Affect. Disord. 6: 341-350.
13. LINNOILA, M., M. VIRKKUNEN, M. SCHEININ, A. NUUTILA, R. RIMOND & F. K. GOODWIN. 1983. Low cerebrospinal fluid 5-hydroxyindoleacetic acid concentration differentiates impulsive from non-impulsive violent behavior. Life Sci. 33: 2609-2614.
14. VIRKKUNEN, M., A. NUUTILA, F. K. GOODWIN & M. LINNOILA. CSF monoamine metabolites in arsonists. Arch. Gen. Psychiatry. (In press.)
15. ASBERG, M., G. EDMAN, E. RYDIN, D. SCHALLING, L. TRASKMAN-BENDZ & A. WAGNER. 1984. Biological correlates of suicidal behavior. Clin. Neuropharmacol. 7: 758-759.

16. SCHALLING, D., M. ASBERG, G. EDMAN & S. LEVANDER. 1984. Impulsivity, nonconformity and sensation seeking as related to biological markers for vulnerability. Clin. Neuropharmacol. **7:** 746-747.
17. YASUEA, N., M. A. GREER & T. AIZAWA. 1982. Corticotropin-releasing factor. Endocrinol. Rev. **3:** 123-140.
18. VIRKKUNEN, M. 1985. Urinary free cortisol secretion in habitually violent offenders. Acta Psychiatr. Scand. **72:** 40-44.
19. VIRKKUNEN, M. 1982. Reactive hypoglycemic tendency among habitually violent offenders: a further study by means of the glucose tolerance test. Neuropsychobiology **8:** 35-40.
20. VIRKKUNEN, M. 1984. Reactive hypoglycemic tendency among arsonists. Acta Psychiatr. Scand. **69:** 445-452.
21. VIRKKUNEN, M. 1983. Insulin secretion during the glucose tolerance test in antisocial personality. Br. J. Psychiatry **142:** 598-604.
22. VIRKKUNEN, M. Insulin secretion during the glucose tolerance test among habitually violent and impulsive offenders. Aggressive Behav. (In press.)
23. VIRKKUNEN, M. Reactive hypoglycemic tendency among habitually violent offenders. Nutrition Rev. (In press.)
24. YAMAMOTO, H., K. NAGAI & H. NAKAGAWA. 1985. Lesions involving the suprachiasmatic nucleus eliminate the glucagon response to intracranial injection of 2-deoxy-D-glucose. Endocrinology **117:** 468-473.
25. MILES, C. 1977. Conditions predisposing to suicide: a review. J. Nerv. Ment. Dis. **104:** 231-246.
26. ROY, A. & M. LINNOILA. 1986. Suicide and alcoholism. J. Life Threat. Behav. **16:** 244-273.
27. ROBINS, E., G. E. MURPHY, R. M. WILKINSON, JR., S. GASSNER & J. KAYES. 1959. Some clinical considerations in the prevention of suicide based on a study of 184 suicides. Am. J. Public Health **49:** 888-899.
28. DORPAT, T. & H. RIPLEY. 1960. A study of suicide in the Seattle area. Compr. Psychiatry **1:** 349-359.
29. BARRACLOUGH, B., J. BUNCH, B. NELSON & P. SAINSBURY. 1974. A hundred cases of suicide: clinical aspects. Br. J. Psychiatry **125:** 355-373.
30. BESKOW, J. 1979. Suicide and mental disorders in Swedish men. Acta Psychiatr. Scand. Suppl. 227.
31. CHYNOWETH, R., J. TONGE & J. ARMSTRONG. 1980. Suicide in Brisbane—a retrospective psychosocial study. Aust. N. Z. J. Psychiatry **14:** 37-45.
32. SAINSBURY, P. 1986. The epidemiology of suicide. *In* Suicide. A. Roy, Ed. Williams & Wilkins. Baltimore, Md.
33. EFFRON, V., M. KELLER & C. GURIOLI. 1972. Statistics on Consumption of Alcohol and on Alcoholism. Rutgers University Center of Alcohol Studies. New Brunswick, N.J.
34. SAINSBURY, P. 1978. Clinical aspects of suicide and its prevention. Br. J. Hosp. Med. **19:** 156-164.
35. ROY, A. 1985. Suicide and psychiatric patients. Psychiatr. Clin. North Am.: 227-241.
36. RITSON, E. 1968. Suicide amongst alcoholics. Br. J. Med. Psychol. **41:** 235-242.
37. MURPHY, G., J. ARMSTRONG, S. HERMELE, J. FISCHER & W. CLENDENIN. 1979. Suicide and alcoholism. Arch. Gen. Psychiatry **36:** 65-69.
38. KESSEL, W. & G. GROSSMAN. 1961. Suicide in alcoholics. Br. Med. J. **2:** 1671-1672.
39. TASHIRO, M. & W. LIPSCOMB. 1964. Mortality experiences of alcoholics. Q. J. Studies Alcoholism **24:** 203-212.
40. GILLIS, L. 1969. The mortality rate and causes of death of treated chronic alcoholics. S. Afr. Med. J.: 230-232.
41. VIRKKUNEN, M. 1971. Alcoholism and suicides in Helsinki. Psychiatr. Fennica: 201-207.
42. SCHMIDT, W. & J. DELINT. 1972. Causes of death of alcoholics. Q. J. Studies Alcohol **33:** 171-185.
43. NICHOLLS, P., G. EDWARDS & E. KYLE. 1974. A study of alcoholics admitted to four hospitals. II. General and cause-specific mortality during follow-up. Q. J. Studies Alcohol **35:** 841-855.
44. GOODWIN, D. 1982. Alcoholism and suicide: associated factors. *In* Encyclopedic Handbook of Alcoholism. E. Mansell Pattison & E. Kaufman, Eds.: 655-662. Gardner Press. New York, N.Y.

45. WILSNACK, S. 1982. *In* Encyclopedic handbook of Alcoholism. E. Mansell Pattison & E. Kaufman, Eds.: 718-735. Gardner Press. New York, N.Y.
46. LINNOILA, M., C. ERWIN, D. RAMM, P. CLEVELAND & A. BRENDLE. 1980. Effects of alcohol on psychomotor performance of women: interaction with menstrual cycle. Alcoholism Clin. Exp. Res. **4:** 302-305.
47. SCHUCKIT, M. & E. MORRISSEY. 1976. Alcoholism in women: some clinical and social perspectives with an emphasis on possible subtypes. *In* Alcoholism Problems in Women and Children. H. Greenblatt & M. Schuckit, Eds. Grune and Stratton. New York, N.Y.
48. CLONINGER, C., M. BOHMAN & S. SIGVARDSSON. 1981. Inheritance of alcohol abuse: cross-fostering analysis of adopted men. Arch. Gen. Psychiatry **38:** 861-868.
49. BOHMAN, M., S. SIGVARDSSON & C. CLONINGER. 1981. Maternal inheritance of alcohol abuse: cross fostering analysis of adopted women. Arch. Gen. Psychiatry **38:** 965-969.
50. CADORET, R., W. O'GORMAN, E. TROUGHTON & E. HEYWOOD. 1985. Alcoholism and antisocial personality. Interrelationships, genetic, and environmental factors. Arch. Gen. Psychiatry **42:** 161-167.
51. VIRKKUNEN, M. 1979. Alcoholism and antisocial personality. Acta Psychiatr. Scand. **59:** 493-501.
52. HERRERO, E. 1980. Monoamine metabolism in rat brain regions following long term alcohol treatment. J. Neural Transm. **47:** 227-236.
53. BADAWY, A. & H. EVANS. 1974. Alcohol and tryptophan metabolism. J. Alcoholism **9:** 97-116.
54. REIS, J. 1973. A possible role of central noradenergic neurons in withdrawal states from alcohol. Ann. N.Y. Acad. Sci. **215:** 249-252.
55. TABAKOFF, B. & W. BOGGAN. 1974. Effects of ethanol on serotonin metabolism in brain. J. Neurochem. **22:** 759-764.
56. TABAKOFF, B. & R. RITZMANN. 1975. Inhibition of the transport of 5-hydroxyindoleacetic acid from brain by ethanol. J. Neurochem. **24:** 1043-1051.
57. ELLINGBOE, J. 1978. Effects of alcohol on neurochemical processes. *In* Psychopharmacology. A Generation of Progress. M. Lipton, A. DiMascio & K. Killman, Eds.: 1654-1664. Raven Press. New York, N.Y.
58. TRUITT, E. 1973. A biogenic amine hypothesis for alcohol tolerance. Ann. N.Y. Acad. Sci. **215:** 177-182.
59. EICHELMAN, B. 1979. Role of biogenic amines in aggressive behaviours. *In* Psychopharmacology of Aggression. M. Sandler, Ed.: 61-93. Raven Press. New York, N.Y.
60. TAKAHASHI, S., H. YAMANE, H. KONDO & N. TANI. 1974. CSF monoamine metabolites in alcoholism, a comparative study with depression. Folia Psychiatr. Neurol. J. **28:** 347-354.
61. BALLENGER, J., F. GOODWIN, L. MAJOR & G. BROWN. 1979. Alcohol and central serotonin metabolism in man. Arch. Gen. Psychiatry **36:** 224-227.
62. BANKI, C. 1981. Factors influencing monoamine metabolites and tryphophan in patients with alcohol dependence. J. Neural Transm. **50:** 98-101.
63. ROSENTHAL, N., Y. DAVENPORT, R. COWDRY, M. WEBSTER & F. GOODWIN. 1980. Monoamine metabolites in cerebrospinal fluid of depressive subgroups. Psychiatry Res. **2:** 113-119.
64. LIDBERG, L., J. TUCK, M. ASBERG, G. SCALIA-TOMBA & L. BERTILSSON. 1985. Homicide, suicide and CSF 5-HIAA. Acta Psychiatr. Scand. **71:** 230-236.
65. ASBERG, M. 1986. Biological factors in suicide. *In* Suicide. A. Roy, Ed. Williams and Wilkins. Baltimore, Md.
66. GOTFRIES, C., L. ORELAND, A. WIBERG & B. WINBLAD. 1975. Lowered monoamine oxidase activity in brains from alcohol suicides. J. Neurochem. **25:** 667-673.
67. COCHRAN, E., E. ROBINS & S. GROTE. 1976. Regional serotonin levels in brain, a comparison of depressive and alcoholic suicides with controls. Biol. Psychiatry **11:** 283-294.

Aminergic Studies and Cerebrospinal Fluid Cations in Suicide

CSABA M. BANKI,[a,c] MIHÁLY ARATÓ,[b] AND CLINTON D. KILTS[a]

[a]*Department of Psychiatry*
Duke University Medical Center
Durham, North Carolina 27710

[b]*National Institute of Nervous and Mental Diseases*
Post Office Box 1, Budapest 27
1281 Hungary

INTRODUCTION

There is a large and growing body of data suggesting that suicidal behavior in man may have measurable biological correlates. Since the first report from Sweden on the association of low cerebrospinal fluid (CSF) 5-hydroxyindoleacetic acid (5-HIAA) with suicidal gestures,[1] there have been several confirmatory observations which also suggested that this relationship was not limited to patients suffering from major, or endogenous, depression.[2-4] CSF 5-HIAA was mainly found to be lower in subjects attempting suicide by violent (i.e. aggressive) methods,[2] and this coincides with the observation that outward aggression in individuals with personality disorders may also have decreased CSF 5-HIAA.[5] These CSF findings are in remarkable accordance with the postmortem findings which also indicated decreased serotonin and/or 5-HIAA concentrations in some brain regions of suicide victims.[6,7] The data have been interpreted as evidence for central serotonin deficiency as a trait marker in certain individuals which, in turn, may render them vulnerable to either affective disorders or aggressive-suicidal behavior or both.[8,9] CSF homovanillic acid (HVA) was also found to be related to the same suicidal acts,[10] which is not surprising given the usually significant correlation between the two metabolites in the CSF.

Most aminergic studies have been undertaken primarily to investigate relationships with the clinical concept of affective disorders within the framework of the monoamine hypotheses.[11-13] Among the various biological markers proposed for these disorders, CSF calcium[14,15] and calcitonin[16] provided an interesting link between cations regulating a multiplicity of enzymes and transport processes relevant to the central neurotransmission and the brain neuropeptides modulating several aspects of mood and behavior.[16] While calcium has been suggested to be mainly involved in bipolar or "biphasic" conditions, another cation, magnesium, is known to affect both aminergic and catecholaminergic transmission,[17] and was suggested to be involved in the pathogenesis of various psychiatric disorders.[18,19]

---

[c]Permanent affiliation: Department of Psychiatry, Regional Neuropsychiatric Institute, H-4321 Nagykallo, P.O. Box 37, Hungary.

During the past decade we performed extensive studies to identify biological correlates of suicidal behavior in recently hospitalized psychiatric patients. One reason for this type of investigation was the primary importance of suicide as a mental health problem in Hungary[20] where all these studies were conducted; as a matter of fact, for almost seven decades Hungary has had the highest suicide rates among all countries that provide statistics.[21] The present paper is an extension of the earlier observations providing further confirmatory evidence for CSF 5-HIAA and magnesium changes in patients displaying suicidal behavior.

PATIENTS AND METHODS

All subjects investigated were hospitalized patients in the Regional Neuropsychiatric Institute, Nagykallo, Hungary. Between 1980 and 1983, we only studied female patients between 21 and 71 years of age (mean of 141 subjects was 42 ± 11 years), suffering from unambiguous clinical conditions which were concordantly diagnosed by at least two psychiatrists on subsequent days using either *Diagnostic and Statistical Manual*, 3rd edition (DSM III) criteria, or its published antecedents. This population actually consisted of three separate samples, whose clinical and background details have been published elsewhere.[22-24] Fifty-two individuals in this combined patient population were admitted following a recent suicide attempt, 18 of which had been made using violent means like neck cutting, drowning, fire setting, etc. All subjects investigated had been previously detoxified and were in stable physical condition at the time of the CSF studies; detailed medical and laboratory examinations excluded all patients with serious physical, endocrine, metabolic, or neurological diseases.

With regard to the known sources of variances,[25,26] CSF was obtained in a strictly standardized setting, i.e., between 8:00 and 9:00 A.M. after an overnight controlled fast and bed rest, at the 4th intervertebral disc with the patient in sitting position. CSF was collected in 6-ml fractions, and CSF amine metabolite measurements were always performed using the first portion; samples were stored in the dark at $-60°C$ until assayed.

The last two patient groups consisted of 84 and 50 individuals, respectively; the first group consisted exclusively of females admitted to the same psychiatric unit where the previous groups were studied, while the second group also included 11 male patients. In the first population, investigated between October 1984 and February 1985, 35 patients had major depression by DSM III criteria and 14 of them had attempted suicide within one week prior to hospitalization. Among the nondepressed patients, 14 had schizophrenic disorder and the other 35 subjects suffered from personality disorders and various forms of an adjustment disorder; 10 of them were admitted because of a recent suicide attempt. Age in this group ranged from 20 to 66 years, and, as before, only individuals without any major physical disease were included. All patients gave informed consent; moreover, none of them had been treated with major psychotropic drugs, such as neuroleptics, antidepressants, lithium, or massive doses of tranquilizers, within at least two weeks prior to admission (however, we did not carry out plasma drug measurements to control for the information received from the patients and their relatives). The second group consisted of 23 patients with major depressive disorder (5 males) and 27 patients with other psychiatric problems (anxiety disorder, personality disorder, alcohol-related problems) which did not include schizophrenia or other psychotic condition. In this second group there were 6 suicide attempters (1 male).

CSF sampling was performed as described above. While, however, the amine metabolites were measured by fluorometric procedures in the earlier groups, the recent combined samples were assayed by liquid chromatography with electrochemical detection (LCEC) using on-line trace enrichment,[27] which allows the use of small (125 μl) CSF samples and requires minimal sample pretreatment.

CSF calcium and magnesium measurements were again obtained from two different patient populations; details of the first group have been given previously.[28] The second group consisted of 34 women hospitalized for either major depression ($n = 16$) or for various nonpsychotic conditions with or without a personality disorder ($n = 18$). Five of the depressed subjects in this second sample had attempted suicide before admission, all using tranquilizer overdoses; in the first sample we obtained data from 11 suicidal patients, 4 of whom used violent methods. Calcium and magnesium were measured by atomic absorption spectrometry.

The statistical analysis of the data involved analysis of variance and t-tests where appropriate.

RESULTS

TABLE 1 shows means and standard deviations of the violent and nonviolent suicidal and the nonsuicidal patients in four diagnostic groups of the three previous studies combined. It was found that violent suicide attempters had clearly and significantly lower mean CSF 5-HIAA levels than did the nonsuicidal patients, and this proved to be remarkably consistent in all the four different diagnostic categories. Two-way analyses of variance yielded significant results for the effect of suicide for both 5-HIAA and HVA, but the significance of the latter was weaker and resulted from a different pattern: it can be seen from the table that the mean HVA levels tended to be higher in the nonviolent suicide attempters while the violent subgroups had only slightly lower levels than the nonsuicidal patients. It is not shown in the table but seems to be important to note that the decrease of 5-HIAA in the violent or combined violent-nonviolent suicidal patients was consistently and repeatedly demonstrable in the original separate studies[22,23] even if statistical significance was not always established because of the small sample sizes.

CSF 5-HIAA and HVA values in the first recent patient population are shown in FIGURES 1 and 2. The highly specific LCEC procedure yielded lower mean 5-HIAA values than did the previous fluorometric technique together with smaller variances; apart from this it is remarkable that the same pattern was again replicated, i.e., both the depressed and the nondepressed suicide attempters had clearly and significantly lower CSF 5-HIAA levels. The only difference from the earlier results seems to be that in this group, both the violent and the nonviolent suicidal patients had lower levels of 5-HIAA, although the violent subgroup tended to have even lower mean values. CSF HVA, which was strongly correlated with the 5-HIAA values ($r = 0.67$, $n = 84$), showed a similar tendency in the nondepressed group, but among the patients with major depression no difference was found. It must be noted, however, that if one outlier was excluded from the analysis then similar statistical significance would be found as with 5-HIAA.

Combined means and standard deviations for all the 134 patients studied in the last year using the LCEC assay are given in TABLE 2. Again it was found that CSF 5-HIAA, but not HVA, was significantly lower in the suicide attempters both in patients with major depression and with other clinical diagnoses.

TABLE 1. Means and Standard Deviations of CSF 5-HIAA and HVA in Violent and Nonviolent Suicidal and Nonsuicidal Patients in Four Diagnostic Groups[a]

	Depression	Schizophrenia	Alcoholism	Adjustment D.
CSF 5-HIAA				
Violent	14.3 ± 4.8 (4)	17.8 ± 3.3 (5)	16.8 ± 4.0 (3)	16.3 ± 8.4 (6)
Nonviolent	27.9 ± 6.9 (13)	18.6 ± 6.5 (4)	22.2 ± 9.9 (9)	26.4 ± 11.5 (8)
Nonsuicidal	30.6 ± 6.9 (19)	24.1 ± 6.8 (37)	31.0 ± 11.9 (23)	28.8 ± 9.6 (10)
	ANOVA: $F_{diagn}(3,128) = 2.81$ (< 0.05); $F_{suic}(2,128) = 14.11$ (< 0.001)			
CSF HVA				
Violent	16.4 ± 9.4	28.9 ± 5.3	20.7 ± 14.0	26.4 ± 9.2
Nonviolent	40.9 ± 19.3	40.7 ± 15.4	32.3 ± 15.2	31.3 ± 15.3
Nonsuicidal	28.0 ± 13.3	31.3 ± 18.5	31.8 ± 15.4	29.4 ± 11.1
	ANOVA: $F_{diag}(3,128) = 0.15$ (NS); $F_{suic}(2,128) = 3.73$ (< 0.05)			

[a] Case numbers in parenthesis; measurements in ng/ml units; NS is not significant.

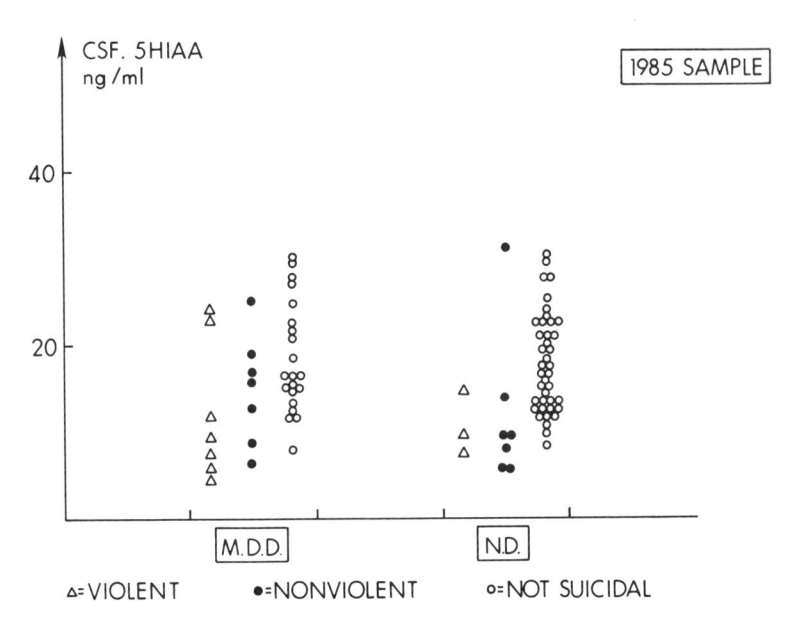

FIGURE 1. CSF 5-HIAA in depressed (M.D.D.) and nondepressed (N.D.) psychiatric inpatients with and without suicidal behavior.

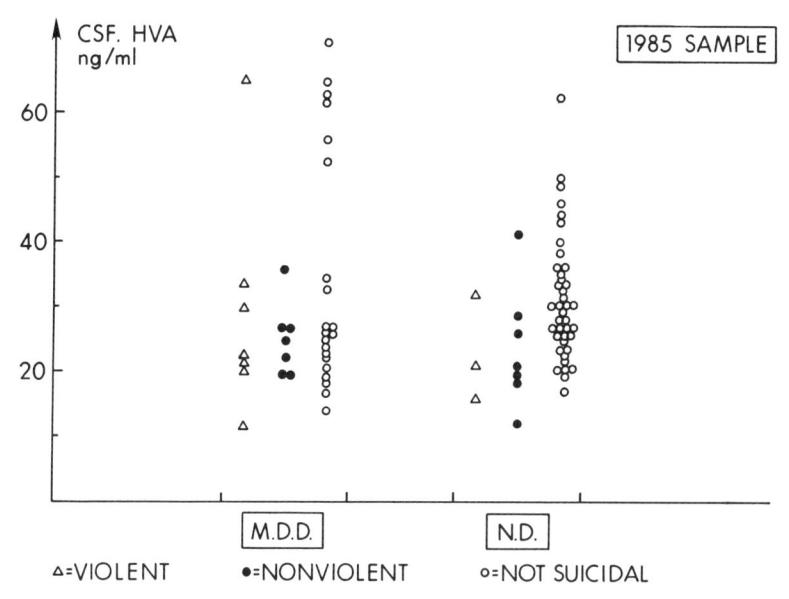

FIGURE 2. CSF HVA in depressed (M.D.D.) and nondepressed (N.D.) psychiatric inpatients with and without suicidal behavior.

In order to see the effects of some other common variables, we performed multiple regression analyses of both 5-HIAA and HVA with age, sex, body height, the diagnosis of major depression, and suicide as independent variables (TABLE 3). As expected, the two metabolites had similar patterns: both were correlated to body height, and both were related to suicidal behavior *after* partialling out the effects of the preceding variables. There was no difference in the partial coefficients representing the effect of violent and nonviolent suicide attempts.

In an earlier study we reported significantly lower CSF magnesium levels in both violent and nonviolent suicide attempters as compared to nonsuicidal psychiatric

TABLE 2. CSF 5-HIAA and HVA in Depressed and Nondepressed Patients with and without Recent Suicide Attempt[a]

	5-HIAA		HVA	
	Depressed	Nondepressed	Depressed	Nondepressed
Suicidal	13.7 ± 6.8 (18)	13.4 ± 8.2 (12)	26.4 ± 9.9	23.6 ± 8.8
Nonsuicidal	16.1 ± 6.1 (40)	18.1 ± 6.2 (64)	28.4 ± 10.6	29.1 ± 9.7
	F_{depr} = 1.64 (NS)		F_{depr} = 0.02 (NS)	
	F_{suic} = 6.30 (< 0.02)		F_{suic} = 1.74 (NS)	

[a] Data from a recent patient sample (n = 134). Means and standard deviations, using ng/ml units.

TABLE 3. Multiple Regression Analysis of CSF 5-HIAA and HVA on Some Hierarchically Evaluated Background Factors

	5-HIAA				HVA			
	R^2	p	ΔR^2	p	R^2	p	ΔR^2	p
Age	0.021	NS	—	—	0.030	NS	—	—
Sex	0.024	NS	0.003	NS	0.041	NS	0.011	NS
Height	0.117	< 0.05	0.093	< 0.01	0.099	< 0.05	0.058	< 0.05
Depression	0.132	< 0.05	0.015	NS	0.102	NS	0.003	NS
Suicide	0.334	< 0.001	0.202	< 0.001	0.266	< 0.01	0.164	< 0.001
Violent			0.132	< 0.001			0.096	< 0.001
Nonviolent			0.110	< 0.001			0.082	< 0.01

patients and in neurological controls;[28] when the suicidal subjects were excluded, there was no significant difference between depressed and nondepressed patients with respect to their mean CSF magnesium levels. CSF calcium did not differ significantly among either diagnostic or suicidal subgroups. In another population of 34 female patients we could replicate this finding in spite of the very small number of suicidal patients (FIGURE 3): it was clearly demonstrable that the 5 suicidal subjects had lower CSF magnesium, but not calcium, values than did the nonsuicidal patients. CSF calcium showed a slight, nonsignificant tendency to be higher in major depression ($t = 0.97$), but there was no relationship to suicide attempts. CSF calcium and magnesium correlated only weakly ($r = 0.31$); on the other hand, there was a pronounced and significant positive correlation between CSF magnesium and 5-HIAA ($r = 0.41$). CSF calcium or magnesium did not correlate significantly with age, body measures, severity of depression, or CSF HVA ($r = 0.30$).

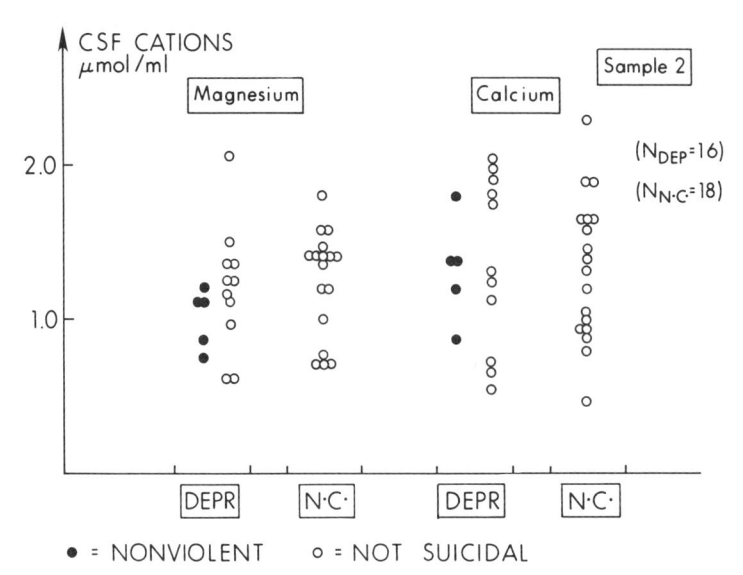

FIGURE 3. CSF magnesium and calcium in depressed (DEPR) and neurological control (N.D.) patients with and without suicidal behavior.

DISCUSSION

In accordance with the majority of studies investigating the relationship between the serotonin metabolite 5-HIAA in the CSF and suicidal behavior,[2,8,12] we have observed consistently low 5-HIAA levels in 82 suicidal psychiatric inpatients (almost exclusively females) among a total population of 275 individuals; moreover it appears even more important that this relationship was found to be replicable in five separate patient groups. Decrease of 5-HIAA in the suicidal patients does not appear to be limited to depressed subjects; in another study the same relationship was found among schizophrenic patients.[29] With certain limitations,[25,26] CSF 5-HIAA may be regarded as a global index of the central serotonin turnover; it follows that suicidal behavior[2,8] and/or other types of aggressive behaviors[5] may be related to central serotonin hypoactivity. There is evidence that low CSF 5-HIAA may be a permanent characteristic of the individual, i.e., a trait factor,[9,12] which may then indicate vulnerability toward impulsive, aggressive acts and/or certain types of affective disorders.[9,11] In this respect it is remarkable that one of the very few negative results concerning suicidal behavior and CSF 5-HIAA was reported in bipolar patients,[30] which disfavors the argument that serotonin hypoactivity is only related to depression and that suicidal behavior is just a symptom of the affective disorder. Although many of our patients diagnosed as having an adjustment disorder (the corresponding European terms "reactive depression," "neurotic reaction," etc., making it even clearer) did actually have one or more depressive symptoms at the time of their suicide attempt, this was quite clearly not the case for the schizophrenic patients, except for the fact that suicide itself qualifies as a depressive symptom. We therefore suggest that suicidal behavior may be related to an underlying, probably permanent, central serotonergic hypoactivity without necessarily involving the presence of a full major depressive syndrome. It must be noted, however, that all our suicidal patients had attempted killing themselves shortly before admission so that we have no evidence to assess whether low 5-HIAA was in fact a trait factor in these individuals or was only associated with the suicidal episode.

It is of interest that the decrease of CSF 5-HIAA in suicidal patients appears to be somewhat specific insofar as HVA is much more variable in this respect. The two metabolites are usually strongly correlated, and this is more evident when using better analytical techniques; even so, the correlation coefficient as high as $r = 0.70$ means that one variable "explains" less than 50% of the variation of the other. CSF HVA showed, of course, a similar tendency in our patients as was found earlier,[10] but the larger variance abolished statistical significance.

CSF calcium appears to be unrelated to suicidal behavior. Earlier studies suggested that CSF calcium may be higher in the depressive episode of bipolar disorder than in the manic phase within the same individual,[14,15] but no reports could demonstrate group differences; in this respect our negative results appear to be consistent with the majority of observations. On the other hand, there are only scarce data concerning CSF magnesium: Gattaz et al. found higher CSF magnesium in schizophrenic patients,[31] while Bech et al. reported no differences across a variety of diagnoses.[32] We are not aware of any other data concerning CSF magnesium in suicidal patients; this area therefore clearly requires further investigation. Magnesium deficiency may be related to several conditions including various psychiatric disorders;[18] specifically, the relationship between magnesium and the affective disorders is prompted by the well-known interaction between magnesium and lithium therapy.[32,33] Our data are, at first sight, also consistent with a decreased magnesium level in the CSF of depressed patients, but controlling for suicidal behavior this difference disappears; suicide therefore seems to be the more important factor in this respect. In addition, we found an interesting association between magnesium and 5-HIAA concentration in the CSF in both suicidal and nonsuicidal patients. The relationship between central serotonergic activity and magnesium availability, suggested by these data, is to our knowledge largely unexplored in man; indirect evidence based on the ability of lithium to both increase magnesium levels[19] and facilitate serotonergic transmission[34] may, however, indicate that this interaction would deserve further investigation.

In conclusion, we found consistent evidence for patients with suicidal behavior to have a lower mean 5-HIAA level in the CSF (although with wide overlapping between the suicidal and nonsuicidal subjects' individual values), which appeared to be uniformly present in all clinical diagnostic categories studied. CSF HVA showed a similar tendency but with much larger variance which abolished statistical significance of the results. CSF magnesium was also found to be lower in the suicidal patients and was also correlated with CSF 5-HIAA, while CSF calcium showed no similar relationships. We believe that further study of the interrelationships of bivalent cations and the monoaminergic transmission in the human central nervous system may yield important additional information to the understanding of some behavioral disorders that do not appear to be sufficiently explainable by the classical amine hypotheses.

SUMMARY

Cerebrospinal fluid 5-hydroxyindoleacetic acid (5-HIAA) and homovanillic acid (HVA) measurements have been collected over six years from 275 drug-free, recently hospitalized psychiatric patients, almost exclusively females. In accord with other observations from various countries, patients who had attempted suicide shortly before admission had significantly lower mean CSF 5-HIAA concentration and this was particularly true for those using violent methods. This finding could be replicated in five subsequent samples of patients evaluated separately and using different assay procedures, and proved to be independent of the clinical diagnoses. CSF HVA also showed similar tendencies but it had much larger variance with respect to suicide attempts and therefore fell short of statistical significance.

In two patient populations CSF calcium and magnesium measurements have been obtained. CSF calcium did not prove to be related to either suicidal behavior or the diagnosis of major depression; on the other hand, CSF magnesium was found to be significantly lower in the suicide attempters and also correlated with CSF 5-HIAA. Nonsuicidal depressives had comparable CSF calcium and magnesium levels to the controls.

REFERENCES

1. ASBERG, M., L. TRASKMAN & P. THOREN. 1976. 5-HIAA in the cerebrospinal fluid—a suicide predictor? Arch. Gen. Psychiatry **33:** 1193-1197.
2. ASBERG, M., L. BERTILSSON, E. RYDIN, D. SCHALLING, P. THOREN & L. TRASKMAN. 1981. Monoamine metabolites in cerebrospinal fluid in relation to depressive illness, suicidal behavior and personality. *In* Recent Advances in Neuropsychopharmacology. B. Angrist, G. D. Burrows, M. Lader, O. Lingjoerde & D. Wheatley, Eds.: 257-271. Pergamon Press. Oxford, England.

3. ORELAND, L., A. WIBERG, M. ASBERG, L. TRASKMAN, L. SJOSTRAND, P. THOREN & G. TYBRING. 1981. Platelet MAO activity and monoamine metabolites in CSF in depressed and suicidal patients and in healthy controls. Psychiatry Res. **4:** 21-29.
4. TRASKMAN, L., M. ASBERG, L. BERTILSSON & L. SJOSTRAND. 1981. Monoamine metabolites in cerebrospinal fluid and suicidal behavior. Arch. Gen. Psychiatry **38:** 631-637.
5. BROWN, G. L., M. H. EBERT, P. F. GOYER, D. C. JIMERSON, W. J. KLEIN, W. E. BUNNEY & F. K. GOODWIN. 1982. Aggression, suicide and serotonin, relationships to CSF amine metabolites. Am. J. Psychiatry **139:** 741-746.
6. LLOYD, K. G., I. J. FARLEY, J. H. N. DECK & O. HORNYKIEWICZ. 1974. Serotonin and 5-HIAA in discrete areas of the brainstem of suicide victims and control patients. Adv. Biochem. Psychopharmacol. **11:** 387-397.
7. BIRKMAYER, W. & P. RIEDERER. 1975. Biochemical postmortem findings in depressed patients. J. Neural Transm. **37:** 95-109.
8. ASBERG, M., D. SCHALLING, E. RYDIN & L. TRASKMAN-BENDZ. 1983. Suicide and serotonin. *In* Depression and Suicide. J. P. Soubrier & J. Vedrinne, Eds.: 367-404. Pergamon Press. Paris, France.
9. VAN PRAAG, H. M. 1984. Depression, suicide, and serotonin metabolism in the brain. *In* Neurobiology of Mood Disorders. R. M. Post & J. C. Ballenger, Eds.: 601-618. Williams & Wilkins. Baltimore, Md.
10. AGREN, H. 1980. Symptom patterns in unipolar and bipolar depression correlating with monoamine metabolites in the cerebrospinal fluid. II. Suicide. Psychiatry Res. **2:** 225-236.
11. ASBERG, M., L. BERTILSSON, B. MARTENSSON, G. P. SCALIA-TOMBA, P. THOREN & L. TRASKMAN. 1984. CSF monoamine metabolites in melancholia. Acta Psychiatr. Scand. **69:** 201-219.
12. VAN PRAAG, H. M. 1977. Depression and Schizophrenia, a Contribution on Their Chemical Pathologies. Spectrum Publishing. New York, N.Y.
13. BANKI, C. M. 1983. Evidence of disturbance of monoamines in depression. *In* Management of Depression with Monoamine Precursors. H. M. van Praag & J. Mendlewicz, Eds.: 176-199. Karger. Basel, Switzerland.
14. CARMAN, J. S. & R. J. WYATT. 1979. Calcium: bivalent cation in the bivalent psychoses. Biol. Psychiatry **14:** 295-333.
15. JIMERSON, D. C., R. M. POST, J. S. CARMAN, D. P. VAN KAMMEN, J. H. WOOD, F. K. GOODWIN & W. E. BUNNEY, JR. 1979. CSF calcium: clinical correlates in affective illness and schizophrenia. Biol. Psychiatry **14:** 37-50.
16. CARMAN, J. S., E. S. WYATT, W. SMITH, R. M. POST & J. C. BALLENGER. 1984. Calcium and calcitonin in bipolar affective disorder. *In* Neurobiology of Mood Disorders. R. M. Post & J. C. Ballenger, Eds.: 340-355. Williams & Wilkins. Baltimore, Md.
17. ALEXANDER, P. E., D. P. VAN KAMMEN & W. E. BUNNEY, JR. 1979. Serum calcium and magnesium in schizophrenia: possible relationship to extrapyramidal symptoms. Arch. Gen. Psychiatry **133:** 143-149.
18. ANANTH, J. & R. YASSA. 1979. Magnesium in mental illness. Compr. Psychiatry **20:** 475-482.
19. PAVLINAC, D., R. LANGER, L. LENHARD & L. DEFTOS. 1979. Magnesium in affective disorders. Biol. Psychiatry **14:** 657-661.
20. BUDA, B. 1983. Suicide in Hungary. *In* Depression and Suicide. J. P. Soubrier & J. Vedrinne, Eds: 23-27. Pergamon Press. Paris, France.
21. MARIS, R. 1985. The adolescent suicide problem. Suicide Life-Threat. Behav. **15:** 91-109.
22. BANKI, C. M. & M. ARATO. 1983. Amine metabolites and neuroendocrine responses related to depression and suicide. J. Affect. Disord. **5:** 171-177.
23. BANKI, C. M., M. ARATO, Z. PAPP & M. KURCZ. 1984. Cerebrospinal fluid amine metabolites and neuroendocrine changes in psychoses and suicide. *In* Catecholamines: Neuropharmacology and Central Nervous System. E. Usdin, A. Carlsson, A. Dahlstrom & J. Engel, Eds. C: 153-159. Alan R. Liss, Inc. New York, N.Y.
24. BANKI, C. M., M. ARATO, Z. PAPP & M. KURCZ. 1984. Cerebrospinal fluid amine metabolites and neuroendocrine findings: biochemical markers in suicidal patients? J. Affect. Disord. **6:** 341-350.
25. BANKI, C. M. & G. MOLNAR. 1981. CSF 5HIAA as an index of central serotonergic processes. Psychiatry Res. **5:** 23-32.

26. POST, R. M. 1984. Cerebrospinal fluid concentrations of amines and metabolites: clinical and methodological perspectives. *In* Catecholamines: Neuropharmacology and Central Nervous System. E. Usdin, A. Carlsson, A. Dahlstrom & J. Engel, Eds. C: 115-122. Alan R. Liss, Inc. New York, N.Y.
27. KILTS, C. D., M. D. GOOCH & K. D. KNOPES. 1984. Quantitation of plasma catecholamines by on-line trace enrichment high performance liquid chromatography with electrochemical detection. J. Neurosci. Methods **11**: 257-273.
28. BANKI, C. M., M. VOJNIK, Z. PAPP, K. Z. BALLA & M. ARATO. 1985. CSF magnesium and calcium related to amine metabolites, diagnosis, and suicide attempts. Biol. Psychiatry **20**: 163-171.
29. NINAN, P. T., D. P. VAN KAMMEN, M. SCHEININ, M. LINNOILA, W. E. BUNNEY & F. K. GOODWIN. 1984. CSF-5-hydroxyindoleacetic acid levels in suicidal schizophrenic patients. Am. J. Psychiatry **141**: 566-601.
30. ROY-BYRNE, P., R. M. POST, D. R. RUBINOW & M. LINNOILA. 1983. CSF 5-HIAA and personal and family history of suicide in affectively ill patients: a negative study. Psychiatry Res. **10**: 263-274.
31. GATTAZ, W. F., R. KATTERMANN, D. GATTAZ & H. BECKMANN. 1983. Magnesium and calcium in the CSF of schizophrenic patients. Biol. Psychiatry **18**: 935-941.
32. BECH, P., C. KIRKEGAARD, E. BOCK, M. JOHANNESEN & O. J. RAFAELSEN. 1978. Hormones, electrolytes, and cerebrospinal fluid proteins in manic-melancholic patients. Neuropsychobiology **4**: 99-112.
33. HERZBERG, L. & B. HERZBERG. 1977. Mood change and lithium, a possible interaction between magnesium and lithium? J. Nerv. Ment. Dis. **165**: 423-426.
34. MELTZER, H. Y., M. LOWY, A. ROBERTSON, P. GOODNICK & R. PERLINE. 1984. Effects of 5-hydroxytryptophan on serum cortisol in major affective disorders. III. Effects of antidepressants and lithium carbonate. Arch. Gen. Psychiatry **41**: 391-399.

Studies of Amine Metabolites in Depressed Patients[a]

Relationship to Suicidal Behavior

STEVEN K. SECUNDA,[b] CHRISTINE K. CROSS,[c]
STEPHEN KOSLOW,[c] MARTIN M. KATZ,[d]
JAMES H. KOCSIS,[e] AND JAMES W. MAAS[f]

[b]*Springfield Professional Park
1050 Baltimore Pike
Springfield, Pennsylvania 19064*

[c]*Neurosciences Branch
Parklawn Building, Room 11-105
National Institute of Mental Health
5600 Fishers Lane
Rockville, Maryland 20852*

[d]*Albert Einstein College of Medicine
Montifiore Medical Center
1300 Morris Park Avenue
New York, New York 10467*

[e]*Department of Psychiatry
Cornell University Medical School
525 East 68th Street
New York, New York 10021*

[f]*Department of Psychiatry
University of Texas Health Science Center
7703 Floyd Carl Drive
San Antonio, Texas 78284*

INTRODUCTION

In recent years, several reports of altered biochemistry in depressed patients who subsequently commit suicide or who have previously attempted suicide have appeared in the psychiatric literature. Most prominent among these, perhaps, are reports of lowered 5-hydroxyindoleacetic acid (5-HIAA) in both suicide attempters and com-

---

[a]The research was supported by grants U01 MH38034, U01 MH26975, U01 MH26977, U01 MH26979, U01 MH26978, U01 MH31921, and U01 MH36232 from the National Institute of Mental Health.

pleters. Reduced cerebrospinal fluid (CSF) concentrations of this monoamine (MA) metabolite have been found in depressed suicide attempters[1,2]—most notably those making violent attempts,[3-5]—suicidal schizophrenics,[5,6] and nondepressed suicides.[2,7] A relationship between CSF concentrations of 3-methoxy-4-hydroxphenylglycol (MHPG) and suicidal behavior has also been reported, with both low and high levels of this MA metabolite predictive of increased suicidal symptomatology in depressed patients.[1]

Given the implications of these findings, which suggest a biochemical basis and potential biological markers for suicidal behavior, establishing their replicability and generalizability is of some importance. The present study was undertaken to explore further the relationship between MA functioning and suicidal behavior in depressed patients. The subjects of this study were participants in the National institute of Mental Health-Clinical Research Branch (NIMH-CRB) Collaborative Program on the Psychobiology of Depression-Biological Studies. Suicide attempters from this group were compared to nonattempters on a variety of biochemical variables including CSF MA metabolites MHPG, 5-HIAA, and homovanillic acid (HVA); urinary MAs norepinephrine (NE) and epinephrine (E) and their respective metabolites MHPG, vanillylmandelic acid (VMA), normetanephrine (NM), and metanephrine (M); plasma measures of MHPG. In addition, the suicide attempter and nonattempter groups were compared in terms of clinical history, course, symptomatology, and behavioral characteristics.

METHODS

The study design and procedures of the collaborative study have been described in detail in previous reports.[8,9] Aspects relevant to this report follow.

Sample

One hundred thirty-two depressed patients were selected for study after extensive psychiatric and medical screening. All patients required hospitalization for treatment of their depression and were admitted to one of the six university hospital centers participating in the collaborative study (see Acknowledgments).

All patients were diagnosed as primary major depressives using the Schedule for Affective Disorders and Schizophrenia (SADS)[10] and Research Diagnostic Criteria (RDC).[11] Of the total sample, 85 were classified as unipolar (39 males, 46 females) and 47 as bipolars (31 males, 16 females), with bipolar Is and IIs represented in approximately equal numbers.

Protocol

On admission patients received psychiatric screening, physical examination, and a battery of standard laboratory tests. All were placed on a low VMA diet and restricted from alcohol and caffeine. Subjects remained drug free for a 14-day baseline testing period, during which biological measurements were made. Antidepressant treatment was initiated on day 15. After four weeks of treatment, patients were categorized as recovered or nonrecovered on the basis of specific behavioral and symptomatic criteria.[12]

Clinical Measures

Specific SADS items were used to assess suicidal thoughts and the number, seriousness, and lethality of suicide attempts made during the current and past episodes (see Appendix A). The SADS was also used to obtain information concerning duration of current episode, age at onset, number of previous episodes, the presence of psychotic features, and outcome. Severity of depression was assessed using the Hamilton Depression Rating Scale (HDRS)[13] and two measures from the SADS—the SADS-C Scale 1, a sum of depressive symptoms, and the Global Assessment of Severity (GAS), a measure of coping mechanisms and degree of impairment.[14]

On the basis of SADS data, patients were assigned to one of three groups:

1. A suicide attempter group (SA; $n = 28$) defined as those patients who had made at least one suicide attempt during the current episode that could be considered significant with regard to the seriousness of its intent (SADS item $249 \geq 4$) and/or its medical lethality (SADS item $250 \geq 4$).
2. A nonattempter group (NA; $n = 60$) defined as those patients with no history of suicide attempts for either the current or past episodes.
3. An unclassified group (UC; $n = 44$) consisting of patients who either had made a suicide attempt during the current episode that did not meet the established "significance" criteria or had a history of suicide attempts for prior episodes.

The UC group was excluded from data analysis.

Biochemical Measures and Procedures

Sample collection and assay procedures used in the measurement of CSF and urinary MAs and metabolites are described in Koslow et al.[15]

Blood samples to be assayed for free and total MHPG were drawn at approximately 0830 hours on study days 9 and 10, prior to meals. Samples consisted of 10 ml of blood drawn into an EDTA tube, which were then centrifuged in an ice bath at 1600 $\times$ g for 15 minutes. After adding 0.5 mg of metabisulfate per ml plasma, 1.5 ml of plasma were aliquoted to each of two tubes containing 300 ng of deuterated MHPG. Samples were coded and stored at $-70°C$ until shipment to the assaying center.

All plasma MHPG assays were done in a single laboratory on coded replicate samples and as blind duplicate using gas chromatography-mass spectrometry (GC-MS) as the method of analysis. Free MHPG was determined in one aliquot and total MHPG, following overnight incubation with a sulfatase-glucuronidase enzyme preparation, in the second. Measurements were conducted on a Finnegan 3200 GC-MS interfaced with a computer automation L15 computer using the Washington University Program System for Selected Ion Monitoring.

Behavioral Measures

Baseline assessments of patient behavior and affect were conducted on day 10 using a multivantaged approach. This consists of combining several observational scales from patient self-report, nurses' observations of ward behaviors, physician-administered rating scales, and videotaped interviews. The definition, reliability, and validity of the 14 behavioral constructs derived from these measures are described in Katz et al.[12]

Data Analysis

Between-group comparisons of continuous variables were made using t-tests or analyses of covariance (ANCOVAS) when correction for age was required. Between-group comparisons of categorical data were made using Fisher's Exact Test. Quadratic regression models were used to test the strength of subsets of biochemical variables as predictors of previous suicide attempts.

RESULTS

Suicide Attempters versus Nonattempters

The demographic, clinical, and behavioral characteristics of the SA and NA groups are presented in TABLE 1. With regard to the demographic and clinical variables, the SA group differed from the NA group only in being significantly younger and having an earlier age at onset. Behaviorally, NA showed more depressive symptoms than did SA, as revealed by their higher SADS-C Scale 1 scores, and displayed higher levels of anxiety, somatization, and psychomotor retardation.

ANCOVAS performed on the biochemical measures revealed few differences between the SA and NA groups (see TABLE 2). Of the three CSF and six urinary MAs and metabolites measured, only urinary MHPG differed between the two groups, being significantly lower in the SA. Both free and total plasma MHPG were also lower in the SA group.

The results of Fisher's Exact Tests performed on median splits of the MAs and metabolites (adjusted for sex) were consistent with those of the ANCOVAS. Only urinary MHPG differed between SA and NA, with more SA showing lower levels. Results of selected tests relevant to previously reported findings are presented in TABLE 3.

Unipolar-Bipolar Analyses

Although the unipolar-bipolar composition of the SA and NA groups did not differ significantly, the proportion of bipolars was higher in the SA group. Therefore, data analyses were repeated for each diagnostic group to ensure that the diagnostic disproportion was not obscuring group differences. The pattern of SA-NA differences

TABLE 1. Demographic, Clinical, and Behavioral Characteristics of Suicide Attempters and Nonattempters

	Suicide Attempters ($n = 28$)	Nonattempters ($n = 60$)
Male/female	15/13	32/28
Age[a]	39 ± 2.3[b]	50.9 ± 1.8
Unipolar/bipolar	16/12	44/16
Severity measures[a]		
HDRS	24.6 ± 1.4	29.5 ± 1.2
SADS-C Scale 1	2.5 ± 0.11[c]	2.8 ± 0.07
GAS	41.8 ± 3.0	41 ± 1.6
Duration of current episode (weeks)[a]	34.2 ± 5.9	34.7 ± 4.0
Previous episodes 0/1-2/3+	2/12/14	12/27/21
Age at onset[a]	28.1 ± 2.1[b]	40.2 ± 2.0
Presence of psychotic features (yes/no)	6/22	8/52
Recovery status (recovered/nonrecovered)	13/4	25/11
Behavioral measures[a]		
Depressed mood	4.74 ± 0.36	4.86 ± 0.22
Anxiety	3.48 ± 0.32[c]	4.52 ± 0.20
Psychomotor retardation	2.90 ± 0.20[c]	3.45 ± 0.16
Agitation	2.18 ± 0.16[c]	2.65 ± 0.12
Somatization	2.86 ± 0.17[c]	3.75 ± 0.16
Distressed expression	2.25 ± 0.33	2.73 ± 0.19
Interpersonal sensitivity	1.87 ± 0.30	1.81 ± 0.26
Positive adaptation	3.48 ± 0.33	4.14 ± 0.26
Congitive impairment	2.76 ± 0.17	2.98 ± 0.16
Sleep disorder	4.68 ± 0.56	6.09 ± 0.31
Depressed scale	3.39 ± 0.31	3.49 ± 0.17
General psychopathology	3.13 ± 0.19	3.34 ± 0.14

[a] Mean ± standard error of the mean (SEM).
[b] Results of t-test: $p > 0.001$.
[c] Results of ANCOVA: $p < 0.05$.

in demographic, clinical, and behavioral variables that emerged from these analyses was remarkably similar to that found in the total group, despite the reduced sample size.

While no new between-group differences appeared with regard to the biochemical variables, the reduction of urinary MHPG observed was found to be restricted to the bipolar SA (bipolar SA 1508.1 ± 167 vs. bipolar NA 2581.1 ± 500.76, $p < 0.05$) (see TABLE 4). Fisher's Exact Tests performed on median splits of the biochemical

TABLE 2. Monoamine, MA Metabolite, and Cortisol Concentrations in the CSF, Urine, and Plasma of Suicide Attempters and Nonattempters

	Suicide Attempters (mean ± SEM)	Nonattempters (mean ± SEM)
CSF measures (pmol/ml)		
MHPG	42.5 ± 2.0	47.7 ± 1.8
5-HIAA	117.3 ± 7.5	120.7 ± 6.5
HVA	198.1 ± 16.9	203.1 ± 12.7
Cortisol	0.89 ± .07	1.04 ± 0.05
Urinary measures (μg/24 hours)		
MHPG	1679.8 ± 103.8[a]	2230.0 ± 165.9
VMA	3257.5 ± 248.6	3691.9 ± 353.2
NM	241.3 ± 31.0	283.8 ± 26.4
M	126.1 ± 8.6	137.8 ± 8.8
NE	37.9 ± 4.4	38.8 ± 4.2
E	18.8 ± 2.7	22.1 ± 1.8
Free cortisol	111.7 ± 16.5	147.9 ± 19.7
Plasma cortisol[b] (μg/dl)		
Morning	15.6 ± 1.1	18.4 ± 0.77
Evening	5.2 ± 1.3[a]	7.0 ± 0.66
Plasma MHPG		
Free	17.7 ± 3.0[a]	31.4 ± 3.1
Total	45.0 ± 9.8[a]	100.3 ± 9.0

[a] ANCOVA results: $p < 0.05$.
[b] Pre-dexamethasone suppression test (DST).

variables revealed that the bipolar SA were significantly more likely to be lower than bipolar NA in urinary MHPG (91% vs. 45%, $p < 0.05$), NM (83% vs. 42%, $p < 0.05$), and E (89% vs. 40%, $p < 0.05$). Unipolar SA, on the other hand, were significantly more likely to be high in urinary NE than were unipolar NA (91% vs. 42%, $p < 0.01$).

Regression Analyses

The quadratic regressions of SADS Suicidal Ideation and Behavior Scale Scores (see Appendix A) on the CSF and urinary MAs and metabolites were significant only for CSF MHPG ($r = 0.35$; $p < 0.05$). As the sign of the quadratic coefficient was negative, this model would predict very high or low MHPG to be associated with less suicidal symptomatology. (This result is the reverse of that reported by Agren.[1] The apparent discrepancy can be at least partially resolved, however, by noting that most regression models are less reliable at the extremes. Thus, both models indicate a monotonically increasing relationship between CSF MHPG and suicidal symptomatology throughout most of the range of the dependent variable.)

DISCUSSION

In our sample, suicide attempters were clearly differentiated from nonattempters by including in the attempter group only those patients whose attempts could be considered significant with regard to seriousness of intent and/or medical lethality, and by restricting the nonattempter group to patients with no history of attempted suicide. The clinical characteristics of our suicidal patients were similar to those previously reported in the literature;[16-20] suicide attempters were significantly younger and had an earlier age at onset; bipolars were more likely to be suicide attempters than were unipolars; and suicide attempters were more likely to display psychotic features than were nonattempters.

In contrast to the previous reports, we found no relationship between CSF 5-HIAA concentrations and suicidal behavior. No significant differences between suicide attempters and nonattempters in mean 5-HIAA concentrations were found (TABLE 2), nor were the proportions of attempters and nonattempters different in "high" and "low" 5-HIAA categories (TABLE 3). A plot of CSF 5-HIAA concentrations for our depressed patient population is depicted in FIGURE 1 with the distribution of suicide attempters noted. As can be seen, there is no clustering of suicide attempters at the lower end.

TABLE 3. Results of Analyses Performed on Categorized Biochemical Variables

	Post-DST Plasma < 5 mg/dl (suppressor)	Cortisol Levels > 5 mg/dl (nonsuppressor)	
Suicide attempters	18	7	
Nonattempters	30	23	$\chi^2 = 1.70$, $p > 0.15$
	Cortisol hypersecreters[a]		
	Yes	No	
Suicide attempters	7	15	
Nonattempters	22	24	FET = 1.56, $p > 0.20$
	CSF 5-HIAA concentration[b]		
	Low	High	
Suicide attempters	11	8	
Nonattempters	16	22	$\chi^2 = 1.27$, $p > 0.25$
	Urinary MHPG concentration[b]		
	Low	High	
Suicide attempters	18	7	
Nonattempters	21	25	$\chi^2 = 4.54$, $p < 0.05$
	CSF MHPG concentration[b]		
	Low	High	
Suicide attempters	15	7	
Nonattempters	18	22	$\chi^2 = 3.06$, $p < 0.10$

[a] Hypersecretion is defined as a urinary free cortisol (UFC) level of > 133 mg/24 hours.
[b] Based on median splits for the combined groups where 132.6 = female 5-HIAA median and 101.1 = male 5-HIAA; 1949.5 = urine MHPG median; and 47.5 = CSF MHPG median.

TABLE 4. Urinary Monoamine and Metabolite Concentrations[a] in Suicidal and Nonsuicidal Depressed Patients by Diagnosis

	Unipolars		Bipolars	
	Suicide Attempters	Non-attempters	Suicide Attempters	Non-attempters
NE	51.5 (4.1)	40.0 (5.0)	21.3 (3.8)	34.1 (7.1)
E	53.9 (4.2)	22.8 (2.2)	12.6 (1.6)	19.8 (2.9)
MHPG	1814.6 (124.6)	2119.7 (152.3)	1508.1[b] (167.0)	2581.1 (500.6)
VMA	3310.7 (300.7)	3363.1 (318.6)	3183.0 (422.0)	4678.3 (1022.1)
NM	331.4 (47.0)	279.0 (30.6)	159.4 (23.6)	299.6 (54.3)
M	134.3 (10.5)	130.2 (9.8)	116.5 (14.0)	162.5 (18.6)

[a] Mean (SEM).
[b] Bipolar suicide attempters < nonattempters ($p < 0.05$).

Significant correlations between attempting suicide and the biogenic amines were limited to the catecholamines. Low urinary and plasma MHPG measures were significantly correlated with suicide attempts, while CSF MHPG showed a trend in the same direction. This finding was limited to the bipolar attempters. Median splits on the biochemical variables within this bipolar group supported the finding of low urinary MHPG and revealed low levels of NM and E as well. All of the above correlations were at a $p < 0.05$ level. Given the number of correlations examined, chance alone could account for this finding. The MHPG results, however, appear more robust as they are confirmed in several different biological fluids, i.e., urine, plasma, and CSF. Agren also reported an association between low levels of CSF MHPG and the seriousness of previous suicide attempts in depressed patients.[1]

We have previously reported an association between a decrease in baseline CSF and urinary MHPG and a positive response to drug therapy.[21,22] In the present study all 10 of our bipolar SA patients recovered while only 7 of the 12 bipolar NA patients responded to treatment. While this difference does not reach significance, the trend is supportive of the previous finding.

No difference in MHPG levels was found between the unipolar and bipolar patients, overall, though male patients in both groups had higher concentrations than did female patients.[15] Increased catecholamine functioning has been associated with increases in anxiety and agitation. In a study of normals, Fibiger et al. (1984) reported a positive correlation between urinary catechol levels (NE and E) and behavioral measures of anxiety, tension, stress, and arousal.[23] Given that our suicide attempter group had significantly lower levels of these behavioral variables, this might also contribute to the above findings.

Brown et al. in earlier studies found that the expression of human aggression was associated with lower levels of CSF 5-HIAA.[24] They subsequently reported that a history of aggressive behavior and a history of suicide attempts were significantly associated with each other and each was significantly associated with lower 5-HIAA levels.[25] In a study of 141 female psychiatric patients, Banki *et al.* found that CSF 5-HIAA was significantly lower in violent attempters in four diagnostic categories (major depression, schizophrenia, alcohol dependence, or adjustment disorder).[5] Biochemical changes were independent of clinical diagnoses. Roy *et al.*, however, in a population of chronic schizophrenic patients found no significant differences between either the violent or nonviolent attempters and those without a history of attempted suicide in CSF 5-HIAA, MHPG, or HVA.[26] Linnoila *et al.* studied two equally violent groups of criminals and found a relatively low 5-HIAA concentration in the CSF of impulsive violent offenders, but not in those offenders who had premeditated their acts.[27] Thus, they felt a low CSF 5-HIAA concentration maybe a marker of impulsivity rather than violence per se.

We are unable to directly compare our work with the studies quoted above as we had no similar measures of hostility in relationship to the suicide attempts rated. In concordance with the above studies, using our overall clinical measure of hostility, our suicide attempter group did trend higher than the nonattempter group, though not significantly so.

In the present study, the suicide *nonattempters* were more depressed and showed more anxiety, psychomotor retardation, agitation, and somatization. One possible explanation is that the nonattempters are more able to tolerate and/or express distressed feeling states, whereas the suicide attempter group is more likely to act out when these feeling states build up. Given that we are examining the SA patients after their attempt, an alternative explanation is that the act of attempting to end one's life relieves distressed feeling states.

It is clear that no unitary clinical or biochemical relationship exists between a clinical diagnosis, e.g., depression and a behavior—suicide. The most recent work attempting to define the impact of alterations in the biogenic amine system on aggression and impulsivity is interesting and invites much speculation as regards one final

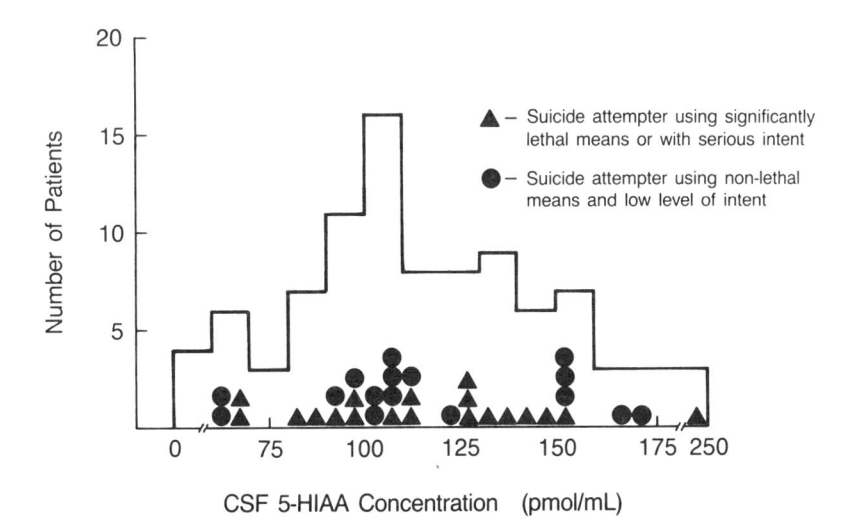

FIGURE 1. Distribution of suicide attempters relative to distribution of CSF 5-HIAA values in depressed patients.

common pathway behavior—suicide. However, the work remains too sketchy and it must be for future authors to provide the necessary linkage.

ACKNOWLEDGMENTS

From the National Institute of Mental Health-Clinical Research Branch Collaborative Program on the Psychobiology of Depression-Biological Studies. The above study was completed with the cooperation and participation of the collaborative program investigators: S. H. Koslow (project director); S. Secunda (deputy project director); M. M. Katz (senior investigator); I. Hanin (consultant); B. Harris-Larkin (protocol monitor) (National Institute of Mental Health); J. W. Maas (chairman) (University of Texas Health Science Center at San Antonio); D. E. Redmond, Jr., A. Swann (Yale University School of Medicine); J. M. Davis, R. Casper, S. Chuang, D. Garver, J. Javaid (Illinois State Psychiatric Institute); J. Mendels, D. Brunswick, A. Frazer, A. Ramsey, S. Stern (Philadelphia Veterans Administration Medical Center); P. E. Stokes, J. Kocsis (Cornell University Medical College); E. Robins (Washington University School of Medicine, St. Louis); J. Croughan (Washington University School of Medicine and Jewish Hospital, St. Louis); C. Bowden, R. Shulman (the University of Texas Health Science Center at San Antonio).

REFERENCES

1. AGREN, H. 1980. Symptom patterns in unipolar and bipolar depression correlating with monoamine metabolites in the cerebrospinal fluid. II. Suicide. Psychiatry Res. **3:** 225-236.
2. ASBERG, M. & L. TRASKMAN. 1981. Studies of CSF 5-HIAA in depression and suicidal behavior. Exp. Med. Biol. **133:** 739-752.
3. ASBERG, M., L. TRASKMAN & P. THOREN. 1976. 5-HIAA in the cerebrospinal fluid. Arch. Gen. Psychiatry **33:** 1193-1197.
4. BANKI, C. M. & M. ARATO. 1983. Amine metabolites, neuroendocrine findings, and personality dimension as correlates of suicidal behavior. Psychiatry Res. **10:** 253-261.
5. BANKI, C. M., M. ARATO & M. KURCY. 1980. Biochemical markers in suicidal patients: investigations with cerebrospinal fluid amine metabolites and neuroendocrine tests. J. Affect. Disord. **6:** 341-350.
6. NINAN, P. T., D. P. VAN KAMMEN, M. SCHEININ, M. LINNOILA, W. E. BUNNEY & F. K. GOODWIN. 1984. CSF 5-hydroxyindoleacetic acid levels in suicidal schizophrenic patients. Am. J. Psychiatry **141:** 566-569.
7. TRASKMAN, L., M. ASBERG & L. BERTILSSON. 1981. Monoamine metabolites in cerebrospinal fluid and suicidal behavior. Arch. Gen. Psychiatry **38:** 631-636.
8. MAAS, J. W., S. H. KOSLOW, J. M. DAVIS, M. M. KATZ, J. MENDELS, E. ROBINS, P. E. STOKES & C. L. BOWDEN. 1980. Biological component of the NIMH Clinical Research Branch Collaborative Program on the psychobiology of depression. I. Background and theoretical considerations. Psychol. Med. **10:** 759-776.
9. SECUNDA, S. K., S. H. KOSLOW, D. E. REDMOND, D. GARVER, A. RAMSEY, J. CROUGHAN, J. KOCSIS, I. HANIN, K. LIEBERMAN & R. CASPER. 1980. Biological component of the NIMH Clinical Research Branch Collaborative Program on the psychobiology of depression. II. Methodology and data analysis. Psychol. Med. **10:** 777-793.
10. SPITZER, R. L. & J. ENDICOTT. 1979. Schedule of Affective Disorders and Schizophrenia. Biometric Research, New York State Psychiatric Institute. New York, N.Y.

11. SPITZER, R. L., J. ENDICOTT & E. ROBINS. 1977. Research Diagnostic Criteria (RDC) for a Selected Group of Functional Disorders. 3rd edit. Biometrics Research, New York State Psychiatric Institute. New York, N.Y.
12. KATZ, M. M., S. H. KOSLOW, N. BERMAN, S. K. SECUNDA, J. W. MAAS, R. CASPER, J. KOCSIS & P. STOKES. 1984. A multivantaged approach to the measurement of behavioral and affect states for clinical and psychobiological research. Psychol. Rep. 55 (Suppl. 1): 619-671.
13. HAMILTON, M. 1960. A rating scale for depression. J. Neurol. Neurosurg. Psychiatry 23: 56-62.
14. ENDICOTT, J. & R. L. SPITZER. 1978. The schedule for affective disorders and schizophrenia. Arch. Gen. Psychiatry 35: 837-844.
15. KOSLOW, S. H., J. W. MAAS, C. L. BOWDEN, J. M. DAVIS, I. HANIN & J. JAVAID. 1983. CSF and urinary biogenic amines and metabolites in depression and mania: a controlled, univariate analysis. Arch. Gen. Psychiatry 40: 999-1010.
16. GUZE, S. & E. ROBINS. 1970. Suicide and primary affective disorder. Br. J. Psychiatry 117: 437-438.
17. GARVEY, M. J., V. B. TUASON, N. HOFFMAN & J. GHASTEK. 1983. Suicide attempters, non-attempters, and neurotransmitters. Comp. Psychiatry 24: 331-336.
18. JOHNSON, G. F. & G. HUNT. 1979. Suicidal behavior in bipolar manic-depressive patients and their families. Comp. Psychiatry 20: 159-164.
19. WOODRUFF, R., S. GUZE & P. CLAYTON. 1971. Unipolar and bipolar primary affective disorder. Br. J. Psychiatry 119: 33-38.
20. ROOSE, S. P., A. H. GLASSMAN, B. T. WALSH, S. WOODRING & J. VITAL-HERNE. 1983. Depression, delusions, and suicide. Am. J. Psychiatry 140: 1159-1162.
21. MAAS, J. W., J. H. KOCSIS, C. L. BOWDEN, J. M. DAVIS, D. E. REDMOND, I. HANIN & E. ROBINS. 1982. Pre-treatment neurotransmitter metabolites and response to imipramine or amitriptyline treatment. Psychol. Med. 12: 37-43.
22. MAAS, J. W., S. H. KOSLOW, M. M. KATZ, C. L. BOWDEN, R. L. GIBBONS, P. E. STOKES, E. ROBINS & J. M. DAVIS. 1984. Pretreatment neurotransmitter metabolite levels and response to tricyclic antidepressant drugs. Am. J. Psychiatry 141(10): 1159-1171.
23. FIBIGER, W., G. SINGER, A. J. MILLER, S. ARMSTRONG & M. DATAR. 1984. Cortisol and catecholamines changes as functions of time-of-day and self-reported mood. Neurosci. Behav. Rev. 8: 523-530.
24. BROWN, G. L., F. K. GOODWIN, J. C. BALLENGER, P. F. GOYER & L. F. MAJOR. 1979. Aggression in human correlates with cerebrospinal fluid amine metabolites. Psychiatry Res. 1: 131-139.
25. BROWN, G. L., M. H. EBERT, P. F. GOYER, D. C. JIMERSON, W. J. KLEIN, W. E. BUNNEY & F. K. GOODWIN. 1982. Aggression, suicide, and serotonin: relationships to CSF amine metabolites. Am. J. Psychiatry 139: 741-746.
26. ROY, A., P. NINAN, A. MAZONSON, D. PICKAR, D. VAN KAMMEN, M. LINNOILA & S. M. PAUL. 1985. CSF monoamine metabolites in chronic schizophrenic patients who attempt suicide. Psychol. Med. 15: 335-340.
27. LINNOILA, M., M. VIRKKUNEN, M. SCHEININ, A. NUUTILA, R. RIMON & F. K. GOODWIN. 1983. Low cerebrospinal fluid 5-hydroxyindoleacetic acid concentration differentiates impulsive from nonimpulsive violent behavior. Life Sci. 23: 2609-2614.

APPENDIX A. SADS Items Related to Suicidal Ideation and Behavior for Current Episodes[a]

Number	Item	Current Episodes Ratings
246	Suicidal tendencies, including preoccupation with thoughts of death or suicide	0–No information. 1–Not at all. 2–Slight, e.g., occasional thoughts of his death (without suicidal thoughts), "I would be better off dead" or "I wish I were dead." 3–Mild, e.g., frequent thoughts that he would be better off dead or occasional thoughts of suicide but has not thought of a specific method. 4–Moderate, e.g., often thinks of suicide or has thought of a specific method. 5–Severe, e.g., often thinks of suicide and has thought of, or mentally rehearsed, a specific plan or has made a suicidal gesture of a communicative rather than a potentially medically harmful type. 6–Extreme, e.g., has made preparations for a potentially serious suicidal attempt. 7–Very extreme, e.g., suicidal attempt with definite intent to die or potentially medically.
247	Past week	0 1 2 3 4 5 6 7
248	Number of discrete suicidal gestures or attempts during the present episode (up to 1 year) or if no current episode, in the last year.	0 1 2 3 4 5 6 7 8 9+
249	Seriousness of suicidal intent to kill self as judged by overall circumstances including likelihood of being rescued, precautions against discovery, action to gain help during or after attempt, degree of planning and the apparent purpose of attempt (manipulative versus killing self).	0–No information. 1–Obviously no intent, purely manipulative gestures. 2–Not sure or only minimal intent. 3–Definite but very ambivalent. 4–Serious. 5–Very serious. 6–Extreme (every expectation of death).
250	Medical lethality. Actual medical threat to life or physical condition following the most serious suicide gesture, taking into account the method (gunshot wound more serious than knife wound, impaired consciousness at or during time of rescue, seriousness of lesion, toxicity of ingested materials, expected for complete recovery) and amount of treatment required.	0–No information. 1–No danger, e.g., no effects, held pills in hand. 2–Minimal, e.g., scratch on wrist. 3–Mild, e.g., took 10 aspirins, mild gastritis. 4–Moderate, e.g., took 10 Seconals. 5–Severe, e.g., cuts throat. 6–Extreme, e.g., respiratory arrest or prolonged coma.

[a] Sum of items 246 through 250 represents score on SADS Suicidal Ideation and Behavior Scale.

Cerebrospinal Fluid Studies in Suicide[a]

An Overview

MARIE ÅSBERG, PETER NORDSTRÖM, AND LIL TRÄSKMAN-BENDZ[b]

Department of Psychiatry and Psychology
Karolinska Hospital
S-104 01 Stockholm 60, Sweden

In the chain of events that terminates in a suicide, biological factors may be more important than previously thought. Recent research has identified two clusters of biological factors that tend to correlate with suicidal behavior, namely, variables associated with monoaminergic neurotransmission and variables associated with certain neuroendocrine functions.

The most convincing evidence for an involvement of monoamines in suicide stems from measurements of serotonin and its main metabolite, 5-hydroxyindoleacetic acid (5-HIAA), in brains from suicide victims and in cerebrospinal fluid (CSF) from patients who have attempted suicide.[1] Initially, such investigations were performed in order to study the biological correlates of depressive disorders, but more recently, interest has focused on the possible biological background of suicidal behavior as such.

The present article will review CSF studies of monoamine metabolites in suicidal individuals, published until 1984, and also discuss some possible mechanisms for the relationship between suicide and serotonin.

METHODOLOGICAL ASPECTS—MONOAMINE METABOLITES

An underlying assumption behind the CSF studies is that the concentrations of neurotransmitter metabolites in CSF will reflect functionally important aspects of the parent transmitters in the brain. There has been some discussion as to whether concentrations of, e.g., the serotonin metabolite 5-hydroxyindoleacetic acid in CSF reflects serotonin turnover in the spinal cord rather than in the brain itself.[2] The

---

[a] Financial support has been received from the Swedish Medical Research Council (5454), the Fredrik and Ingrid Thuring Foundation, the Söderström-König Foundation, the Torsten and Ragnar Söderberg Foundation, and funds from the Karolinska Institute.

[b] Present affiliation: Department of Psychiatry, Lund University Hospital, 5-22185 Lund, Sweden.

demonstration by Stanley and co-workers that 5-HIAA in CSF drawn after death correlates strongly with 5-HIAA in brain cortex[3] suggests, however, that brain events are indeed reflected in CSF metabolite concentrations.

A main advantage of the CSF technique is that spinal fluid is comparatively easy to obtain at little discomfort to the patient. There are many disadvantages as well. The concentrations of 5-HIAA and of the dopamine metabolite homovanillic acid (HVA) depend, inter alia, on the subject's sex (men have lower concentrations), age (concentrations increase with age), and body height (the taller the subject, the lower the metabolite concentrations).[4] The dependence on body height is presumably due to an active removal from CSF of the acid metabolites as they flow from the brain ventricles down to the lumbar sac where the CSF is sampled. Metabolite concentrations also vary seasonally[5] and with the time of the day.[6]

Most important in clinical studies, the monoamine metabolite concentrations are drastically altered by treatment with certain psychotropic drugs. The classical tricyclic antidepressants, for instance, reduce the CSF concentrations of the noradrenaline metabolite 4-hydroxy-3-methoxyphenyl glycol (HMPG). Many antidepressants also lower the concentrations of 5-HIAA, and the interference with serotonin turnover appears to affect HVA concentrations as well.[7] The importance of an appropriate washout period before an individual is admitted to a research project is underlined by these findings. Lingering effects of previously given treatment might otherwise be misinterpreted as evidence of biological disturbances when patients are compared to healthy control subjects.

METHODOLOGICAL ASPECTS—ASSESSMENT OF SUICIDAL BEHAVIOR

The method used to assess "suicidality" in studies of monoamine metabolites varies from dichotomizing groups of subjects into those who have and those who have not made a suicide attempt to assessment of present or past suicidal tendencies in various rating instruments. In the rating scales, suicidal ideation and suicide attempts are usually considered as indicators of increasing severity of an underlying variable, "suicidality." Although this may make sense in the assessment of suicide risk, it may create problems in biological studies, since the biological correlates of recurring thoughts may differ profoundly from those of manifest action.

The observation period under consideration also varies between studies. While the earlier studies focused on recent suicide attempts, later studies have often investigated lifetime suicidal behavior. When lifetime suicidal behavior is correlated to a biological marker, the implicit assumption would seem to be that the biological variable is a trait marker, rather than state dependent. Although there is some evidence of a relative stability of CSF monoamine metabolite concentrations in normal people over short time periods, this may not always be so over longer periods and in psychiatric patients, as will be discussed below.

An even more problematic issue is the selection of subjects for research projects. Most research in biological psychiatry is performed in highly specialized clinics, which admit patients via a referral system. The extent to which such patients are representative of the population is rarely known, but problematic cases and treatment failures (which may be biologically deviant) are likely to be overrepresented. This should be borne in mind, e.g., when large-scale treatment programs are based on research findings.

LOW CSF 5-HIAA AND ATTEMPTED SUICIDE IN DEPRESSION

The first description of a relationship between suicide and a biological substance in CSF was a serendipitous finding in the course of a CSF study of 5-HIAA in depressive illness.[8] The concentrations of the serotonin metabolite appeared to be bimodally distributed in depression, both when baseline values[9] and accumulation after probenecid administration[10] were considered. The bimodal distribution suggested that depressive disorder might be a heterogeneous condition on the biochemical level, which in turn stimulated the search for clinical differences between patients in the two modes of the CSF 5-HIAA distribution.

In their attempts to find clinical correlates to a low concentration of CSF 5-HIAA in depressed patients, Åsberg and co-workers unexpectedly found an increased incidence of suicide attempts in the low CSF 5-HIAA subgroup.[8] Forty percent of the low 5-HIAA patients had attempted suicide during their present illness, as compared with 15% in the normal 5-HIAA patients. Furthermore, the suicide attempts were of a more determined nature with a preference for active, violent methods in the low 5-HIAA patients, while those in the high 5-HIAA group were confined to drug overdoses. Two deaths from suicide occurred during the study period, both in low 5-HIAA patients.

The relationship between CSF 5-HIAA and suicidal behavior was first confirmed by Ågren.[11] He studied depressed patients and measured suicidal behavior by means of the Schedule for Affective Disorder and Schizophrenia (SADS) scales for suicidal behavior. These scales do not differentiate between suicidal ideation and suicidal acts, which may have weakened the correlation. In the Åsberg et al. study, there was no association between low CSF 5-HIAA and suicidal ideation, or rated suicide risk.[8]

These early studies did not take the relationship between CSF 5-HIAA and such interference factors as sex and body height into account. The sex factor could, however, be ruled out in a subsequent confirmatory study by Träskman et al.[12]

More recently, the relationship has been confirmed in Dutch depressed patients studied by van Praag, who found a very highly significant increase in suicidal behavior in patients with low probenecid-induced accumulation of 5-HIAA.[13] Lower 5-HIAA concentrations in suicidal than in nonsuicidal depressed patients were also reported by Montgomery and Montgomery in British patients.[14] Palanappian and co-workers found a significant correlation between suicidal tendencies (estimated by the item Suicide in the Hamilton Rating Scale) and CSF 5-HIAA concentrations in Indian depressed patients.[15] Banki and co-workers demonstrated a relationship between low CSF 5-HIAA and violent suicide attempts in Hungarian female patients.[16] Pérez de los Cobos et al. have reported a relationship between suicide attempts and low CSF 5-HIAA in Spanish depressed patients, regardless of the method used in the suicide attempt.[17]

There is also one well-designed, nonconfirmatory study by Roy-Byrne and co-workers, who mainly studied treatment-resistant affectively ill American patients, referred to a research center specializing in the study of depressive disorders.[18] No significant relationship was found between lifetime suicidal behavior and CSF 5-HIAA, possibly owing to the high proportion of bipolar (manic depressive) patients in the group. When their unipolar cases were examined separately, the suicidal unipolars tended to have lower CSF 5-HIAA than did other unipolars. The biological correlates of suicidal behavior may thus differ in bipolar and unipolar disorder. A similar conclusion was reached by Ågren.[19]

LOW CSF 5-HIAA AND SUICIDE ATTEMPTS IN OTHER DISORDERS

Although depressive disorder is the single largest diagnostic category in completed suicide, other psychiatric disorders are also connected with an increased suicide risk. Several groups have studied the relationship between suicidal behavior and CSF 5-HIAA in other diagnostic categories. Träskman *et al.* found low CSF 5-HIAA in comparison with normals also in *nondepressed* psychiatric inpatients who had recently made a suicide attempt (mainly patients with personality disorders and minor affective disorders).[12] Brown *et al.* studied two groups of men with *personality disorders* and found more lifetime suicide attempts in those with low CSF 5-HIAA.[20]

van Praag[21] and Ninan and co-workers[22] found a similar association between lifetime suicide attempts and 5-HIAA in *schizophrenia*. Both studies are well designed with carefully chosen, matched controls. Lower CSF 5-HIAA in suicidal patients among subjects with schizophrenia has also been reported by Banki *et al.*[16]

Banki and co-workers also found that CSF 5-HIAA was significantly lower in female violent attempters than in nonattempters with *alcoholism* and *adjustment disorder*. The relationship between low CSF 5-HIAA and suicide attempts thus appears to be surprisingly robust.

HVA IN CSF AND SUICIDAL BEHAVIOR

The concentrations of the dopamine metabolite homovanillic acid in CSF are reduced in depression,[23,24] and more consistently so than CSF 5-HIAA. HVA and 5-HIAA in CSF are strongly correlated. Whether the correlation between the two metabolites is due to their sharing the same transport mechanism or to a functional connection between the parent amines is not known.

If suicidal behavior is correlated with a low 5-HIAA concentration, there is reason to expect a correlation with HVA as well. Low concentrations of HVA in suicidal depressed patients were indeed reported by Träskman *et al.*,[12] by Montgomery and Montgomery,[14] and by Ågren.[19] In a follow-up study of depressed patients by Roy *et al.*, a low level of HVA was an even better predictor than 5-HIAA of subsequent suicide.[25] Banki *et al.* found a less clear-cut relationship between suicide and HVA than with 5-HIAA.[16] In particular, their depressed patients who had taken drug overdoses had significantly higher HVA than did nonsuicidal patients, while HVA in violent attempters was very low.

In the Träskman *et al.* study, only the suicide attempters who were also depressed had lower than normal HVA concentrations.[12] This may suggest that the reduced HVA concentrations may be more closely related to some particular aspect of depressive illness than to suicidal behavior in general. Only depressive suicide attempters were included in the Montgomery and Montgomery, the Ågren, and the Roy et al. studies. The failure of Ninan et al. to find any difference in CSF HVA between their suicidal and nonsuicidal schizophrenic subjects[26] is in line with this.

HMPG IN CSF

In comparison with the evidence relating suicide to serotonin, the relationships with noradrenaline are less clear. Ågren reported a negative correlation between the noradrenaline metabolite HMPG and suicidal tendencies in his depressed patients.[27] Brown and co-workers found a positive correlation in subjects with personality disorders,[28] which was not reproduced in their study of borderline patients.[20]

Ostroff and associates have measured the ratio between noradrenaline and adrenaline in urine in two studies of mixed diagnostic groups, and found a relationship between low ratio and suicidal behavior.[29,30]

POSTMORTEM CSF STUDIES

The CSF studies summarized above all concerned survivors of a suicide attempt. In one study by Kauert et al. suboccipital CSF concentrations of the monoamines serotonin, adrenaline, noradrenaline, and dopamine were measured after death by suicide.[31] Serotonin levels were *increased* in the suicide victims. It cannot be excluded, however, that this unexpected difference may reflect differences in the time of death in suicides and controls. In monkeys, CSF serotonin concentrations are almost doubled during the night, and the daytime mean concentration is only 5% of the peak concentration at night.[32]

INTERRELATIONS BETWEEN MONOAMINES AND ENDOCRINE VARIABLES

Activation of the hypothalamic-pituitary-adrenal axis (HPA axis) is a consistent finding in depressive disorder with melancholia.[33] It is reflected in a disturbed secretion pattern of cortisol, high urinary output of cortisol and its metabolites, high CSF concentrations of cortisol, and a reduced ability to suppress cortisol secretion after dexamethasone administration.

There is relatively good agreement that HPA activation is more common in suicidal than in nonsuicidal depressed patients.[34–36] In nondepressed suicide attempters, the findings are conflicting. Thus Träskman and co-workers found normal CSF cortisol concentrations in suicide attempters who were not depressed.[37]

Abnormalities of the thyroid-stimulating hormone (TSH) response to injection of thyrotropin-releasing hormone (TRH) have also been described in suicidal patients, and a blunted TRH/TSH response has been associated with an increased incidence of completed suicide.[38]

Monoaminergic neurons are known to be involved in the chain of events that leads to release of many hormones, including cortisol. The details of the sequence have not yet been worked out, but the data from the Meltzer et al. study of 5-hydroxytryptophan-induced release of cortisol[39] strongly suggest a functional connection between the serotonin system and the HPA axis.

The available data in man do not, however, show any negative correlations between markers of the systems, such as might be expected if they reflect an identical risk factor for suicide. Thus CSF concentrations of cortisol and of 5-HIAA have been shown to correlate positively, though weakly,[37] or not at all.[40] Carroll et al.[41] and Banki and Arató[42] found a positive correlation between postdexamethasone cortisol and 5-HIAA. The interpretation of the results from Carroll et al. is, however, complicated by the fact that spinal fluid was drawn after the administration of dexamethasone, which raises CSF 5-HIAA concentrations.[43]

Gold and co-workers report an inverse correlation between the magnitude of the TSH reaction to TRH and CSF 5-HIAA.[44] The negative correlation between the TRH/TSH test and CSF 5-HIAA appears also in the study by Banki and co-workers,[16] where it is compatible with their finding of more normal TRH/TSH responses in suicidal than in nonsuicidal patients.

CSF 5-HIAA AS A PREDICTOR OF SUICIDE

With one exception, the studies reviewed so far focus on suicide attempts, rather than completed suicide. However, those who attempt and those who commit suicide are well known to differ in many important respects, even if there is an extensive overlap between the two populations.[45] In several studies, subsequent mortality from suicide among suicide attempters has amounted to about 2% within a year after the attempt.[46] Although this is a considerable increase in suicide compared to the general population, suicide is a rare event even in this group.

Estimating suicide risk and taking appropriate precautions in the individual case is one of the most difficult tasks of the practicing psychiatrist. It is therefore of clinical interest to increase the precision of risk evaluation, and there have been many attempts to create rating scales and inventories for the purpose. These have not usually been very successful.[47] Could the measurement of CSF 5-HIAA be of any help?

There is some evidence that this may be so. A one-year follow up of 76 patients who were hospitalized in our clinic after a suicide attempt showed that those with low CSF 5-HIAA were 10 times more likely to die from suicide than were the remainder. Twenty-one percent of the low 5-HIAA patients had died from suicide, as compared to 2% of the patients with normal or high CSF 5-HIAA.[1] A similar increase in suicide mortality after a suicide attempt in patients who had low CSF 5-HIAA was found by Roy and co-workers.[25]

CSF 5-HIAA—STATE OR TRAIT MARKER?

In the follow-up study mentioned above,[1] the suicide deaths were concentrated to a six-month period after the index attempt. This finding raises the question of the stability of the disturbance of serotonin function that is reflected in a low CSF 5-HIAA.

The bulk of the evidence suggests that 5-HIAA concentrations in CSF remain fairly stable over limited periods in normal subjects, and in depressed patients readmitted for relapse of depression.[48]

Recovered depressives whose 5-HIAA concentrations are normal during illness also remain stable over prolonged periods, whereas in depressives with low 5-HIAA during illness the situation is not so clear. van Praag, who has studied a large group of patients with the probenecid technique, reports that initially low 5-HIAA concentrations remained low after recovery in about 50% of the patients.[49] Träskman et al. found a significant average increase of CSF 5-HIAA in recovered depressives whose 5-HIAA had been low during illness, although the concentrations did not reach the normal range.[48]

It should be pointed out that CSF studies of recovered depressives are necessarily rare. Such patients are often maintained on drugs for extended periods, and those who are not, even if available for lumbar puncture studies, may well be a biased sample of the depressed population.

A possible interpretation of the existing data is that there is a subgroup of depressed patients, characterized by concentrations of CSF 5-HIAA that are not only low but also less stable over time. If this type of unstable serotonin system is associated with an increased vulnerability to illness, and with a further decrease in release during illness, the emergence of bimodal distributions in diseased populations is easily explained.

On the whole, CSF 5-HIAA concentrations tend to remain similar from one illness episode to another. We have, however, performed repeated lumbar punctures in two patients who subsequently committed suicide. In both cases, there was a substantial *reduction* in CSF 5-HIAA from one puncture to the next. Taken together with the finding that in patients whose CSF 5-HIAA is low during illness, its concentration increases on recovery, the observation suggests that failure to maintain a stable serotonin transmission may be of pathophysiological significance.

TOWARDS A PSYCHOBIOLOGY OF SUICIDE?

Apparently, both a low CSF 5-HIAA and an activation of the HPA axis are associated with an increased risk for suicide. The absence of reports of negative correlations between the two markers suggests that they may be independent and associated with suicide through different mechanisms.

Although the nature of these mechanisms is far from clear, the available data do allow some speculation. The HPA activation, for instance, has long been regarded as a consequence of emotional stress and failing defenses.[50] Recently, strong support for the stress hypothesis was provided in a study by Ceulemans et al., who found almost 50% abnormal dexamethasone suppression tests (DSTs) immediately prior to surgery for herniated discs in otherwise healthy, nondepressed individuals.[51] The nonsuppressors had higher scores in inventories for state anxiety, whereas their trait anxiety scores were similar to those of the suppressors, suggesting that anticipatory anxiety prior to surgery was indeed the reason for the HPA activation.

If the HPA activation reflects the emotional suffering and subjective helplessness associated with depressive illness, the relationship with suicide makes intuitive sense.

The abnormal DST may function as an alert signal that the emotional pain is approaching unbearable levels.

With a low CSF 5-HIAA, the situation is slightly different. Low 5-HIAA concentrations occur also in mentally healthy people who have never been depressed or contemplated suicide. This has led to the hypothesis that 5-HIAA is a marker of vulnerability to affective disorder and to suicide.

In most individuals with a low CSF 5-HIAA, the vulnerability will never be manifested in a suicide attempt. A suicide attempt is unlikely to occur unless the individual finds himself in a situation that he conceives of as desperate, or when he is without hope for the future. Adverse events may have created this situation, or the individual's perception of the situation may be colored by depressive illness. Whether this state of affairs leads to a suicide attempt is partially determined by the quality of the person's social support net, which may attenuate the effect of adverse events, or render the sufferings of depressive illness more tolerable. Previous experience of adverse events (e.g., early parental loss) is likely to render the interpretation of current adversity more ominous.

A low output serotonin system (or perhaps even more likely, a low stability one) might render an individual more vulnerable to self-destructive or impulsive action in times of crisis. This characteristic of the serotonin system might have a genetic basis, or it might be acquired. There are suggestions that "learned helplessness" situations in rats may lead to functional changes in the monoamine systems,[52] and that prolonged social isolation in mice consistently reduces serotonin turnover.[53]

If serotonin transmission is permanently low or unstable in suicide-prone individuals, it is conceivable that this may be manifested in other ways than in suicidal tendencies. The often quite unpremeditated, impulsive, and violent character of many of the suicide attempts in low 5-HIAA patients suggests that they might have difficulties with impulse control, particularly perhaps in the control of aggressive impulses. What, then, is the evidence of a connection between serotonin and aggression in man?

SEROTONIN AND AGGRESSIVE BEHAVIOR

Early psychoanalytic authors stressed the aggressive component in suicidal behavior, and in depressive illness.[54] Serotonin neurons are involved in the control of aggressive behavior in animals.[53]

In an investigation of the hypothesis that aggression dyscontrol was the link between serotonin turnover and suicidal behavior, Brown and associates studied men with personality disorders.[28] These men were rated for aggression on the basis of lifetime history of overt hostile and destructive behavior. A significant inverse correlation was found between CSF 5-HIAA and overt aggression.

Brown et al. gave personality inventories to their subjects in an extended study, and found an inverse relationship between CSF 5-HIAA and the Psychopathic Deviate (Pd) scale from the Minnesota Multiphasic Personality Inventory (MMPI).[20] They did not, however, find any significant relationship between CSF 5-HIAA and self-reported aggressive feelings, as measured by the Buss Durkee Inventory. Rydin and co-workers compared hostility, rated on the basis of Rorschach protocols, in otherwise matched pairs of psychiatric patients with low vis-à-vis high CSF 5-HIAA.[55] Low CSF 5-HIAA patients scored significantly higher in hostility, but also on several anxiety measures, which is in agreement with Banki's findings,[56] based on anxiety ratings.

The finding by Åsberg and co-workers that suicide *acts*, but not suicide *ideation*, are related to a low CSF 5-HIAA[8] is paralleled in an interesting way in the studies of aggressive *feelings* and aggressive *acts*, respectively. Three studies of homicide offenders suggest that serotonin turnover may be of importance to aggressive acts. Linnoila and co-workers found lower CSF 5-HIAA in impulsive violent offenders than in other types of murderers.[57] Lidberg *et al.* found lower CSF 5-HIAA in those homicide offenders who had killed a spouse or a lover than in those who had killed someone less emotionally cathected (most often a drinking buddy).[58] Lidberg and co-workers also examined three suicide attempters who had killed, or attempted to kill, a child as well.[59] In all three, the CSF 5-HIAA concentrations were very low.

The findings in murderers may be relevant for the suicide-serotonin association, since having committed a murder is probably the strongest risk factor of all for ultimate suicide, at least in Western Europe. In Great Britain, a 30% suicide incidence is reported after a murder, and it is precisely in those cases where the victim was a spouse that the risk of suicide is greatest.[60] (In the United States the suicide rate after murder is lower, around 4%, according to Wolfgang.)[61]

SEROTONIN AND DISINHIBITORY PERSONALITY TRAITS

The finding that low CSF 5-HIAA appears more closely related to aggressive or self-destructive acts than to ideation or feelings suggests that difficulties in the suppression of impulses to act may be a key problem. This raises the issue of the possible relationships between serotonin and other, less pathological aspects of disinhibitory and impulsive behavior. Available evidence (e.g., from personality questionnaire studies) supports a relationship between low CSF 5-HIAA and impulsivity[62] and the Validity scale, in the Marke-Nyman Temperament Scales (Banki and Arató 1983),[42] and between CSF 5-HIAA and the Pd scale from the MMPI.[20] There are also weak, but consistent, correlations with Eysenck's scale Psychoticism, which reflects schizoid, nonconforming, nonempathetic, hostile personality traits.[62]

IMPLICATIONS FOR SUICIDE PREVENTION

The association with a heightened risk of suicide suggests that markers of serotonin and HPA activation may be valuable in the clinic. Low concentrations of CSF 5-HIAA in suicide attempters, for instance, were connected with a 20% mortality from suicide within a year, which suggests that the two markers in combination may be one of the strongest suicide predictors hitherto identified.

A dexamethasone test is easy to perform and is unaffected by current antidepressant treatment. In contrast, spinal taps for 5-HIAA measurements require hospitalization and highly standardized procedures, and the patient must not be taking any antidepressant or neuroleptic drugs. There is an obvious need for new, more easily accessible markers of the state of the serotonin system.

A better understanding of the biological and psychological links between serotonin turnover and suicidal behavior might also open up new approaches to the prevention of suicide. Serotonin transmission can be influenced with drugs or amino acid precursors, and possibly by dietary changes, and it would seem important to test such treatment strategies in patients with a high suicide potential. It is also plausible that a better understanding of the psychological processes in suicide that are controlled by serotonin neurons could be used to develop more specific psychotherapeutic techniques than has hitherto been accomplished.

ACKNOWLEDGMENTS

The authors wish to thank Ms. Marie Skjöldebrand for secretarial assistance.

REFERENCES

1. ÅSBERG, M., P. NORDSTRÖM & L. TRÄSKMAN-BENDZ. 1986. Biological factors in suicide. In Suicide. A. Roy, Ed.: 47-51. Williams and Wilkins. Baltimore, Md.
2. BULAT, M. & B. ZIVKOVIĆ. 1971. Origin of 5-hydroxyindoleacetic acid in the spinal fluid. Science 173: 738-40.
3. STANLEY, M., L. TRÄSKMAN-BENDZ & K. DOROVINI-ZIS. 1985. Correlations between aminergic metabolites simultaneously obtained from human CSF and brain. Life Sci. 37: 1279-1286.
4. ÅSBERG, M. & L. BERTILSSON. 1979. Serotonin in depressive illness—studies of CSF 5-HIAA. In Neuropsychopharmacology. B. Saletu, Ed.: 105-115. Pergamon Press. Oxford & New York.
5. ÅSBERG, M., L. BERTILSSON, E. RYDIN, D. SCHALLING, P. THORÉN & L. TRÄSKMAN-BENDZ. 1981. Monoamine metabolites in cerebrospinal fluid in relation to depressive illness, suicidal behaviour and personality. Biosci. 31: 257-271.
6. NICOLETTI, F., R. RAFFAELE, A. FALSAPERLA & R. PACI. 1981. Circadian variation in 5-hydroxyindoleacetic acid levels in human cerebrospinal fluid. Eur. Neurol. 20: 834-838.
7. BERTILSSON, L., M. ÅSBERG & P. THORÉN. 1974. Differential effects of chlorimipramine and nortriptyline on cerebrospinal fluid metabolites of serotonin and noradrenaline in depression. Eur. J. Clin. Pharmacol. 7: 365-368.
8. ÅSBERG, M., L. TRÄSKMAN & P. THORÉN. 1976. 5-HIAA in the cerebrospinal fluid—a biochemical suicide predictor? Arch. Gen. Psychiatry 33: 1193-1197.
9. ÅSBERG, M., P. THORÉN, L. TRÄSKMAN, L. BERTILSSON & V. RINGBERGER. 1976. "Serotonin depression"—a biochemical subgroup within the affective disorders? Science 191: 478-480.
10. VAN PRAAG, H. M. & J. KORF. 1971. Endogenous depressions with and without disturbances in the 5-hydroxytryptamine metabolism: a biochemical classification? Psychopharmacologia 19: 148-152.
11. ÅGREN, H. 1980. Symptom patterns in unipolar and bipolar depression correlating with monoamine metabolites in the cerebrospinal fluid. II. Suicide. Psychiatry Res. 3: 225-236.
12. TRÄSKMAN, L., M. ÅSBERG, L. BERTILSSON & L. SJÖSTRAND. 1981. Monoamine metabolites in CSF and suicidal behavior. Arch. Gen. Psychiatry 38: 631-636.
13. VAN PRAAG, H. M. 1982. Depression, suicide and the metabolism of serotonin in the brain. J. Affect. Disord. 4: 275-290.
14. MONTGOMERY, S. A. & D. B. MONTGOMERY. 1982. Pharmacological prevention of suicidal behaviour. J. Affect. Disord. 4: 291-298.

15. PALANAPPIAN, V., V. RAMACHANDRAN & O. SOMASUNDARAM. 1983. Suicidal ideation and biogenic amines in depression. Indian J. Psychiatry **25:** 286-292.
16. BANKI, C. M., M. ARATÓ, Z. PAPP & M. KURCZ. 1984. Biochemical markers in suicidal patients. Investigations with cerebrospinal fluid amine metabolites and neuroendocrine tests. J. Affect. Disord. **6:** 341-350.
17. PÉREZ DE LOS COBOS, J. C., J. J. LÓPEZ-IBOR ALINO, JR. & J. SAIZ-RUIZ. 1984. Correlatos biológicos dél suicidio y la agresividad en depresiones mayores (con melancolía); 5-HIAA en LCR, DST, y respuesta terapéutica a 5-Htp. Paper presented to the First Congress of the Spanish Society for Biological Psychiatry, Barcelona, October 17-19, 1984.
18. ROY-BYRNE, P., R. M. POST, D. R. RUBINOW, M. LINNOILA, R. SAVARD & D. DAVIS. 1983. CSF 5HIAA and personal and family history of suicide in affectively ill patients: a negative study. Psychiatry Res. **10:** 263-274.
19. ÅGREN, H. 1983. Life at risk: markers of suicidality in depression. Psychiatr. Dev. **1:** 87-104.
20. BROWN, G. L., M. H. EBERT, P. F. GOYER, D. C. JIMERSON, W. J. KLEIN, W. E. BUNNEY & F. K. GOODWIN. 1982. Aggression, suicide, and serotonin: relationships to CSF amine metabolites. Am. J. Psychiatry **139:** 741-746.
21. VAN PRAAG, H. M. 1983. CSF 5-HIAA and suicide in non-depressed schizophrenics. Lancet ii: 977-978.
22. NINAN, P. T., D. P. VAN KAMMEN, M. SCHEININ, M. LINNOILA, W. E. BUNNEY, JR & F. K. GOODWIN. 1984. CSF 5-hydroxyindoleacetic acid in suicidal schizophrenic patients. Am. J. Psychiatry **141:** 566-569.
23. POST, R. M., J. C. BALLENGER & F. K. GOODWIN. 1980. Cerebrospinal fluid studies of neurotransmitter function in manic and depressive illness. In J. H. Wood, Ed. Neurobiology of Cerebrospinal Fluid **1:** 685-717. Plenum Press. New York, N.Y.
24. ÅSBERG, M., L. BERTILSSON, B. MÅRTENSSON, G.-P. SCALIA-TOMBA, P. THORÉN & L. TRÄSKMAN-BENDZ. 1984. CSF monoamine metabolites in melancholia. Acta psychiatr. Scand. **69:** 201-219.
25. ROY, A., H. ÅGREN, D. PICKAR, M. LINNOILA, A. R. DORAN, N. R. CUTLER & S. M. PAUL. Reduced cerebrospinal fluid concentrations of homovanillic acid and homovanillic acid to 5-hydroxyindoleacetic acid ratios in depressed patients: relationship to suicidality and dexamethasone nonsuppression. Am. J. Psychiatry. (In press.)
26. NINAN, P. T., D. P. VAN KAMMEN & M. LINNOILA. 1985. Letter to the editor. Am. J. Psychiatry **142:** 148.
27. ÅGREN, H. 1981. Biological markers in major depressive disorders. A clinical and multivariate study. Academic Dissertation. Acta Universitatis Upsaliensis, Abstracts of Uppsala Dissertations from the Faculty of Medicine 405. Uppsala, Sweden.
28. BROWN, G. L., F. K. GOODWIN, J. C. BALLENGER, P. F. GOYER & L. F. MAJOR. 1979. Aggression in humans correlates with cerebrospinal fluid amine metabolites. Psychiatry Res. **1:** 131-139.
29. OSTROFF, R. B., E. GILLER, K. BONESE, E. EBERSOLE, L. HARKNESS & J. MASON. 1982. Neuroendocrine risk factors of suicidal behavior. Am. J. Psychiatry **139:** 1323-1325.
30. OSTROFF, R. B., E. GILLER, L. HARKNESS & J. MASON. 1985. The norepinephrine-to-epinephrine ratio in patients with a history of suicide attempts. Am. J. Psychiatry **142:** 224-227.
31. KAUERT, G., T. GILG, W. EISENMENGER & W. SPANN. 1984. Post mortem biogenic amines in CSF of suicides and controls. Presented to the Collegium Internationale Neuro-Psychopharmacologicum on its 14th Congress in Florence 1984.
32. GARRICK, N. A., L. TAMARKIN, P. L. TAYLOR, S. P. MARKEY & D. L. MURPHY. 1983. Light and propranolol suppress the nocturnal elevation of serotonin in the cerebrospinal fluid of rhesus monkeys. Science **221:** 474-476.
33. CARROLL, B. J. 1982. The dexamethasone suppression test for melancholia. Br. J. Psychiatry **140:** 292-304.
34. CARROLL, B. J., J. F. GREDEN & M. FEINBERG. 1981. Suicide, neuroendocrine dysfunction and CSF 5-HIAA concentrations in depression. Adv. Biosci. **31:** 307-313.
35. CORYELL, W. & M. A. SCHLESSER. 1981. Suicide and the dexamethasone suppression test in unipolar depression. Am. J. Psychiatry **138:** 1120-1121.

36. TARGUM, S. D., L. ROSEN & A. E. CAPODANNO. 1983. The dexamethasone suppression test in suicidal patients with unipolar depression. Am. J. Psychiatry **140:** 877-879.
37. TRÄSKMAN, L., G. TYBRING, M. ÅSBERG, L. BERTILSSON, O. LANTTO & D. SCHALLING. 1980. Cortisol in the CSF of depressed and suicidal patients. Arch. Gen. Psychiatry **37:** 761-767.
38. LINKOWSKI, P., J. P. VAN WETTERE, M. KERKHOFS, F. GREGOIRE, H. BRAUMAN & J. MENDLEWICZ. 1984. Violent suicidal behavior and the thyrotropin-releasing hormone-thyroid-stimulating hormone test: a clinical outcome study. Neuropsychobiology **12:** 19-22.
39. MELTZER, H. Y., R. PERLINE, B. J. TRICOU, M. LOWY & A. ROBERTSON. 1984. Effect of 5-hydroxytryptophan on serum cortisol levels in major affective disorders. II. Relation to suicide, psychosis, and depressive symptoms. Arch. Gen. Psychiatry **41:** 379-387.
40. BANKI, C. M., M. VOJNIK, Z. PAPP, K. Z. BALLA & M. ARATÓ. 1985. Cerebrospinal fluid magnesium and calcium related to amine metabolites, diagnosis and suicide attempts. Biol. Psychiatry **20:** 163-171.
41. CARROLL, B. J., J. F. GREDEN, R. HASKETT, M. FEINBERG, A. A. ALBALA, F. I. R. MARTIN, R. T. RUBIN, B. HEATH, P. T. SHARP, W. L. MCLEOD & M. F. MCLEOD. 1980. Neutrotransmitter studies of neuroendocrine pathology in depression. Acta Psychiatr. Scand. **61**(Suppl. 280): 183-198.
42. BANKI, C. M. & M. ARATÓ. 1983. Relationship between cerebrospinal fluid amine metabolites, neuroendocrine findings and personality dimensions (Marke-Nyman scale factors) in psychiatric patients. Acta Psychiatr. Scand. **67:** 272-280.
43. BANKI, C. M., M. ARATO, Z. PAPP & M. KURCZ. 1981. The influence of dexamethasone on cerebrospinal fluid monoamine metabolites and cortisol in psychiatric patients. Pharmacopsychiatria **16:** 77-81.
44. GOLD, P. W., F. K. GOODWIN, T. WEHR & R. REBAR. 1977. Pituitary thyrotropin response to thyrotropin-releasing hormone in affective illness: relationship to spinal fluid amine metabolites. Am. J. Psychiatry **134:** 1028-1031.
45. STENGEL, E. & N. C. COOK. 1958. Attempted Suicide. Chapman & Hall. London, England.
46. ETTLINGER, R. 1975. Evaluation of suicide prevention after attempted suicide. Acta Psychiatr. Scand. (Suppl. 260.)
47. POKORNY, A. D. 1983. Prediction of suicide in psychiatric patients. Arch. Gen. Psychiatry **40:** 249-257.
48. TRÄSKMAN-BENDZ, L., M. ÅSBERG, L. BERTILSSON & P. THORÉN. 1984. CSF monoamine metabolites of depressed patients during illness and after recovery. Acta Psychiatr. Scand. **69:** 333-342.
49. VAN PRAAG, H. M. 1977. Significance of biochemical parameters in the diagnosis, treatment, and prevention of depressive disorders. Biol. Psychiatr **12:** 101-131.
50. BUNNEY, W. E., JR. & J. A. FAWCETT. 1965. Possibility of a biochemical test for suicide potential. Arch. Gen. Psychiatry **13:** 232-239.
51. CEULEMANS, D. L. S., H. G. M. WESTENBERG & H. M. VAN PRAAG. 1985. The effect of stress on the dexamethasone suppression test. Psychiatry Res. **14:** 189-195.
52. ANISMAN, H., A. PIZZINO & L. S. SKLAR. 1980. Coping with stress, norepinephrine depletion, and escape performance. Brain Res. **191:** 583-588.
53. VALZELLI, L. 1981. Psychobiology of Aggression and Violence. Raven Press. New York, N. Y.
54. ABRAHAM, K. 1927. Versuch einer Entwicklungsgeschichte der Libido auf Grund der Psychoanalyse seelischer Störungen. *In* Neue Arbeiten zur ärztlichen Psychoanalyse, 2. Internationaler Psychoanalytischer Verlag. Leipzig, Germany.
55. RYDIN, E., D. SCHALLING & M. ÅSBERG. 1982. Rorschach ratings in depressed and suicidal patients with low levels of 5-hydroxyindoleacetic acid in cerebrospinal fluid. Psychiatry Res. **7:** 229-243.
56. BANKI, C. M. 1977. Correlation of anxiety and related symptoms with cerebrospinal fluid 5-hydroxyindoleactic acid in depressed women. J. Neural Transm. **41:** 135-143.
57. LINNOILA, M., M. VIRKKUNEN, M. SCHEININ, A. NUUTILA, R. RIMON & F. K. GOODWIN. 1983. Low cerebrospinal fluid 5-hydroxyindoleacetic acid concentration differentiates impulsive from nonimpulsive violent behavior. Life Sci. **33:** 2609-2614.

58. LIDBERG, L., J. R. TUCK, M. ÅSBERG, G.-P. SCALIA-TOMBA & L. BERTILSSON. 1985. Homicide, suicide and CSF 5-HIAA. Acta Psychiatr. Scand. 71: 230-236.
59. LIDBERG, L., M. ÅSBERG & U. B. SUNDQVIST-STENSMAN. 1984. 5-Hydroxyindoleacetic acid levels in attempted suicides who have killed their children. Lancet ii: 928.
60. WEST, D. J. 1965. Murder followed by Suicide. Heinemann. London, England.
61. WOLFGANG, M. E. 1958. Patterns in Criminal Homicide. Oxford University Press. London, England.
62. SCHALLING, D., M. ÅSBERG & G. EDMAN. Personality and CSF monoamine metabolites. (In preparation.)

Neuroendocrine Studies in Depression

Relationship to Suicidal Behavior

JAMES H. KOCSIS, SARA KENNEDY,
RICHARD P. BROWN, J. JOHN MANN,
AND BARBARA MASON

Department of Psychiatry
New York Hospital-Cornell Medical Center
525 East 68th Street
New York, New York 10021

Suicide is a major world public health hazard.[1] However, the incidence of suicide, even within identified psychiatric populations, is low enough that clinical techniques have proven notoriously imperfect in predicting actual suicide behavior. The recent development of potential biological markers for psychiatric illnesses has led to a number of investigations of the possibility that these markers can be used as valid predictors of suicidal acts.[2-12]

Several previous studies have examined relationships between abnormalities of the hypothalamic-pituitary-adrenocortical (HPA) axis and occurrence of suicide attempts. Six investigations have reported on relationships between urinary corticosteroid levels and suicide attempts. Three of these found elevated levels of 24-hour urinary 17-hydroxycorticosteroids or urinary free cortisol in patients who had been severely suicidal or who later completed suicide.[2-4] Two other studies, however, reported low or normal urinary cortisol levels in patients attempting or completing suicide.[5,6] Investigations of relationships between suicidal behavior and plasma cortisol levels, both before and after administration of dexamethasone, have yielded contradictory results. Most have found higher rates of nonsuppression on the dexamethasone suppression test (DST) in patients who have attempted or completed suicide compared to non-suicide attempters.[7-10] However, one recent study has reported no association of recent suicidal behavior and nonsuppression of the DST.[11]

Only one study to date has assessed the relationship between cerebrospinal fluid (CSF) cortisol and suicidal behavior.[12] Increased CSF cortisol levels were found in depressed patients; however, levels in depressed patients who had made a suicide attempt were not significantly higher than in depressed nonattempters. Normal CSF cortisol values were present in nondepressed suicide attempters.

The purpose of the current report is to summarize results of two additional investigations of relationships between suicidal behavior and HPA function,[13,14] to relate these findings to results of prior studies, and to discuss practical and theoretical implications.

NATIONAL INSTITUTE OF MENTAL HEALTH STUDY METHODS

One hundred thirty-two hospitalized patients with a diagnosis of major depressive disorder as determined by the schedule for Affective Disorders and Schizophrenia (SADS)[15] and the Research Diagnostic Criteria (RDC)[16] were selected for inclusion in the NIMH-Clinical Research Branch Collaborative Study-Biology of Depression. Eighty-two were classified as unipolar depressives and 47 as bipolar depressives. Patients were admitted to one of six university hospital centers participating in the collaborative study between 1975 and 1980. Full details about the rationale and methods of the study have been published.[17,18]

Specific SADS items were used to assess suicidal thoughts and the number, seriousness, and lethality of previous suicide attempts during the current episode. On the basis of SADS data, patients were assigned to one of three groups: (1) a suicide attempter group (SA), defined as those patients who had made at least one suicide attempt during the current episode that could be considered significant with regard to the seriousness of its intent and/or its medical lethality; (2) a nonattempter group (NA), defined as those patients with no history of suicide attempts for either the current or past episodes; and (3) an unclassified group (UC) consisting of patients who had made a suicide attempt during the current episode that did not meet the established "significant" criteria and patients who had a history of suicide attempts during prior episodes. Except where noted, the UC group was excluded from data analyses. Severity of depression was assessed using the Hamilton Depression Rating Scale (HDRS) and the Global Assessment of Severity (GAS),[19] a measure of coping mechanisms and degree of impairment.

Within two weeks of admission three successive morning and one evening plasma cortisol level, a 24-hour urine collection for urinary free cortisol, and a CSF cortisol level were obtained. Subsequently, 1 mg of dexamethasone was given orally in liquid solution, under observation of a nurse at 10:40 P.M. The following day, post-DST plasma cortisol levels were obtained at 8:30 A.M., 4 P.M., and 10 P.M. During the 24-hour period following dexamethasone administration, urine was collected to measure urinary cortisol. DST nonsuppression was defined as an A.M. postdexamethasone plasma cortisol of 5 μg/dl or more. Urine free cortisol hypersecretion was defined as more than 133 μg/24 hours.[20]

NEW YORK STUDY METHODS

Sixty-six inpatients, who participated in depression research protocols on the clinical research unit at the Payne Whitney Psychiatric Clinic during 1982-84, and also met *Diagnostic and Statistical Manual,* third edition (DSM III)[21] criteria for primary major depressive disorder were included. Patients were categorized as attempters if a suicide attempt requiring medical intervention or hospitalization had been made within four weeks prior to hospitalization. Ten patients had a past history but no recent history of suicide attempts, and were dropped from the analysis. A further evaluation of suicidal ideation was completed at the time of the administration of dexamethasone and at the time of drawing cortisol levels. Severity of depression was assessed using the HDRS. Blood samples were collected at 9 A.M. and 4 P.M. on the day before and the day after administration of 1 mg of dexamethasone orally at 11 P.M. under observation by a nurse. DST nonsuppression was defined as either the 9 A.M. or 4 P.M. plasma cortisol greater than 5 μg/dl.[14]

No patient in either sample had major medical illnesses or was taking medication known to affect cortisol levels or DST results. Patients were not treated with antidepressant medication until after cortisol measures were obtained. CSF plasma and urinary free cortisol for both studies were measured in one laboratory by radioimmunoassay by methods previously described in detail.[20]

RESULTS FROM THE NIMH STUDY

The demographic and clinical characteristics of the suicide attempters and nonattempters have been reported.[13] No differences were found with regard to sex, polarity, duration of current episodes, number of previous episodes, presence of psychotic

TABLE 1. NIMH Study—CSF, Urine and Plasma Cortisol Concentrations of Suicide Attempters and Nonattempters

	Suicide Attempters[a]	Nonattempters[a]
CSF cortisol (pmol/ml)	0.89 ± 0.07	1.04 ± 0.05
Urinary Free Cortisol (μg/24 hrs)	111.7 ± 16.5	147.9 ± 19.7
Plasma cortisol[b] (μg/dl)		
Morning	15.6 ± 1.1	18.4 ± 0.77
Evening	5.2 ± 1.3[c]	7.0 ± 0.66

[a] Mean ± standard error of the mean.
[b] Pre-DST.
[c] ANCOVA results: p < 0.05.

features, or recovery status. Suicide attempters were significantly younger and had an earlier age at onset than nonattempters. Nonattempters showed more depressive symptoms, higher levels of anxiety, agitation, and somatization, and greater psychomotor retardation than did the suicide attempter group.

Analyses of covariance performed on the various HPA measures revealed few differences between the attempter and nonattempter groups (TABLE 1). Among the plasma, CSF, and urinary cortisol comparisons made, only the pre-DST evening plasma cortisol sample was significantly different, being lower in the suicide attempter group. The results of statistical analyses performed on the post-DST plasma cortisol levels (i.e., suppressors versus nonsuppressors) and on urine free cortisol hypersecreters versus normal secreters did not reveal significant differences between attempters and nonattempters (see TABLE 2).

Pearson product moment correlations between the HPA variables and scores on the SADS Suicidal Ideation and Behavior Scale and the individual items that comprise the scale were performed on the entire depressed population (including the UC group). None of these achieved the 0.05 level of significance.

TABLE 2. NIMH Study: Results of Analyses Performed on Categorized Biochemical Variables

	Post-DST Plasma Cortisol Levels		
	< 5 µg/dl (suppressor)	> 5 µg/dl (nonsuppressor)	
Suicide attempters	18	7	
Nonattempters	30	23	$\chi^2 = 1.70$, p > 0.15

	Cortisol Hypersecreters (UFC 133 µg/24 hours)		
	Yes	No	
Suicide attempters	7	15	
Nonattempters	22	24	$\chi^2 = 1.56$, p > 0.20

RESULTS FROM THE NEW YORK STUDY

The mean age of attempters was 63 ± 11 (standard deviation, SD) years and of nonattempters was 61 ± 14. Female:male ratios were approximately two to one for attempters and nonattempters. Baseline mean HDRS scores were 34 ± 11 for attempters and 32 ± 9 for nonattempters. None of these differences were significant.

Morning and evening cortisol levels before and after dexamethasone did not differ significantly between groups (TABLE 3). There was also no significant difference between attempters and nonattempters in frequency of cortisol suppression in the morning or afternoon following dexamethasone (TABLE 4). Furthermore, no significant differences were found in cortisol levels between those patient groups rated as currently having active suicidal intent, passive suicidal ideation, or no suicidal ideation.

Correlations among cortisol levels and other variables possibly related to suicidality were also calculated. Significant positive correlations included the following: presence of delusions and postdexamethasone morning and afternoon cortisol levels ($r = 0.41$, p = 0.001, $r = 0.43$, p = 0.001, respectively), age and morning and afternoon postdexamethasone cortisols ($r = 0.39$, p = 0.001, $r = 0.48$, p = 0.001, respectively).

TABLE 3. New York Study: Pre- and Postdexamethasone Plasma Cortisol Levels (µg/dl)

	Mean Plasma Cortisol Levels (± SD)	
	Attempters (n)	Nonattempters (n)
Predexamethasone		
9 A.M.	20 ± 9 (13)	21 ± 9 (42)
4 P.M.	11 ± 4 (12)	14 ± 6 (36)
Postdexamethasone		
9 A.M.	11 ± 9 (12)	10 ± 8 (43)
4 P.M.	8 ± 5 (11)	10 ± 6 (38)

DISCUSSION

The possibility that hyperactivation of the pituitary-adrenal axis might have a special relationship to suicidal behavior was initially suggested by the empirical observation of elevated urinary corticosteroids in patients who later committed suicide.[2] Several subsequent studies investigating this association have yielded mixed results.[3-11] Thus, further research is merited to clarify these issues.

The current report summarizes findings from two recent studies done in hospitalized depressed patients comparing results of measures of HPA function in suicide attempters versus nonattempters. The main findings are a lack of significant HPA differences in these two subgroups. One significant difference was found in the two studies, and this was in the direction opposite of what was predicted. Evening plasma cortisol concentrations in the collaborative study were higher in nonattempters on the day prior to administration of dexamethasone. ($p < 0.05$ by ANCOVA).

Relationships between HPA function and suicidal acts are clearly not simple. Clinical research in this area is likely to have been confounded by numerous interacting

TABLE 4. New York Study: Results of the Dexamethasone Suppression Test in Attempters and Nonattempters

	n	Percent Nonsuppressors (5 μg/dl)
9 A.M. post-DST		
Attempters	12	59
Nonattempters	43	65
4 P.M. post-DST		
Attempters	11	73
Nonattempters	38	79

variables, which are difficult to control in any single study. These would include age, presence or absence of psychosis, recent weight loss, levels of anxiety and agitation, psychiatric diagnosis, method of suicide attempt, and proximity of the biological sampling to the suicidal act.

The New York study patient ages were similar in the attempter and nonattempter groups. However, in the NIMH study attempters were younger than nonattempters. The latter situation would work against finding increased HPA activity in the attempter sample, because increased age is a known correlate of higher HPA activity.[22] Presence of psychosis in depression has also been associated with both HPA activation and suicidality in some but not all previous studies.[23,24] The current study from New York did find an association between delusions and higher cortisol levels. However, neither study reported significant differences in suicidality between delusional and nondelusional patients. HPA studies conducted separately in psychotic and nonpsychotic depressed patients will help to resolve these questions.

Weight loss, anxiety, and agitation were all found to correlate with HPA measures in the NIMH study.[22] Unfortunately data on these possibly confounding variables were not compared between attempters and nonattempters in the present studies. Such analyses are suggested for future research.

Psychiatric diagnoses were carefully established in both of the current studies by research psychiatrists who had established diagnostic reliability. All subjects were diagnosed as having major depressive disorders by RDC or DSM III criteria. It is possible that suicide attempters and nonattempter samples in other studies have contained either mixed or unreliable diagnoses. Such samples might create a bias for both suicide and abnormal HPA function to cluster in the subgroups with major depressive disorders, and thus yield a spurious impression that suicidal behavior has a special association with the endocrine findings.

Method of suicide attempt may also be an important variable because previous research has suggested links between inwardly and outwardly directed aggression and brain serotonin systems in humans, based on CSF studies in patients who used violent methods of attempting suicide.[25] Although prior studies of suicide and HPA function have not reported linkage with method of suicide act, this remains at least a theoretical possibility.

Whether associations between suicidal behavior and biology are confounded by the proximity between the times of the biological sampling and the suicide attempt would depend on whether the putative biological marker is state or trait related. For example, low CSF serotonin has been suggested as a trait marker for aggressive acts and violent suicide attempts[25] because the altered biochemistry appears to persist long after a suicide act. On the other hand behavioral assessments performed in suicidal subjects before and after their attempts have demonstrated distinctive patterns prior to suicidal behavior with reversion back toward patterns seen in nonsuicidal patients following an attempt.[26] This kind of observation raises important questions about the longitudinal patterns of potential biological markers for suicidality. Specifically, in the case of HPA function, increased activation associated with a state of arousal prior to a suicide attempt could theoretically revert to normal following the attempt. All of the HPA measures in the current studies were obtained in subjects who had attempted suicide earlier during their current illness episode. Thus, some prior studies, which have evaluated HPA function in patients who later suicided, might have their discrepant findings explained on the basis of different temporal sequences between biological sampling and the suicidal act.

In conclusion, this brief review has summarized results from two recent studies of relationships between suicidal behavior and adrenocortical activity in depressed psychiatric inpatients. Hopefully a consideration of these findings and the discussion of previous studies and of factors that can influence these relationships will help to alert investigators in the biology of suicide to methodological considerations and important unresolved questions to be answered in future studies.

REFERENCES

1. 1975. Mortality and Morbidity Trends 1962-1972. WHO Cron. **29:** 377-386.
2. BUNNEY, W. E., JR. & J. A. FAWCET. 1965. Possibility of a biochemical test for suicidal potential. Arch. Gen. Psychiatry **13:** 232-239.
3. BUNNEY, W. E., JR., J. A. FAWCET, J. M. DAVIS & S. GIFFORD. 1969. Further evaluation of urinary 17-hydroxycorticosteroids in suicidal patients. Arch. Gen. Psychiatry **21:** 138-150.
4. OSTROFF, R., E. GILLER, K. BONESE, et al. 1982. Neuroendocrine risk factors of suicide. Am. J. Psychiatry **139:** 1323-1325.

5. KRIEGER, G. 1970. Biochemical predictors of suicide. Dis. Nerv. Syst. **31:** 478-482.
6. LEVY, B. & E. HANSEN. 1969. Failure of the urinary test for suicidal potential. Arch. Gen. Psychiatry **20:** 415-418.
7. CARROLL, B. J., J. F. GREDEN & M. FEINBERG. 1981. Suicide, neuroendocrine dysfunction and CSF 5-HIAA concentrations in depression. *In* Recent Advances in Neuropsychopharmacology. B. Angrist, Ed.: 307-313. Pergamon Press. Oxford & New York.
8. CORYELL, W. & M. A. SCHLESSER. 1981. Suicide and the dexamethasone suppression test in unipolar depression. Am. J. Psychiatry **138:** 1120-1121.
9. TARGUM, S. D., L. ROSEN & A. E. CAPODANNO. 1981. The dexamethasone suppression test in suicidal patients with unipolar depression. Am. J. Psychiatry **140:** 877-879.
10. BANKI, C. M. & M. ARATO. 1983. Amine metabolites and neuroendocrine response related to depression and suicide. J. Affect. Disord. **5:** 223-232.
11. VAN WETTERE, J. P., G. CHARLES & J. WILMOTTE. 1983. Test de function a la dexamethasone et suicide. Acta Psychiatr. Belg. **83:** 569-578.
12. TRASKMAN, L., G. TYBRING, M. ASBERG, *et al.* 1980. Cortisol in the CSF of depressed and suicidal patients. Arch. Gen. Psychiatry **37:** 761-767.
13. SECUNDA, S. K., C. CROSS, S. KOSLOW, *et al.* 1986. Biochemical predictors of suicide. Biol. Psychiatry **21:** 756-767.
14. BROWN, R. P., B. MASON, P. STOLL, *et al.* 1986. Hypothalamic-pituitary-adrenal axis function and suicidal behavior in depressed patients. Psychiatry Res. **17:** 317-323.
15. SPITZER, R. L. & J. ENDICOTT. 1978. Collaborative Depressive Study-Clinical SADS-RDC. New York State Psychiatric Institute. New York, N.Y.
16. SPITZER, R. L., J. ENDICOTT & E. ROBINS. 1978. Research diagnostic criteria for a selected group of functional disorders. New York State Psychiatric Institute. New York, N.Y.
17. MAAS, J. W., S. H. KOSLOW, J. DAVIS, *et al.* 1980. Biological component of the NIMH clinical research branch collaborative program on the psychobiology of depression. I. Background and theoretical considerations. Psychol. Med. **10:** 759-776.
18. SECUNDA, S., S. H. KOSLOW, D. E. REDMOND, *et al.* 1980. Biological component of the NIMH clinical research branch collaborative program on the psychobiology of depression II. Methodology and data analysis. Psychol. Med. **10:** 777-793.
19. ENDICOTT, J., R. SPITZER, J. L. FLEISS, *et al.* 1976. The Global Assessment Scale, a procedure for measuring overall severity of psychiatric disturbance. Arch. Gen. Psychiatry **33:** 766-771.
20. STOKES, P. E., P. M. STOLL, S. H. KOSLOW, *et al.* 1984. Pretreatment DST and hypothalamic-pituitary-adrenocortical function in depressed patients and comparison groups. Arch. Gen. Psychiatry **41:** 257-267.
21. 1980. Diagnostic and Statistical Manual of Mental Disorders. 3rd edit. American Psychiatric Association, Washington, D.C.
22. KOCSIS, J. H., J. M. DAVIS, M. M. KATZ, *et al.* 1985. Depressive behavior and hyperactive adrenocortical function. Am. J. Psychiatry **143:** 1291-1298.
23. SCHATZBERG, A. F., A. J. ROTHCHILD, J. B. STAHL, *et al.* 1983. The dexamethasone suppression test: identification of subtypes of depression. Am. J. Psychiatry **140:** 88-91.
24. KOCSIS, J. H., J. L. CROUGHAN, M. M. KATZ, *et al.* Clinical and biological features of psychotic depression. (Unpublished manuscript.)
25. ASBERG, M. & L. TRASKMAN. 1981. Studies of CSF 5-HIAA in depression and suicidal behavior. Exp. Med. Biol. **133:** 739-752.
26. MASON, B. J., J. E. EXNER & J. B. COHEN. The fallacy of studying suicide potential after the attempt. J. Pers. Assess. (In press.)

Hypothalamic-Pituitary-Adrenal Axis and Suicide

MIHÁLY ARATÓ,[a] CSABA M. BANKI,[b] CHARLES B. NEMEROFF,[b] AND GARTH BISSETTE[b]

[a]*Research Department*
National Institute for Nervous and Mental Diseases
Budapest 27, Pf. 1 1281 Hungary

[b]*Department of Psychiatry*
Duke University Medical Center
Durham, North Carolina 27710

Adrenal steroid hormones are essential to human life and play a central role in maintaining survival in times of stress.[1] Indices of hypothalamic-pituitary-adrenal (HPA) axis function have been extensively evaluated in various psychiatric disturbances. There are at least three reasons for studying adrenal function in pathological emotional states:

1. An objective indicator of excessive stress/distress may inform us about a subjective unpleasant or hardly bearable affect.
2. According to another interpretation, the activated HPA may reflect a disturbance of limbic-hypothalamic monoamine metabolism, something that has been implicated in the pathophysiology of affective disorders.
3. A third, and comparatively neglected, aspect is the possible effect of steroids on the central nervous system (CNS) and mental functioning.[2] Adrenal steroids have a regulatory role in adrenergic and opiate receptor mechanisms.[3-5] Instead of looking for the solution to the "egg or chicken dilemma," we should face the complex interplay between steroid hormonal systems and CNS neurotransmitter functions.

Several lines of evidence suggest an association between HPA axis dysregulation, affective disorders, and suicidal behavior. As early as 1965 Bunney and Fawcett reported high levels of urinary 17-hydroxycorticosteroids in depressed suicidal patients.[6] Subsequently, elevation of plasma total cortisol was suggested as a predictor of suicide.[7] Recently an abnormal dexamethasone suppression test (DST) result has been postulated as a biological marker of suicide by several investigators.[8-12] There are, however, contradictory data regarding both urinary steroid excretion[13] and the DST results[14-16] as they apply to suicidal behavior. Furthermore, cerebrospinal fluid (CSF) cortisol levels did not differ between suicidal and nonsuicidal depressed patients.[17]

The aim of this article is to focus on CSF measurements of HPA axis function in relation to suicidal behavior. CSF data are usually more "respected" than those of other body fluids on the assumption that CSF parameters more closely reflect CNS activity. Most likely this is not the case for cortisol. The source of CSF cortisol is the plasma, and cortisol levels in CSF are correlated with plasma total and free cortisol as well as with urinary free cortisol excretion.[17,18] CSF cortisol levels are reported to be about 10% of the plasma cortisol concentration.[19] Studies on CSF cortisol in depression have been reported with conflicting results.[17,18,20-22]

CSF adrenocorticotropic hormone (ACTH) data are scanty in the psychiatric literature. CSF levels of ACTH are relatively high, in fact exceeding plasma levels.[23] Therefore the origin of the CSF ACTH is thought to be mainly in the CNS.[24] As far as we are aware, no results have been published regarding the relationship between suicide and ACTH secretion.

CSF corticotropin-releasing factor (CRF), the hypothalamic stimulatory peptide of adrenal function, has been found to be elevated in depression.[25] Significant positive correlations between CSF CRF and 3-methoxy-4-hydroxyphenylethylene glycol (MHPG),[26] and 5-hydroxyindoleacetic acid (5-HIAA),[27] respectively, have been described in depressives, providing further evidence for the interaction of monoaminergic mechanisms and HPA function.

The literature on the possible association of HPA dysregulation and suicidal behavior is far from unanimous. We wanted to explore this issue in a comprehensive way. CSF cortisol was measured in different groups of psychiatric patients, including both suicidal and nonsuicidal subjects, as well as in victims of violent suicide and sudden natural or accidental death. We have also measured CSF concentrations of ACTH and CRF in a portion of the patients. We analyzed the relationships of these different indices of HPA function.

Two different patient populations were investigated in two large Hungarian psychiatric institutes. In the Nagykálló Neuropsychiatric Institute, newly admitted, drug-free female patients were included who underwent CSF and neuroendocrine tests in a four-year period. After giving informed consent, all patients remained on placebo and standard hospital diet for two to four days, and had a lumbar puncture at 8:00-9:00 A.M. in a standardized procedure. In a portion of the patients, blood samples were obtained simultaneously for cortisol measurement. One milligram of dexamethasone was administered to the patients on the same day at 10:00 P.M. The postdexamethasone blood samples were collected on the following day at 8:00 and 15:00 hours for estimation of cortisol. Postdexamethasone cortisol levels higher than 5 μg/dL either at 8:00 or 15:00 hours were considered abnormal (nonsuppression, NS). Using this cutoff point, we have found 6% false-positive results in 160 normal controls, and 58% sensitivity in 480 patients with primary major affective disorders. Diagnoses were made using *Diagnostic and Statistical Manual,* third edition (DSM III) categories, and thereafter clustered into three main groups: depression, schizophrenia, and adjustment disorders. Further details are described elsewhere.[28,29]

The same DST procedure was carried out in the National Institute for Nervous and Mental Diseases, Budapest, without CSF sampling. In a retrospective analysis using the DST data base, which includes more than 1000 patients, the relationship of DST results and history of suicide attempt has been investigated in 353 depressives. All patients fulfilled the Research Diagnostic Criteria of primary major affective disorder. The majority of the patients were female (84%). Each patient who had a lifetime history of suicide attempt, regardless of its seriousness or method, was considered as suicidal in this analysis.

In the postmortem study, cisternal and lumbar (5 ml each) CSF was obtained from victims of violent suicide ($n=16$), mostly by hanging, and controls ($n=16$), sudden accidental and natural death, in the first few hours after death. The suicide and control groups were comparable regarding sex, age, postmortem delay, and the time of day of death.

Cortisol was measured using the competitive protein-binding method.[30] ACTH in CSF was quantified with radioimmunoassay using a commercial kit (CIS-SORIN). CSF CRF-like immunoreactivity (CRF) was measured by a specific radioimmunoassay.[25]

The CSF cortisol levels showed a significant correlation with those of the plasma obtained at the same time (FIGURE 1) as well as with both postdexamethasone plasma cortisol values (8:00 hours $r=0.39$, $p<0.05$; 15:00 hours $r=0.44$, $p<0.02$). Female inpatients with depression ($n=18$), schizophrenia ($n=7$), and adjustment disorder ($n=7$) were included in this study. Fifty percent of them were nonsuppressors in DST.

Another finding which further indicates a relationship between CSF cortisol and DST results is that DST nonsuppressors, regardless of the diagnosis, had significantly higher CSF cortisol concentration than did suppressors (FIGURE 2). However, suicidal

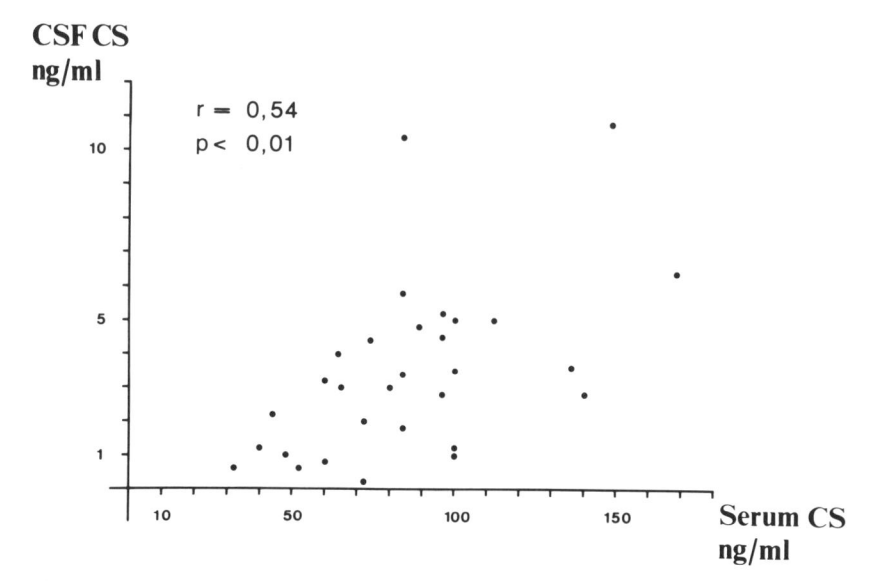

FIGURE 1. Significant positive correlation between CSF and serum cortisol in female patients ($n=30$).

patients did not have higher CSF cortisol levels than did nonsuicidal patients. (Only patients who had attempted suicide immediately before the recent hospitalization were included in this comparison.) Depressed patients had significantly higher CSF cortisol values than did schizophrenics and patients with adjustment disorder (4.1 ± 0.44 vs. 2.9 ± 0.344 and 2.6 ± 0.4 ng/ml, respectively, $p<0.05$ in both cases). This finding is in agreement with the results of three other studies,[17,18,20] while others have not found elevated CSF cortisol in depressives.[21,22] Both Carroll and associates[18] and Gerner and associates[20] have found a positive correlation between CSF cortisol and severity of depression. Gerner and associates hypothesized that high CSF levels of cortisol might alter homeostatic balances of neurotransmitter systems within the brain.[20]

The results of a retrospective analysis of DST and suicide are summarized in TABLE 1. We found no difference in the frequency of suicide attempts between DST suppressor and nonsuppressor depressives.

Depressed patients had significantly higher CRF concentrations than did controls (mixed group of neurologic patients), but this had no relationship to recent or past

CSF CS ng/ml

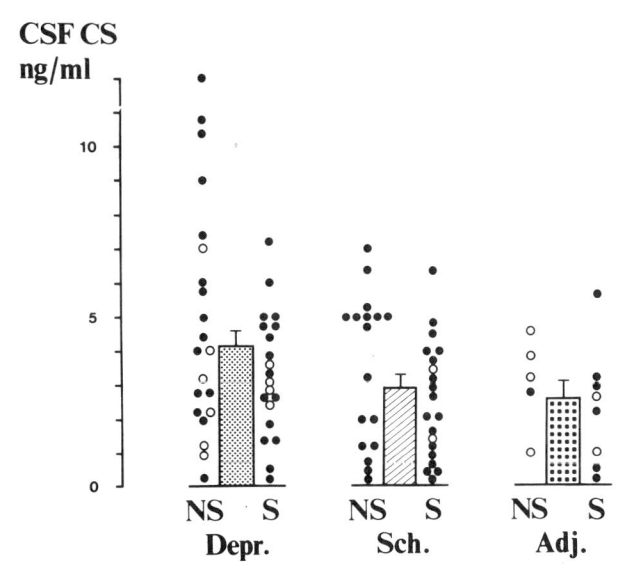

FIGURE 2. CSF cortisol levels of patients with depression ($n=40$), schizophrenia ($n=37$), and adjustment disorder ($n=13$). Nonsuppressors had significantly higher mean value than did suppressors (4.14 ± 0.44 vs. 2.75 ± 0.27 ng/ml; $t=2.87$, $p<0.01$). Patients with a recent suicide attempt were marked with open circles. Cortisol was significantly elevated in the depression group compared to the two other groups ($t=2.14$, and 2.39, respectively; $p<0.05$).

suicidal behavior (FIGURE 3). This finding supports the hypothesis that hyperactivity of the HPA function in depression may be due to hypersecretion of CRF.[25]

In the postmortem study we found that cisternal and lumbar CSF cortisol levels did not differ in the same subjects (FIGURE 4). This finding provides a further evidence of the lack of a gradient for cortisol in the cerebrospinal space.[31]

There was a trend for positive correlation between cisternal CSF and ACTH values in the subjects who had ACTH levels in the normal range (FIGURE 5). There was no

TABLE 1. No Difference in the Frequency of Suicide Attempts between DST Nonsuppressors and Suppressors in Any Group of Depressives

Nonsuppressors	Suicide Attempts	Suppressors
	Unipolar Depression	
$n = 106$	$n = 225$	$n = 119$
39%		50%
	Bipolar-I Depression	
$n = 20$	$n = 38$	$n = 18$
45%		50%
	Bipolar-II Depression	
$n = 50$	$n = 90$	$n = 40$
49%		50%

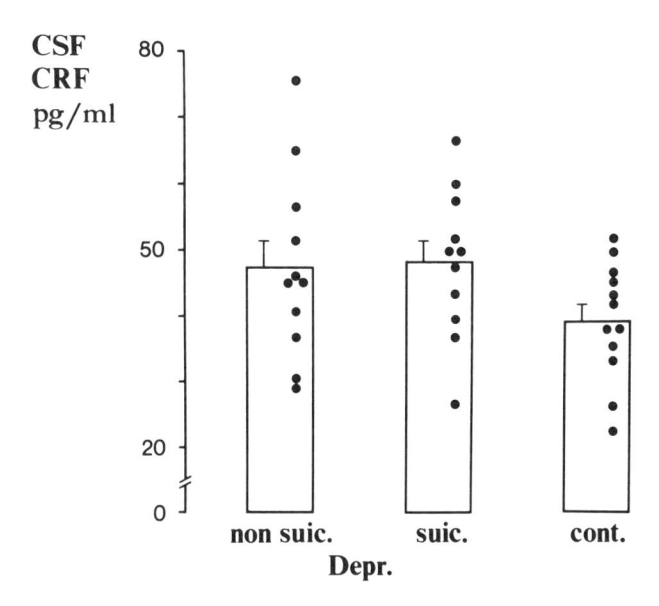

FIGURE 3. Concentration of CSF CRF in depressed patients ($n=22$) and controls ($n=12$). Means ± standard error of the mean: 47.8 ± 4.3 vs. 39.41 ± 2.59 pg/ml, $t = 2.25$, $p < 0.05$. No difference between suicidal and nonsuicidal depressives.

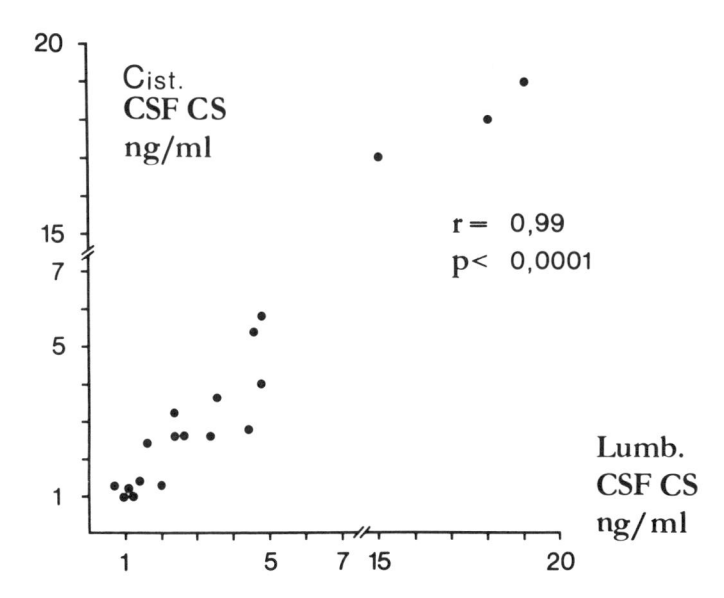

FIGURE 4. Highly significant positive correlation between cisternal and lumbar postmortem CSF cortisol values ($n=19$).

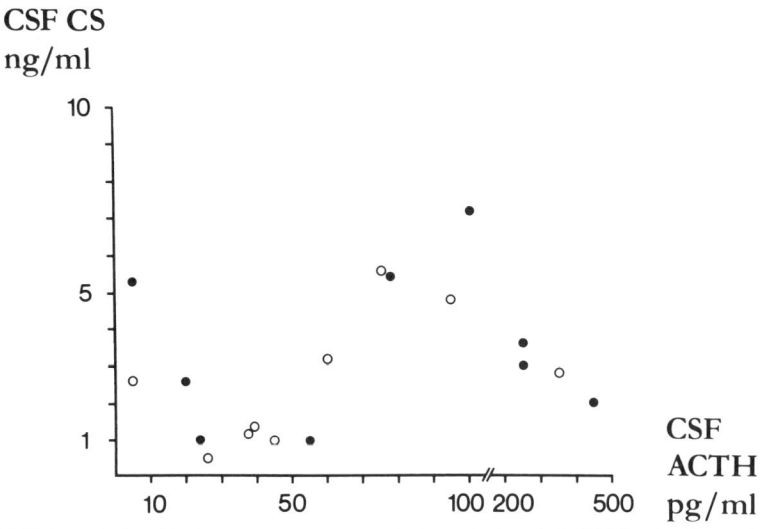

FIGURE 5. Relationship between postmortem CSF cortisol and ACTH levels. Open circles, suicides; solid circles, controls. (Excluding the four highest values: $r=0.56$, $p<0.05$.)

difference between the suicide and control groups in CSF cortisol and ACTH levels (FIGURE 6).

As it was pointed out in the introduction, several studies suggested an association between HPA hyperactivity and suicidal behavior. However, most of these results were not replicated in controlled, follow-up studies on a large number of patients.

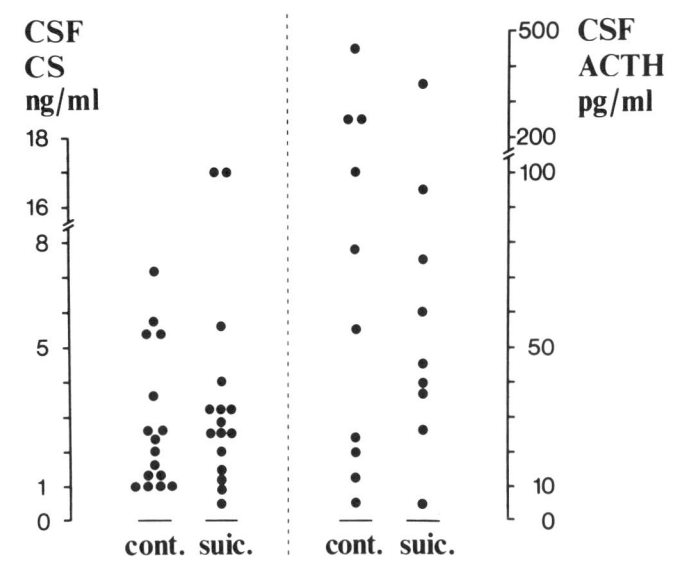

FIGURE 6. Cortisol and ACTH levels in postmortem CSF from suicides and controls.

Our efforts to investigate in a comprehensive way the possible connection between HPA dysregulation and suicidality failed to confirm this association. It is possible that the investigated populations were heterogenous regarding their HPA functions. It can be assumed that in a portion of the patients, as a result of excessive or long-lasting distress, high cortisol levels can be found. On the other hand exhaustion of the HPA function (and the coping system?) may result in low cortisol levels in others. This speculation needs to be tested in further investigations.

REFERENCES

1. SELYE, H. 1950. Br. Med. J. **1**: 1383-1392.
2. CARPENTER, W. T. & P. H. GRUEN. 1982. J. Clin. Psychopharmacol. **2**: 91-101.
3. MOBLEY, P. L. & F. SULSER. 1980. Nature **286**: 608-609.
4. DAVIES, A. O. & R. J. LEFKOWITZ. 1984. Annu. Rev. Physiol. **46**: 119-130.
5. KANYICSKA, B., M. I. K. FEKETE, A. SIMONYI, T. SZENTENDREI & E. STARK. 1984. In Stress: the Role of Catecholamines and Other Transmitters. E. A. Usdin, Ed.: 345-351. Gordon and Breach Science Publications. New York, N.Y.
6. BUNNEY, W. E. & J. A. FAWCETT. 1965. Arch. Gen. Psychiatry **13**: 232-239.
7. KRIEGER, G. 1974. Dis. Nerv. Syst. **35**: 237-240.
8. CARROLL, B. J., J. F. GREDEN & M. FEINBERG. 1981. In Recent Advances in Neuropsychopharmacology. B. Angrist, Ed.: 307-313. Pergamon Press. Oxford, England.
9. CORYELL, W. & M. A. SCHLESSER. 1981. Am. J. Psychiatry **138**: 1120-1121.
10. AGREN, H. 1983. Psychiatry Dev. **1**: 87-104.
11. TARGUM, S. D., L. ROSEN & A. E. CAPODANNO. 1983. Am. J. Psychiatry **140**: 877-879.
12. BERGER, M., K.-M. PIRKE, P. DOERR, J.-C. KRIEG & D. VON ZERSSEN. 1984. Br. J. Psychiatry **145**: 372-382.
13. LEVY, B. & E. HANSEN. 1969. Arch. Gen. Psychiatry **20**: 415-418.
14. CORYELL, W. 1982. Am. J. Psychiatry **139**: 1214.
15. KRONFOL, Z., J. F. GREDEN, R. GARDNER & B. J. CARROLL. 1982. Am. J. Psychiatry **139**: 1214-1215.
16. DAM, H., E. T. MELLERUP & O. J. RAFAELSEN. 1985. J. Affect. Disord. **8**: 95-103.
17. TRASKMAN, L., G. TYBRING, M. ASBERG, L. BERTILSSON, O. LANTTO & D. SCHALLING. 1980. Arch. Gen. Psychiatry **37**: 761-767.
18. CARROLL, B. J., G. C. CURTIS & J. MENDELS. 1976. Psychol. Med. **6**: 235-244.
19. UETE, T., S. NISHIMURA, H. OHYA, T. SHIMOMURA & Y. TATEBAYASHI. 1970. J. Clin. Endocrinol. Metab. **30**: 208-214.
20. GERNER, R. H. & J. N. WILKINS. 1983. Am. J. Psychiatry **140**: 92-94.
21. COPPEN, A., B. W. L. BROOKSBANK, R. NOGUERA & D. A. WILSON. 1971. J. Neurol. Neurosurg. Psychiatry **34**: 432-435.
22. JIMERSON, D. C., R. M. POST, D. P. VAN KAMMEN, J. S. SKYLER, G. L. BROWN & W. E. BUNNEY. 1980. Am. J. Psychiatry **137**: 979-980.
23. ALLEN, J. P., J. W. KENDALL, R. MCGILVRA & C. VANCURE. 1974. J. Clin. Endocrinol. Metab. **38**: 586-593.
24. POST, R. M., P. GOLD, D. R. RUBINOW, J. C. BALLENGER, W. E. BUNNEY & F. K. GOODWIN. 1982. Life Sci. **31**: 1-15.
25. NEMEROFF, C. B., E. WIDERLÖV, G. BISSETTE, H. WALLEUS, I. KARLSSON, K. EKLUND, C. D. KILTS, P. T. LOOSEN & W. VALE. 1984. Science **226**: 1342-1344.
26. DAVIS, B. M., K. L. DAVIS, R. C. MOHS, A. A. MATHE, W. VALE & D. KRIEGER. 1984. Presented at the Annual Meeting of the American College of Neuropsychopharmacology, Puerto Rico.
27. WIDERLÖV, E., H. WALLEUS, G. BISSETTE, I. KARLSSON, K. EKLUND, C. D. KILTS, P. T. LOOSEN, W. VALE & C. NEMEROFF. 1984. Presented at the 15th Congress of the International Society of Psychoneuroendocrinology, Vienna, Austria.

28. BANKI, C. M. & M. ARATÓ. 1983. J. Affect. Disord. **5:** 223-232.
29. BANKI, C. M., M. ARATÓ, Z. PAPP & M. KURCZ. 1984. J. Affect. Disord. **6:** 341-350.
30. MURPHY, B. E. P. 1967. J. Clin. Endocrinol. Metab. **27:** 973-990.
31. BERTILSSON, L., M. ASBERG, O. LANTTO, G.-P. SCALIA-TOMBA, L. TRASKMAN-BENDZ & G. TYBRING. 1982. Psychiatry Res. **6:** 77-83.

Platelet Markers of Suicidality[a]

H. Y. MELTZER AND R. C. ARORA

Department of Psychiatry
Case Western Reserve University
School of Medicine
2040 Abington Road
Cleveland, Ohio 44106

Although there is extensive evidence relating serotonin (5-HT) to affective disorders,[1-4] the evidence concerning 5-HT and suicide appears to cut across clinical diagnoses and be related to psychological constructs such as aggression and impulsivity.[5] This has been discussed in detail by others in this volume[6,7] and will not be reviewed here. We have been studying the role of 5-HT in depression by neuroendocrine[4,8,9] and biochemical strategies.[10,11] The latter involve, in part, the study of blood platelets which have been considered to provide a model system for studying serotonergic neurons.[12,13]

Blood platelets take up 5-HT from the medium by an active process which appears to be similar to that found in 5-HT nerve terminals.[12,13] This 5-HT is stored in granules and has frequently been measured in psychiatric patients as an index of serotonergic function,[14,15] but results have been inconsistent. Recently, the specific binding of ^{3}H-imipramine to platelet membranes has also been studied extensively, revealing properties very similar to those of the high-affinity ^{3}H-imipramine binding (IB) sites in human brain.[16,17] The IB sites appear to be distinct from but able to modulate the activity of the 5-HT transport system.[18,19] Platelets also contain monoamine oxidase (MAO), which is believed to provide a measure of brain serotonergic activity.[20] The MAO in platelets is type B MAO which has a low affinity for 5-HT as a substrate.[21] The kinetic constants of 5-HT uptake, IB, 5-HT content, and platelet MAO activity were correlated with admission Hamilton Depression Scale suicide ratings[22] and the history of a suicide attempt with a serious intent in the current or previous episodes.

METHODS

All patients were admitted on a voluntary basis to the inpatient research unit of the Laboratory of Biological Psychiatry of the University of Chicago from 1980-1985. Patients were interviewed with the Present State Examination[23] supplemented by additional items from the Schedule for Affective Disorders-Change (SADS-C)[24] to make diagnoses by Research Diagnostic Criteria.[25] The nondepressed group included schizophrenics, manics, and a variety of other psychiatric disorders. A 24-item Hamilton Depression Rating Scale for depression was completed at the end of a drug-free

---

[a] Supported in part by U.S. Public Health Service Grants MH 30059, 41594, and 41684, Research Scientist Award MH 47808, and by a grant from the Cleveland Foundation.

washout period which was a minimum of seven days duration. Information concerning current or previous suicide attempts was obtained from the patient, family, or friends and medical records.

In the results to be reported, the number of subjects varies because not all platelet measures were available for all subjects. Blood was drawn in plastic syringes from the patients and transferred into plastic tubes containing appropriate anticoagulant. All blood samples were obtained between 7 A.M. and 9 A.M. in fasting subjects and processed within one hour of drawing the blood.

MAO activity in blood platelets was determined using benzylamine as a substrate as previously described.[26]

Serotonin uptake in platelets was determined by incubating platelet-rich plasma with ^{14}C-5-HT according to our published method.[27]

^{3}H-Imipramine binding in platelet membranes was studied following the method of Langer et al. with some modification.[28]

TABLE 1. Platelet Serotonin Uptake in Major Affective Disorders

Group	n	K_m (μM)	V_{max} (pmol/10^7 platelets per minute)
Normal controls	140	0.47 ± 0.13	12.5 ± 2.9
Major depression	100	0.43 ± 0.13	9.7 ± 2.9[a]
Unipolar	63	0.43 ± 0.13	10.4 ± 2.9[a]
Bipolar	37	0.43 ± 0.12	8.5 ± 2.9[a]
Psychotic	52	0.43 ± 0.13	9.1 ± 3.2[a]
Nonpsychotic	48	0.44 ± 0.12	10.4 ± 2.6[a]
Unipolar psychotic	23	0.43 ± 0.12	10.1 ± 2.9
Unipolar nonpsychotic	40	0.44 ± 0.13	10.6 ± 2.8
Bipolar psychotic	29	0.43 ± 0.13	8.4 ± 2.9[a]
Bipolar nonpsychotic	8	0.44 ± 0.13	9.0 ± 3.0[a]
Schizoaffective depressed mainly affective	10	0.44 ± 0.14	8.4 ± 2.8[a]
Schizoaffective depressed mainly schizophrenic	13	0.48 ± 0.15	11.1 ± 5.4
Manic	38	0.45 ± 0.13	9.8 ± 2.1[a]
Schizophrenia	84	0.45 ± 0.13	10.9 ± 3.3

[a] Significantly less than normal controls

RESULTS AND DISCUSSION

Platelet 5-HT uptake in normal controls, patients with major affective disorders, and schizophrenia is given in TABLE 1. A significant decrease in V_{max}, the number of uptake sites, was found in blood platelets of major depression and the following subtypes: unipolar, bipolar, psychotic, and nonpsychotic. The lowest levels were in the bipolar and psychotic subgroups. There were no differences in the K_m (inversely related to the affinity for 5-HT) values.

The univariate correlations (Spearman) between K_m, V_{max}, and Hamilton suicide ratings are given in TABLE 2. There was a significant but small negative correlation between K_m and Hamilton suicide ratings for all patients (rho = -0.163, $p < 0.05$). The correlation for nondepressed patients was -0.179, which was also significant.

TABLE 2. Univariate Correlations between Suicide Ratings (Hamilton) and Kinetic Constants of 5-HT Uptake in Blood Platelets

Subjects (n)	K_m (rho)	V_{max} (rho)
All (306)	−0.163[a]	−0.105[b]
Depressed (105)	−0.074	−0.116
Nondepressed (201)	−0.179[a]	−0.044

[a] $p < 0.05$.
[b] $p = 0.10$.

The correlation in depressed patients was not significant. Only 3% of the variance in suicide ratings in the nondepressed group is accounted for by K_m. The negative correlation indicates that the patients with lower K_m, i.e., higher affinity for 5-HT, were more suicidal. There was also a weak trend for V_{max} to be negatively correlated with Hamilton suicide rating for all patients. This reflects the high positive correlation between K_m and V_{max} (rho=0.43, n=117, p=0.0001). A higher affinity for 5-HT would lead to increased 5-HT uptake at the nerve terminal and, thus, less stimulation of 5-HT receptors, if there was increased affinity for 5-HT in brain as well as platelets. There were no significant differences in K_m or V_{max} between the 19 patients who had made suicide attempts prior to the current admission (Hamilton suicide rating of 4) and the 283 patients who had not (TABLE 3). There were too few patients (n=5) who had made violent suicide attempts in the index episode to compare these two groups. We found no significant differences in V_{max} or K_m levels between patients who had made violent suicide attempts, nonviolent suicide attempts, or no attempt of any kind at any time through the course of their illness (TABLE 4).

The kinetic constants, K_d and B_{max}, of IB, in normal controls, major depression, manics, and schizophrenics are given in TABLE 5. An ANOVA showed no differences in K_d or B_{max} between any of the groups, after covarying out age, which in our sample, but not in others, is inversely related to B_{max} in depressed patients.[29] Without covarying age, B_{max} is decreased in unipolar and psychotic depressed patients. However, B_{max} is decreased in psychotic depressed patients even after covarying out age[29] and a mul-

TABLE 3. Platelet Measures in Patients Who Attempted Suicide and Those Who Did Not

Platelet Measure	n	Suicide Attempters	n	No Suicide Attempt
K_m[a]	19	0.43 ± 0.13	283	0.45 ± 0.13
V_{max}[b]	19	9.9 ± 2.5	283	10.5 ± 3.2
K_d[c]	9	1.2 ± 0.8	132	0.96 ± 0.4
B_{max}[d]	9	790 ± 155	132	874 ± 282
MAO[e]	29	10.9 ± 4.3	339	11.3 ± 4.4
5-HT content[f]	15	78.5 ± 43.5	236	75.8 ± 35.8

[a] μM.
[b] pmol/10^7 platelets per minute.
[c] nM.
[d] fmol/mg protein.
[e] nmol benzaldehyde/10^8 platelets per hour.
[f] ng/10^8 platelets.

TABLE 4. K_m, V_{max}, K_d, B_{max}, MAO and 5-HT Content in All Patients as a Function of Lifetime History of Suicide

Group	K_m[a,b]	V_{max}[c]	K_d[d]	B_{max}[e]	MAO[f]	5-HT[g]
No attempt	0.43 (106)	10.8 (106)	0.94 (89)	823 (89)	11.3 (95)	74.1 (84)
Nonviolent attempt	0.43 (19)	12.0 (19)	0.92 (15)	893 (15)	13.8 (16)	70.5 (16)
Violent attempt	0.45 (14)	10.3 (14)	0.94 (9)	869 (9)	11.3 (13)	63.2 (10)

[a] (n). ANOVA for each measure showed no significant differences among groups.
[b] μM.
[c] pmol/10[7] platelets per minute.
[d] nM.
[e] fmol/mg protein.
[f] nmol benzaldehyde/10[8] platelets per hour.
[g] ng/10[8] platelets.

tivariate analysis shows that K_d and B_{max} can discriminate between schizophrenics and normal controls.[30]

The univariate correlations between K_d, B_{max}, and Hamilton suicide ratings are given in TABLE 6. K_d, a measure of the affinity of the platelet for imipramine and for the putative endogenous imipramine-like substances,[31] was positively correlated with Hamilton Depression Scale suicide ratings in 57 depressed patients (rho=0.32, $p<0.05$), but not in the nondepressed or all patients. A significant positive correlation between K_d and suicide ratings was also found for all psychotic depressed (unipolar psychotic, bipolar psychotic, and schizoaffective depressed, mainly affective) patients (rho = 0.45, $n=25$, p=0.02). The correlation was positive but not significant in the nonpsychotic depressed patients (rho = 0.28). The positive correlation between these measures suggests that lesser affinity (higher K_d) for any putative imipramine-like inhibitor of 5-HT uptake is associated with higher suicide ratings. In other words, less inhibition of 5-HT uptake, because of low affinity for an endogenous uptake inhibitor, which could produce more 5-HT uptake and less 5-HT at the synapse, is associated with higher suicide ratings in depression. This assumes that the observed relationship between K_d in the blood platelets and suicide ratings is a reflection of what is present at 5-HT nerve terminals. Thus, about 10% of the variance in suicide rating in depressed patients overall and 20% in psychotic depression is associated with K_d. There was no significant relationship between B_{max} and current episode suicide ratings in any of the subgroups of depressed patients. There was a trend for B_{max} to be negatively correlated with Hamilton Depression Scale suicide ratings in schizophrenic patients (rho=0.27, $n=41$, p=0.09). There was no relation between low B_{max} and a history of violent suicide attempts (TABLE 4).

TABLE 5. K_d, B_{max} of ^{3}H-Imipramine Binding in Major Affective Disorders[a]

Group	n	K_d (nM)	B_{max} (fmol/mg protein)
Normal controls	86	0.91 ± 0.29	926 ± 215
Major depression	73	0.96 ± 0.45	829 ± 227
Mania	26	0.91 ± 0.29	913 ± 331
Schizophrenic	49	0.99 ± 0.37	861 ± 252

[a] No significant differences were observed in K_d or B_{max} between the groups.

TABLE 6. Correlation between Suicide Ratings (Hamilton) and Kinetic Constants of Imipramine Binding in Blood Platelets

Subjects (n)	K_d (rho)	B_{max} (rho)
All (145)	0.13	−0.064
Depressed (57)	0.32[a]	0.180
Nondepressed (88)	0.091	−0.148

[a] $p < 0.05$.

We found no significant differences in platelet MAO activity or 5-HT content between major depression and normal controls (data not presented). No significant correlation between platelet MAO activity or 5-HT content and Hamilton suicide rating was observed (TABLE 7). No significant difference in platelet 5-HT content or MAO activity between all patients who made suicide attempts and those who did not was noted (TABLE 3). However, platelet MAO activity was significantly lower in seven nondepressed patients who made suicide attempts [8.2 ± standard deviation (SD) 2.6 nmol benzaldehyde per hour per 10^8 platelets] compared to 237 patients who did not (11.1 ± 4.4, p=0.025). Of interest is the fact that all seven of the nondepressed subjects who attempted suicide were females who normally have high platelet MAO activity compared to males. Only 45.1% of the 237 patients who had not made suicide attempts were females. There was no difference in platelet MAO activity between the 22 depressed patients who had made suicide attempts prior to this admission and the 102 who had not (11.8 ± 4.4 vs. 11.5 ± 4.5) (TABLE 3). There was no significant relation between a history of violent suicide attempt and low MAO activity, although the violent attempters had the lowest MAO followed by the nonviolent attempters (TABLE 4). Low MAO activity has been proposed to be a marker for low serotonergic activity due to inadequate development of the neuronal system which utilizes 5-HT as a neurotransmitter.[20]

There have been three previous studies reporting a relationship between low platelet MAO activity and suicide. Buchsbaum et al. in 1977 found that low platelet MAO activity in male normal volunteers was associated with a family history of suicide or suicide attempts.[32] Four completed suicides were found among relatives of low MAO probands whereas no high MAO proband had a relative who committed suicide. Gottfries et al. found lower MAO activity in 6 patients who had attempted suicide by active methods (2 gas poisoning, 1 jumping from window, 1 throwing himself in front of a car, 1 electrocution, and 1 wrist cutting) compared to 9 patients who had attempted suicide by passive methods and 59 without any previous history of suicide attempts.[33] They postulated that low MAO activity in platelets was a marker of low

TABLE 7. Univariate Correlations between Suicide Ratings (Hamilton), MAO, and 5-HT in Blood Platelets

Subjects	MAO (rho)	5-HT (rho)
All	−0.019 (369)[a]	0.011 (118)
Depressed	−0.074 (125)	0.13 (65)
Nondepressed	0.081 (244)	−0.032 (53)

[a] (n).

brain serotonergic activity. In a subsequent study, Oreland et al. found no significant difference in platelet MAO activity between 19 suicidal and 14 nonsuicidal patients.[34] There were only 2 patients who had made violent attempts. Thus, our results suggest the association between suicide attempts and low MAO activity may be confined to groups other than major depression and, further, may be strongest in females. This finding must be viewed in light of the fact that it was the only significant finding of this type among 18 such tests and the number of nondepressed subjects who had made suicide attempts was only 7.

We next examined the relationship between the Hamilton suicide ratings and the platelet measures using a series of multivariate analyses. We first examined K_m and V_{max} together for all subjects ($n=306$), then K_d and B_{max} for subjects who had such data ($n=145$), and then all subjects with data on all six measures ($n=76$).

As can be seen in TABLE 8, K_m, with V_{max} covaried, was a significant predictor of Hamilton suicide ratings for all patients. This was due solely to the nondepressed patients. Adjusted K_m had no relation to suicide ratings for the depressed group. Adjusted V_{max} contributed weakly to prediction of suicide ratings in the nondepressed group. The negative relationship between K_m and suicide in nondepressed patients suggests that a higher affinity for the reuptake of 5-HT by the platelets (and perhaps brain), which would be expected to produce less 5-HT at the synapse if the platelet findings were relevant to the brain, is associated with suicidal thoughts and acts.

K_d, with B_{max} covaried, was a slightly more potent predictor of suicide ratings for all patients and particularly for depressed patients. The multivariate analysis showed that B_{max} was negatively correlated with suicide ratings in all subjects. This was entirely due to the nondepressed group. High K_d was associated with high suicide ratings in the depressed group. Wagner et al. have recently reported that depressed patients who had attempted suicide by violent means tended to have higher B_{max} than did nonviolent attempters.[39] We did not replicate this but we had only six patients with B_{max} data who had made violent attempts prior to this admission. The positive relationship between K_d and Hamilton suicide rating suggests that a higher K_d is associated with higher suicidal ratings, as was found in the univariate relationships. As previously indicated, the higher K_d could be associated with less inhibition of 5-HT uptake, that is, more 5-HT uptake and less 5-HT at the synapse, consistent with the hypothesis that suicidal thoughts and acts are related to decreased serotonergic activity. Thus, increased 5-HT uptake appears to be weakly related to Hamilton suicide ratings in both depressed and nondepressed patients. However, this is mediated through the 5-

TABLE 8. Multiple Regression to Determine Which Platelet Measures Predict Suicide

Predictor	All Patients (n)	Depressed (n)	Nondepressed (n)
K_m	-0.15^b (306)	-0.01 (105)	-0.24^b (201)
V_{max}	0.01 (306)	-0.11 (105)	0.14^c (201)
R^2	0.02	0.01	0.04
K_d	0.17^b (145)	0.39^b (57)	0.07 (88)
B_{max}-Age	-0.17^b (145)	0.10 (57)	-0.21^c (88)
R^2	0.02	0.12	0.01

[a] Standardized beta weight.
[b] $p < 0.05$.
[c] $p = 0.1$.

TABLE 9. Multiple Regression to Determine Which Platelet Measures Predict Suicide in Psychiatric Patients

Predictor	Adj R^2	F Value of Equation	p	Standardized Beta Weight of Significant Predictor(s)	p
All Patients					
$K_m + V_{max}$ (76)	0.04	2.50	0.04	K_m, −0.30	0.04
$K_m + V_{max}$ + MAO-sex + $K_d + B_{max}$ + age (76)	0.06	1.64	0.13	K_m, −0.42	0.007
				B_{max}, −0.22	0.09
Nondepressives					
$K_m + V_{max}$ (41)	0.08	2.75	0.08	K_m, −0.40	0.03
				V_{max}, 0.32	0.08
$K_m + V_{max}$ + MAO-sex + $K_d + B_{max}$ + age (41)	0.36	3.85	0.003	V_{max}, 0.45	0.01
				Sex, 1.33	0.002
				MAO-sex, −1.08	0.04
				B_{max}, −0.24	0.09
Depressives					
$K_d + B_{max}$ + age (35)	0.11	2.34	0.09	K_d, 0.39	0.03
$K_m + V_{max}$ + MAO-sex + $K_d + B_{max}$ + age (35)	0.01	0.99	0.46	K_d, 0.37	0.06

HT transporter in the nondepressed patients and the ^{3}H-imipramine binding site in the depressed patients. Additional studies with larger numbers of subjects are necessary to determine whether these associations can be replicated and if they may be stronger in specific diagnostic groups.

Multivariate analysis of the relationship between suicide ratings and all platelet biochemical measures considered together is reported in TABLE 9. As evident from TABLE 9, K_m, with V_{max} covaried, was still a significant predictor of suicide in all patients. With V_{max} plus the four other platelet measures held constant, the beta weight of K_m was increased from −0.30 to −0.42, though the overall F for this model was not significant. K_m, with V_{max} covaried, was also a significant predictor in the two-factor (K_m and V_{max}) model for nondepressed patients. The five-factor model predicted 36% of the variance in Hamilton suicide ratings in the nondepressed patients. V_{max}, being female, and sex-adjusted MAO activity were significant predictors of suicide ratings in this model, with a trend for B_{max} also to be a predictor. The direction of the predictors is again toward effects that would lead to less 5-HT at the synapse if these same relationships occurred at 5-HT nerve terminals. Thus, increased numbers of 5-HT uptake sites, decreased MAO activity (which may indicate low presynaptic serotonergic activity),[20] and fewer IB sites all might lead to decreased 5-HT at the synapse in the nondepressed patients. The low MAO activity-suicide attempt relationship in the univariate analysis or the nondepressed patients indicates that low MAO activity, without considering any other platelet measure, is associated with suicide attempts. The multivariate analysis also indicates that when 5-HT uptake and IB parameters are held constant, decreased MAO activity is a predictor of suicidal tendencies. For the depressed patients, only K_d emerged as a significant predictor of suicide, although the two- and five-factor models in which K_d was included were not significant. Nevertheless, in view of K_d being significantly related to suicidal ratings in the univariate model, it is appropriate to point out this relationship.

Thus, our results suggest that the admission Hamilton suicide rating may be associated with increased 5-HT uptake in blood platelets, which if it occurred in the brain, could be associated with decreased serotonergic activity. Univariate and multivariate analyses indicate that K_d is the best platelet predictor in major depression; V_{max}, K_m, and MAO activity were found to be the best predictors among the platelet measures in nondepressed patients. This is in agreement with evidence for low 5-HT as a vulnerability factor in suicide[6] and the platelet as a marker for central serotonergic properties.[12,20] The evidence suggests this relationships is not specific for depression or violent suicide.

CONCLUSION

The role of brain 5-HT in suicide rests mainly on studies that show lower cerebrospinal fluid (CSF) 5-HIAA levels in patients who have made suicide attempts.[6] There have been few attempts to examine the continuum of suicidal ideation in relation to biological variables. In these analyses, we have examined the relationship between suicidal thoughts or attempts and six serotonergic measures in blood platelets. Although blood platelets have been thought to be potential models for central serotonergic activity, there is little direct evidence of correlates between biochemical measures in brain and platelets. However, decreased ^{3}H-imipramine binding has been reported in both brain[35,36] and platelets[11,37-39] of depressed patients.

The finding of a variety of significant but small correlations between platelet serotonergic biochemical measures and Hamilton suicide ratings could be evidence for the role of 5-HT in suicidal ideation as well as attempts, but this depends on the yet to be proven assumption that the platelet is a model for brain 5-HT neurons and replication in an independent sample. At the current time, the platelet-suicide relationships are best interpreted as possible "markers" of a linkage between the platelet 5-HT regulatory processes and central nervous system (CNS) activity relevant to suicide, not necessarily serotonergic in nature.

The fact that different facets of platelet serotonergic activity relate to the suicide ratings in depressed and nondepressed patients demands caution in interpreting these results, especially since the associations found are very weak. The small magnitude of the observed associations may reflect the multiple factors that affect each platelet measure, assay error during the multiple years of obtaining this data, difficulty obtaining reliable information about suicidal ideation, and the multiple CNS factors that must influence a complex behavior such as suicidal thoughts or attempts.

SUMMARY

Six serotonergic measures in blood platelets, K_m and V_{max} of serotonin (5-HT) uptake, K_d and B_{max} of ^{3}H-imipramine binding, 5-HT content, and MAO activity, were measured in depressed and other psychiatric patients and related to Hamilton Depression Scale suicide ratings. K_m was negatively correlated with the suicide rating while K_d was positively correlated with it. Multivariate analyses showed that K_m, K_d, V_{max}, and MAO activity were significant predictors of Hamilton Depression Scale suicide ratings. Low platelet MAO activity was present in seven nondepressed females who had made suicide attempts in the current episode. The direction of the association between the platelet measures and suicide ratings indicated diminished presynaptic serotonergic activity in patients with high suicide ratings, if the platelet findings could be extrapolated to 5-HT nerve terminals.

REFERENCES

1. COPPEN, A. 1967. The biochemistry of affective disorders. Br. J. Psychiatry **113**: 1237-1264.
2. LAPIN, I. P. & G. F. OXENKRUG. 1969. Intensification of the central serotoneric processes as a possible determinant of the thymoleptic effect. Lancet **1**: 132-136.
3. VAN PRAAG, H. M. 1983. In search of the mode of action of antidepressants: 5-HTP tyrosine mixtures in depression. Neuropharmacology **22**: 433-440.
4. MELTZER, H. Y., M. LOWY, A. ROBERTSON, P. GOODNICK & R. PERLINE. 1984. Effect of 5-hydroxytryptophan on serum cortisol levels in major affective disorders. III. Effect of antidepressants and lithium carbonate. Arch. Gen. Psychiatry **41**: 391-397.
5. BROWN, G. L., M. E. EBERT & P. F. GOYER. 1982. Aggression, suicide, and serotonin: relationship to CSF amine metabolites. Am. J. Psychiatry **139**: 741-746.
6. ASBERG, M., P. NORDSTROM & L. TRASKMAN-BENDZ. Cerebrospinal fluid studies in suicide: an overview. Ann. N.Y. Acad. Sci. (This volume.)
7. TRASKMAN-BENDZ, L., M. ASBERG & D. SCHALLING. Serotonergic function and suicidal behavior in personality disorders. Ann. N.Y. Acad. Sci. (This volume.)
8. MELTZER, H. Y., B. UMBERKOMAN-WIITA, A. ROBERTSON, B. J. TRICOU, M. LOWY & R. PERLINE. 1984. Effect of 5-hydroxytryptophan on serum cortisol levels in major affective disorders. I. Enhanced response in depression and mania. Arch. Gen. Psychiatry **41**: 366-374.
9. MELTZER, H. Y., R. PERLINE, B. J. TRICOU, M. LOWY & A. ROBERTSON. 1984. Effect of 5-hydroxytryptophan on serum cortisol levels in major affective disorders. II. Relation to suicide, psychosis and depressive symptoms. Arch. Gen. Psychiatry **41**: 379-387.
10. MELTZER, H. Y., R. C. ARORA, R. BABER & B. J. TRICOU. 1981. Serotonin uptake in blood platelets of psychiatric patients. Arch. Gen. Psychiatry **38**: 1322-1326.
11. MELTZER, H. Y., R. C. ARORA, A. ROBERTSON & M. LOWY. 1984. Platelet ^{3}H-imipramine binding and platelet 5-HT uptake in affective disorders and schizophrenia. Clin. Neuropharmacol. 7(Suppl. 1): 320-321.
12. SNEDDON, J. M. 1973. Blood platelets as a model for monamine containing neurons. Prog. Neurobiol. **1**: 151-198.
13. STAHL, S. M. 1977. The human platelet: a diagnostic and research tool for the study of biogenic amines in psychiatric and neurologic disorders. Arch. Gen. Psychiatry **34**: 509-516.
14. JACKMAN, H., D. LUCHINS & H. Y. MELTZER. 1983. Platelet serotonin levels in schizophrenia: relationship to race and psychopathology. Biol. Psychiatry **18**: 887-902.
15. QUAN-BUI, K. H. L., O. PLAISANT, M. LEBOYER, C. GAY, L. KAMAL, M-A. DEVEYNCH & P. MEYER. 1984. Reduced platelet serotonin in depression. Psychiatry Res. **13**: 129-139.
16. LANGER, S. Z., M. S. BRILEY, R. RAISMAN, J-P. HENRY & P. L. MORSELLI. 1980. Specific ^{3}H-imipramine binding in human platelets. Naunyn-Schmiedeberg's Arch. Pharmacol. **313**: 189-194.
17. LANGER, S. Z., F. JAVOY-AGID, R. RAISMAN, M. BRILEY & Y. AGID. 1981. Distribution of specific high affinity binding sites for (^{3}H) imipramine in human brain. J. Neurochem. **37**: 267-271.
18. BRILEY, M., S. Z. LANGER & M. SETTE. 1981. Allosteric interaction between the ^{3}H-imipramine binding site and the serotonin uptake mechanism. Proc. Br. Pharmacol. Soc. 817P-818P.
19. WENNOGLE, L. P. & L. R. MEYERSON. 1983. Serotonin modulates the dissociation of ^{3}H-imipramine from human platelet recognition sites. Eur. J. Pharmacol. **86**: 303-307.

20. ORELAND, L., A. WIBERG & C. J. FOWLER. 1981. Monoamine oxidase activity in platelets as related to monoamine oxidase activity and monoamine function in the brain. Adv. Biosci. **31:** 195-201.
21. EDWARDS, D. J. & S. S. CHANG. 1975. Evidence for interacting catalytic sites of human platelet monamine oxidase. Biochem. Biophys. Res. Commun. **65:** 1018-1025.
22. HAMILTON, M. 1960. A rating scale for depression. J. Neurol. Neurosurg. Psychiatry **23:** 56-62.
23. WING, J. K., J. E. COOPER & N. SARTORIUS. 1974. The Measurement and Classification of Psychiatric Symptoms. Cambridge University Press. Cambridge, England.
24. ENDICOTT, J. & R. SPITZER. 1978. A diagnostic interview: a schedule for affective disorders and schizophrenia. Arch. Gen. Psychiatry **35:** 837-844.
25. SPITZER, R. L., J. ENDICOTT & E. ROBINS. 1978. Research diagnostic criteria: rationale and reliability. Arch. Gen. Psychiatry **35:** 733-782.
26. JACKMAN, H., R. C. ARORA & H. Y. MELTZER. 1979. Comparison of platelet count and platelet protein methods for determination of platelet MAO activity. Clin. Chim. Acta **96:** 15-23.
27. ARORA, R. C. & H. Y. MELTZER. 1981. A modified assay method for determining serotonin uptake in human platelets. Clin. Chim. Acta **112:** 225-233.
28. ARORA, R. C., C. TONG, H. L. JACKMAN, D. STOFF & H. Y. MELTZER. 1983. Serotonin uptake and imipramine binding in blood platelets and brain of fawn-hooded and Sprague-Dawley rats. Life Sci. **33:** 437-442.
29. MELTZER, H. Y., A. G. ROBERTSON & R. C. ARORA. Platelet ^{3}H-imipramine binding in affective disorders: relation to age and psychosis. Psychiatry Res. (In press.)
30. ARORA, R. C., J. J. LOCASCIO & H. Y. MELTZER. ^{3}H-imipramine binding in blood platelets of schizophrenic patients. Psychiatry Res. (In press.)
31. BARBACIA, M. L., O. GANDOLFI, D-M. CHUANG & E. COSTA. 1983. Modulation of neuronal serotonin uptake by a putative endogenous ligand of imipramine recognition sites. Proc. Nat. Acad. Sci. USA **80:** 5134-5138.
32. BUCHSBAUM, M. S., R. J. HAIER & D. L. MURPHY. 1977. Suicide attempts, platelet monoamine oxidase and the average evoked response. Acta Psychiatr. Scand. **56:** 69-79.
33. GOTTFRIES, C-G., L. V. KNORRING & L. ORELAND. 1980. Platelet monoamine oxidase activity in mental disorders. 2. Affective psychosis and suicidal behavior. Prog. Neuropsychopharmacol. **4:** 185-192.
34. ORELAND, L., A. WIBERG, M. ASBERG, L. TRASKMAN, L. SJOSTRAND, P. THOREN, L. BERTILLSON & G. TYBRING. 1981. Platelet MAO activity and monoamine metabolites in cerebrospinal fluid in depressed and suicidal patients and in healthy controls. Psychiatry Res. **4:** 21-29.
35. STANLEY, M., J. VIRGILIO & S. GERSHON. 1982. Tritiated imipramine binding sites are decreased in the frontal cortex of suicides. Science **216:** 1337-1339.
36. PERRY, E. K., E. F. MARSHALL, G. BLESSED, B. E. TOMLINSON & R. H. PERRY. 1983. Decreased imipramine binding in the brains of patients with depressive illness. Br. J. Psychiatry **142:** 188-192.
37. BRILEY, M. S., S. Z. LANGER, R. RAISMAN, D. SECHTER & E. ZARIFIAN. 1980. Tritiated imipramine binding sites are decreased in platelets of untreated depressed patients. Science **209:** 303-305.
38. PAUL, S. M., M. REHAVI, P. SKOLNICK, J. C. BALLENGER & F. K. GOODWIN. 1981. Depressed patients have decreased binding of tritiated imipramine to platelet serotonin transporter. Arch. Gen. Psychiatry **38:** 1315-1317.
39. WAGNER, A., A. ABERG-WISTEDT, A. ASBERG, B. EKQUIST, B. MARTENSSON & D. MONTERO. 1985. Lower ^{3}H-imipramine binding in platelets from untreated depressed patients compared to healthy controls. Psychiatry Res. **16:** 131-139.

Personality and Suicide

ALLEN FRANCES, MINNA FYER,
AND JOHN CLARKIN

*Department of Psychiatry
Cornell University Medical College
525 East 68th Street
New York, New York 10021*

Individuals with psychiatric disorders are at greatly increased risk for suicide: Robins et al. found that 94% of suicides had a psychiatric disorder,[1] Barraclough found similar rates in Britain,[2] and Martin et al. found suicide rates to be 15 times higher in psychiatric outpatients than in matched nonpsychiatric controls.[3] Most suicide studies have focused on Axis I disorders: increased risk has been identified for primary affective disorders;[4-8] schizophrenia;[9-11] and alcoholism.[12-15] Although the relationship between Axis II disorders and suicide is less well established, several reports suggest that personality disorder patients represent a significant proportion of completed suicides and even more attempters:[2,3,6,16-19] moreover, the presence of a concurrent personality disorder may increase suicide risk in patients with Axis I disorders.[20-23]

This paper summarizes the literature on the two personality disorders (borderline and antisocial) and on the personality traits most associated with suicide behavior, outlines some of the methodological problems involved in this type of research, and discusses the clinical and research implications of available findings.

PERSONALITY DISORDERS AND SUICIDE

Borderline Personality Disorders

Borderline personality disorder (BPD) patients engage in a great deal of self-destructive behavior, most of which is not considered to be seriously suicidal.[24-28] There has been surprisingly little study of completed suicide in BPD patients. Stone found a 10% mortality from suicide on a 10-15 year follow-up,[28] Akiskal a 4% rate on shorter follow-up,[29] and Pope et al. a 7% rate after 4-7 years.[30]

Several studies suggest that the combination of BPD and affective disorder is particularly lethal. Among 76 adolescent inpatients, Friedman et al. found that patients who met criteria for both BPD and major affective disorder (MAD) made more frequent and more lethal attempts.[20] Friedman et al. also studied 53 inpatient depressives and found that the 36 who also met criteria for BPD made more serious and numerous suicide attempts.[21] Crumly found that among 40 adolescent suicide attempters, 24 suffered from MAD and 22 from BPD.[22] A large percentage were also substance abusers.

Among 180 BPD inpatients, Fyer et al. found a difference in suicidal behavior between those with and those without concurrent affective disorder.[31] For the whole sample, 19% had no history of suicide, 32% made only gestures, and 49% had made serious attempts. However, significantly more of those with affective disorder had made serious attempts (56%) than those without an affective diagnosis (37%) and fewer of the affective BPD had no history of suicide (13% vs. 29%).

Although BPD patients often engage in self-destructive behavior without lethal intent, a substantial proportion (at least 5-10%) do eventually die by suicide. Concurrent major affective disorder increases the risk of suicide in BPD (and vice versa) as does substance abuse.

Antisocial Personality Disorder

Reports of antisocial personality disorder (ASPD) suicide rates vary considerably, and most studies have not used *Diagnostic and Statistical Manual,* third edition (DSM III) criteria. Miles estimated that 5% eventually die by suicide.[9] Maddocks found that 46% made suicide attempts and 5% successfully suicided.[32] On the other hand, Robins found that while 11% of ASPD patients had made suicide attempts, the rate of completed suicide on follow-up was not different from psychiatrically normal controls.[33] In a series of 500 psychiatric patients, Woodruff et al. found that 23% of 71 suicide attempters met ASPD criteria,[17] equivalent to the rate of ASPD for the whole sample. ASPD seems to be uncommon in series of completed suicides.[2,34] It has also been observed that ASPD and criminality are predictors of recurrent attempts.[35,36] Garvey and Spoden found that 72% of 29 ASPD individuals had a total of 63 suicide attempts, but only 3 were serious and none used violent methods.[37] Half of the ASPD attempters indicated that their most recent attempt was preceded by a crisis in a significant relationship. These coauthors conclude that sociopaths usually have no real intention of killing themselves and use suicide attempts to manipulate those around them. Robins et al. found that only 1 of 16 ASPD patients had made a serious suicide attempt compared with 80% affective disorder controls.[38] Attempts were often precipitated by anger and frustration in love or marital relationships. ASPD patients were younger than affective controls, and 85% consumed alcohol just prior to the attempt.

Batchelor studied 42 suicide attempters with "psychopathic states" and also found that the majority of attempts were precipitated by difficulties in relationships, that almost half had made previous attempts, and that most used nonviolent means.[39] However, at least one-third of attempts were felt to be serious.

In summary, suicide attempts in ASPD appear to be common, repetitive, usually not serious, and are often precipitated by difficulties in important relationships. The 5% rate of successfully completed suicide in this group may represent primarily those individuals with ASPD who also have concurrent affective disorder, substance abuse, and/or other personality disorders that increase risk for successful suicide.

Substance Abuse, Personality Disorders and Suicide

Substance abuse is associated with marked increased risk for suicide.[12-14] The suicide rate for male alcoholics is 75 times greater than for the general male population.[40]

The age-adjusted rate of suicide for opiate addicts is estimated to be 5 to 20 times that of the general population.[41] Many patients with personality disorders are substance abusers, and DSM III includes substance abuse among the criteria for both ASPD and BPD.

Ward and Schuckit *et al.* studied suicidal behavior in 155 polydrug abusers of whom 29% received a diagnosis of ASPD.[42] In contrast to the previously mentioned studies of ASPD alone, patients with both drug abuse and ASPD made more serious suicide attempts.

Rounsaville *et al.* found that 37% of 533 treated opiate addicts met Research Diagnostic Criteria (RDC) ASPD criteria; 16.5% for labile personality disorder, and 8.4% had schizotypal features.[43] Using DSM III, they found that 54% met ASPD criteria. Fifty-two percent of the sample had two or more psychiatric diagnoses in addition to opiate addiction. There was a 17% lifetime prevalence of suicide attempts in the whole sample, and 60% of attempters were DSM III ASPD, 32% were "borderline type" (schizotypal, BPD, schizoid, paranoid), 24% were "narcissistic type" (dependent, narcissistic, histrionic), and 7.5% had other personality disorders; 87% of attempters had a diagnosis of depression and 32% had alcoholism. Suicide attempters had significantly more affective disorder, schizophrenia, alcoholism, and borderline and narcissistic personality disorders than did nonattempters. Rates of ASPD and of other personality disorders did not differ between the two groups. These studies represent an early effort to apply rigorous diagnostic assessment and examination of comorbidity to the problem of suicidal behavior. The results confirm that comorbidity of personality disorders and Axis I disorders may interact to increase suicide risk.

PERSONALITY TRAITS AS PREDICTORS OF SUICIDE

Suicide attempters and suicide completers appear to differ in their personality characteristics, and attempters have the more disturbed personality profiles. Suicide attempters are usually women, under 24 years of age, more often receive "neurotic" or personality disorder diagnoses, make their attempts more publicly and impulsively, and often use less serious means. Suicide completers tend to be men, older, more likely to have an Axis I diagnosis (especially depression or alcoholism), make private attempts, and use lethal means.[44] Most of the following literature on personality traits applies to suicide attempters and may not generalize to completers.

There has been a continuing interest in the relationship between suicide and aggression stemming from psychodynamic formulations of depression that emphasize "hostility turned against the self."[45,46] Numerous studies have found increased hostility in suicide attempters,[17,47-57] and a few studies have identified increased impulsivity.[49] Suicidal individuals tend to be socially withdrawn or to experience considerable interpersonal difficulties.[47,57,59-65] A few studies have identified lack of trust and cynicism about other people.[51,55] Lowered or negative self-esteem seems to be characteristic of both suicide attempters and completers.[47,58,66-74] One study found more schizoid features in serious suicide attempters. Increased dependency has also been reported.[48,54,55,75]

Studies of hysterical traits in suicide have yielded conflicting results. Four studies have used the Hysteroid-Obsessoid Questionnaire. Vinoda found a trend for suicidal patients and psychiatric controls to obtain more obsessoid scores than do normal controls.[52] Murthy reported that more nonserious attempters than serious attempters scored in the hysteroid range.[53] Eastwood *et al.* reported that suicide attempters scored in "the direction of obsessoid personality."[76] Goldney found that young women who attempted suicide did not score in a more hysterical range than psychiatric controls.[77] Using the Minnesota Multiphasic Personality Inventory (MMPI) hysteria scale, Farberow[78] and Pallis and Birtchnell[55,79] found no significant differences between suicidal and nonsuicidal subjects. Using the same scale, Leonard found significant elevation in those who subsequently successfully suicided compared to serious attempters and nonsuicidal psychiatric controls.[80]

Studies using the Eysenck Personality Inventory have a fairly consistent result: an increase on Neuroticism and Psychoticism scales and either a lower Extroversion or higher Introversion score.[64,66,81-84]

A number of studies describe the cognitive characteristics of suicidal individuals. Beck found that hopelessness correlated more highly than did depression with suicide.[85-88] Other investigators have also found a relationship between suicide and hopelessness. Powerlessness[93] and external locus of control[29,94] have also been identified in suicidal populations. Suicidal individuals have a rigid cognitive style[52,95,96] and difficulty with problem solving.[90,97]

The many studies using the MMPI to identify, predict, or characterize suicidal individuals have yielded inconsistent results. Eight studies compared MMPI scales in suicidal and nonsuicidal individuals in an attempt to identify "suicidal" scales.[80,86,95,98-103] Eleven of the 13 MMPI scales were identified as suicide related in at least one study, but none of the scales was consistently so related. Two studies attempting to develop an MMPI suicide scale were unsuccessful.[98,103] Several studies have described multiscale MMPI profiles for suicidal patients,[98,104] but one study failed to.[105] Clopton recently found that descriminant function analysis produced only a "modest degree of differentiation" between suicidal and nonsuicidal subjects.[106] Overall, use of the MMPI to study suicide has not been very promising.

BIOLOGICAL FACTORS, PERSONALITY TRAITS, AND SUICIDE

Several biologic factors have been associated with suicidal behavior including increased plasma cortisol and urinary 17 hydroxycorticosteroid (17-OHCS) levels[107,108] and decreased platelet monoamine oxidase (MAO) activity,[109] cerebrospinal fluid (CSF) melatonin, homovanillic acid (HVA),[110] magnesium, and blunted thyrotropin stimulating hormone (TSH) response.[117] The most exciting biological finding is low serotonin turnover, which may provide the first instance of a close tie between a specific biological finding and a particular pattern of behavior. There is consistent evidence for an association between lowered CSF 5-hydroxyindoleacetic acid (5-HIAA) levels, suicide (especially violent suicide), and aggression.[111-116,118-126] CSF 5-HIAA has a modal distribution in depressed patients, but those with low levels commit suicide more often and use more violent means. Studies of low 5-HIAA in recovered depressives suggest that these levels normalize either partially or not at all. Low CSF 5-HIAA correlated both with past[112,118,121] and future suicide attempts[112,116] or history of aggressive acts. An increased incidence of depressive illness has been found in the relatives of both patients[127] and normals[128] with low CSF 5-HIAA. Levels appear to be genetically determined and consistent over time.[129]

There have been two studies of CSF 5-HIAA in patients with personality disorders, without concurrent affective disorder. Brown et al. compared CSF 5-HIAA in 26 personality disorder patients with 26 normal controls.[118] Personality disorder diagnoses were divided into more impulsive (antisocial, explosive, immature, and hysterical) and less impulsive (passive-aggressive, passive dependent, schizoid, obsessive-compulsive, and inadequate). Both personality disorder groups had significantly higher aggression scores (as compared to controls). The more impulsive group had higher mean aggression scores and lower CSF 5-HIAA than did the less impulsive group. Suicidal subjects had higher mean aggression scores and lower 5-HIAA.

Brown et al. also studied 12 BPD subjects without concurrent affective disorder, and found that aggressive and suicide attempts were again significantly associated with each other and with lower CSF 5-HIAA levels.[123] The MMPI psychopathic deviance scale reflecting aggression was negatively correlated with CSF 5-HIAA.[118,123,121,124,125] The level of central serotonergic function may contribute to the individual's characteristic impulse control, aggressivity, and potential for suicidal behavior which is released in the presence of clinical depression.[118,121,123–125] Bioulac found decreased CSF 5-HIAA in six 47-chromosome XYY men who had personality disorders and were institutionalized for aggressivity and violence.[130] Lidberg compared 16 convicted murderers to 22 suicide attempters and 39 controls.[126] Those who had killed a lover or sexual rival had 5-HIAA levels similar to suicide attempters, and these were significantly lower than controls or other murderers.

METHODOLOGICAL ISSUES

The Relationship between Personality Disorders and Suicide

Research on personality disorders and on suicide have each separately been impeded by conceptual and methodologic difficulties so that the study of their interaction presents complex problems. Although it is known that psychiatric patients are at increased risk for suicide and have high rates of personality disorder, very little is as yet known about causal relationships between personality disorders and suicidal behavior. We will briefly present some of the possible ways of conceptualizing the relationship: (1) Suicidal behavior may be an inherent component of certain personality constructs in the same way that suicidal behavior is included in the definition of major depressive disorder. Currently, DSM III includes suicidal acts as criteria for two personality disorders: borderline and histrionic. Whenever suicidal behavior forms part of the definition of a disorder, be it depressive or personality, this necessarily results in an inflated covariation between that disorder and suicide. (2) Personality disorder may predispose to suicidal behavior or to a particularly lethal form of suicide attempt. (3) Personality disorders may predispose to Axis I disorders (e.g., depression), which then independently increase the risk of suicide. (4) Personality disorders might also exert an influence on the expression of an Axis I disorder. Most patients with major depression do not commit suicide. The presence of a personality disorder may help to determine whether a given depressed individual is likely to attempt or succeed at suicide. (5) Since suicide is not diagnostically specific for Axis I disorders, it is perhaps unrealistic to expect it to be so for Axis II disorders which are even less well defined. Combinations of personality traits that cut across traditional diagnostic categories might better predict suicidal behavior. For instance, impulsivity and decisiveness together might make it particularly likely for an individual to commit suicide, especially if he were depressed. Study of specific personality traits may be more useful than study of categories of personality disorders. (6) Axis I conditions that are associated with suicide may predispose to increased prevalence of Axis II disorders, which may or may not then independently contribute to increased risk of suicide. (7) Any association between personality disorder and suicide may be no more than coincidental—that is, not higher than the comorbidity one might expect from the base rates of both conditions in whatever setting is used for study.

A number of studies are necessary to sort out the nature of these relationships. Determining the rate of personality disorders in suicidal as compared to nonsuicidal patients, controlling for diagnosis, would determine whether there is a greater than chance comorbidity. Determining the suicide rate and severity of attempt for various kinds of personality disorder patients, and comparing those with and without accompanying Axis I disorders, would determine the degree of independent contribution of specific personality disorders to suicide. Determining the predictive power of the suicide criterion for BPD and the predictive power of the rest of the BPD criteria set (leaving out this one item) for suicide will determine the degree to which the association is merely definitional. Studies should also compare the ability of the DSM III disorder system vs. an underlying personality trait system to predict suicide.

Types of Suicidal Behavior

An additional problem in exploring the relationship between personality and suicide is that it is difficult to define and classify the very broad spectrum of suicidal behaviors, which range from fleeting ideation to completed suicide.[131-136] No one system has achieved widespread acceptance and considerable controversy continues, making comparison of results difficult or impossible. The one clear distinction is between those who attempt and those who complete suicide. Many studies select one population or the other, while others include both. It is known that a previous attempt carries an increased risk of eventual successful suicide: 2% of attempters will go on to kill themselves within one year, and about 10% eventually will successfully suicide.[44] It remains unclear the degree to which data on attempters (who are obviously much easier to study) are relevant to completers. It is very likely that completers and attempters represent two separate but overlapping populations[38,137] and that the distributions and contribution of personality disorders differ in each. Attempters do not greatly resemble completers in demographic, diagnostic, or psychological variables.[55,137-139]

Technical Problems

The conditions under which most suicide research is done accentuate the difficulty in making reliable and valid personality diagnoses. In the case of completed suicide, postmortem psychological autopsies consist of a review of available records and interviews with those who knew the victim. In studies of attempted suicide, assessments are frequently brief and often made in the emergency room setting. Patients who are not admitted to the hospital are difficult to follow up and frequently do not want to discuss their suicide attempt.[76] Personality assessments take place at variable time intervals[76] from the suicide attempt and may be contaminated by the presence of accompanying Axis I diagnoses and situational stress. It has been clearly demonstrated that the presence of an Axis I disorder, particularly depression, exerts a strong influence on personality assessment.[140]

Few studies have used systematic and rigorous personality disorder diagnoses, and those that do have used a variety of different classification systems. The advent of DSM III Axis II classification should be helpful in this regard. Moreover, most studies, because of their focus on Axis I, have tended to lump all personality disorder diagnoses together, so that knowledge of suicidality in any particular personality disorder is scant. The reporting of concurrent Axis I and II disorders is necessary but has rarely been done.

Studies in this area have also suffered from the effects of retrospective design and biased sample selection which limit the generalizability of results. The prevailing strategy has been to identify and study patients who have made recent suicide attempts. Settings have varied widely (emergency rooms, inpatient, private practice, and outpatient clinics). A variety of different control groups have been used in some studies, but not in others. Because suicide is a relatively rare event, prospective study has presented great difficulties and has not been performed very often. There are extremely few studies of suicidal behavior in an identified personality disorder population. Therefore, although there is some information about personality disorders in suicidal individuals, there is much less about suicide in persons with personality disorders.

Despite all of the technical difficulties, there are grounds for optimism that we will soon have a much fuller understanding of the relationship between personality disorders and suicide. The provision within DSM III of a separate axis for personality disorders and the system of operational diagnostic criteria have greatly increased the attention accorded personality disorder research and the reliability with which diagnoses are made. There are now available three reliable, semistructured, and diagnostic instruments that allow for the systematic assessment of all the DSM III personality disorders.[141-143] These also exist in a format that is suitable for use with family informants that could be made a part of postmortem studies. Undoubtedly we will also soon have a much clearer understanding of the relationship between Axis I and Axis II disorders, prospective longitudinal studies of the rate of completed suicide and attempts in personality disorder patients, and studies of personality diagnoses in suicide attempters.

The current clinical implications of the available findings are clear and demand attention. Clinicians should become especially concerned about those patients who present with several comorbid diagnoses, i.e., especially combinations of BPD or ASPD with MAD and/or substance abuse. Such patients are likely to have an increased frequency and severity of attempts and are especially likely to require hospitalization, antidepressant medication, and detoxification. It is also possible that suicidal patients may benefit preferentially from drugs that work on the serotonin system.

REFERENCES

1. ROBINS, E., S. GASSNER, J. KAYES, et al. 1959. The communication of suicidal intent: a study of 135 cases of successful (completed) suicide. Am. J. Psychiatry 115: 724-733.
2. BARRACLOUGH, B., J. BUNCH, B. NELSON, et al. 1974. A hundred cases of suicide: clinical aspects. Br. J. Psychiatry 125: 355-373.
3. MARTIN, R. L., C. R. CLONINGER, S. B. GUZE, et al. 1985. Mortality in a follow up of

500 psychiatric outpatients. II. Cause-specific mortality. Arch. Gen. Psychiatry **30:** 737-746.
4. GUZE, S. B. & E. ROBINS. 1970. Suicide and primary affective disorder. Br. J. Psychiatry **117:** 437-438.
5. WEISSMAN, M. M. 1974. The epidemiology of suicide attempts: 1960-1971. Arch. Gen. Psychiatry **30:** 737-746.
6. POKORNY, A. D. 1964. Suicide rates in various psychiatric disorders. J. Nerv. Ment. Dis. **139:** 499-506.
7. ROY, A. 1982. Risk factors for suicide in psychiatric patients. Arch. Gen. Psychiatry **39:** 1090-1095.
8. ROY, A. 1983. Suicide in depressives. Compr. Psychiatry **24:** 487-491.
9. MILES, P. 1977. Conditions predisposing to suicide: a review. J. Nerv. Ment. Dis. **164:** 231-246.
10. ROY, A. 1982. Suicide in chronic schizophrenia. Br. J. Psychiatry **141:** 171-177.
11. KRAFT, D. & M. BABIGIAN. 1976. Suicide by persons with and without psychiatric contacts. Arch. Gen. Psychiatry **33:** 209-215.
12. VAILLANT, G. 1966. Twelve-year follow up of New York narcotic addicts. Am. J. Psychiatry **122:** 727-737.
13. JAMES, I. 1967. Suicide and mortality in heroin addicts in Britain. Br. J. Addict. **62:** 391-398.
14. NOBLE, P., T. HART & R. NATION. 1972. Correlates of outcome of illicit drug use by adolescent girls. Br. J. Psychiatry **120:** 497-504.
15. BLACK, D. W., G. WARRACK & G. WINOKUR. 1985. The Iowa record-linkage study. I. Suicide and accidental deaths among psychiatric patients. Arch. Gen. Psychiatry **42:** 71-75.
16. MCHUGH, P. R. & H. GOODELL. 1971. Suicidal Behavior. Arch. Gen. Psychiatry **25:** 456-464.
17. WOODRUFF, R. A. JR., P. J. CLAYTON & S. B. GUZE. 1972. Suicide attempts and psychiatric diagnosis. Dis. Nerv. Syst. **33:** 617-621.
18. URWIN, P. & J. L. GIBBONS. 1979. Psychiatric diagnosis in self-poisoning patients. Psychol. Med. **9:** 501-507.
19. MORRISON, J. R. 1982. Suicide in a psychiatric practice population. J. Clin. Psychiatry **43:** 348-352.
20. FRIEDMAN, R. C., J. F. CLARKIN, R. CORN, et al. 1982. DSM-III and affective pathology in hospitalized adolescents. J. Nerv. Ment. Dis. **170:** 511-521.
21. FRIEDMAN, R. C., M. S. ARONOFF, J. F. CLARKIN, et al. 1983. History of suicidal behavior in depressed borderline inpatients. Am. J. Psychiatry **140:** 1023-1026.
22. CRUMLY, F. E. 1979. Adolescent suicide attempts. J. Am. Med. Assoc. **241**(22): 2404-2407.
23. ALESSI, N. E., M. MCMANUS, A. BRICKMAN & L. GRAPENTINE. 1984. Suicidal behavior among serious juvenile offenders. Am. J. Psychiatry **141**(2): 286-287.
24. GUNDERSON, J. F. & J. E. KOLB. 1978. Discriminating features of borderline patients. Am. J. Psychiatry **135:** 792-796.
25. SPITZER, R. L., J. ENDICOTT & M. GIBBON. 1979. Crossing the border into borderline personality and borderline schizophrenia. Arch. Gen. Psychiatry **36:** 17-24.
26. GUNDERSON, J. F. & M. T. SINGER. 1975. Defining borderline patients: an overview. Am. J. Psychiatry **132:** 1-10.
27. PERRY, J. C. & G. L. KLERMAN. 1978. The borderline patient: a comparative analysis of four sets of diagnostic criteria. Arch. Gen. Psychiatry **35:** 141-150.
28. STONE, M. H. 1986. Exploratory psychotherapy in schizophrenic-spectrum patients: a reevaluation. Bull. Menninger Clin. **50**(3): 287-306.
29. AKISKAL, H. S., S. E. CHEN, G. C. DAVIS, et al. 1985. Borderline: an adjective in search of a noun. J. Clin. Psychiatry **46:** 41-48.
30. POPE, H. G., JR., J. M. JONAS, J. I. HUDSON, et al. 1983. The validity of DSM-III borderline personality disorder. Arch. Gen. Psychiatry **40:** 23-30.
31. FYER, M., A. FRANCES, T. SULLIVAN, et al. Borderline personality disorder and affective disorder: impact of comorbidity on suicide. (Unpublished manuscript.)
32. MADDOCKS, P. D. 1970. A five year follow up of untreated psychopaths. Br. J. Psychiatry **116:** 511-515.

33. ROBINS, L. N. 1966. Deviant Children Grown Up. Williams & Wilkins. Baltimore, Md.
34. ROBINS, E., G. E. MURPHY, R. H. WILKINSON, et al. 1959. Some clinical considerations in the prevention of suicide based on a study of 134 successful suicides. Am. J. Public Health **49**: 888-889.
35. MORGAN, H. G., J. BORTON, L. S. POFFLE, et al. 1976. Deliberate self-harm: a followup study of 279 patients. Br. J. Psychiatry **128**: 361-368.
36. BUGLASS, P. & J. HORTON. 1974. The repetition of parasuicide: a comparison of three cohorts. Br. J. Psychiatry **125**: 168-174.
37. GARVEY, M. J. & F. SPODEN. 1980. Suicide attempts in antisocial personality disorder. Compr. Psychiatry **21**(2): 146-149.
38. ROBINS, E., E. H. SCHMIDT & P. O'NEAL. 1957. Some interrelations of social factors and clinical diagnosis in attempted suicide: a study of 109 patients. Am. J. Psychiatry **114**: 221-231.
39. BATCHELOR, I. R. C. 1954. Psychopathic states and attempted suicide. Br. Med. J. **1**: 1342-1347.
40. KESSEL, N. & G. GROSSMAN. 1961. Suicide in alcoholics. Br. Med. J. **2**: 1671-1672.
41. MURPHY, S. L., B. J. ROUNSAVILLE, S. EYRE & H. D. KLEBER. 1983. Suicide attempts in treated opiate addicts. Compr. Psychiatry **241**: 79-88.
42. WARD, N. G. & M. A. SCHUCKIT. 1980. Factors associated with suicidal behavior in polydrug abusers. J. Clin. Psychiatry **41**(11): 379-385.
43. ROUNSAVILLE, B. J., M. M. WEISSMAN, H. KLEBER & C. WILBER. 1982. Heterogeneity of psychiatric diagnosis in treated opiate addicts. Arch. Gen. Psychiatry **39**: 161-166.
44. CLAYTON, P. J. 1985. Suicide. Psychiatry Clin. North Am. **8**(2): 203-214.
45. FREUD, S. 1916. Mourning and melancholia. In Collected Papers. E. Jones, Ed. **4**: 15-72. Hogarth Press. London, England.
46. ABRAHAM, K. 1927. Notes on the psychoanalytic investigation and treatment of manic-depressive insanity and allied conditions. In Selected Papers. E. Jones, Ed.: 137-156. Hogarth Press. London, England.
47. CROOK, T., A. RASKIN & D. DAVID. 1975. Factors associated with attempted suicide among hospitalized depressed patients. Psychol. Med. **5**: 381-388.
48. PAYKEL, E. S. & M. DIENELT. 1971. Suicide attempts following acute depression. J. Nerv. Ment. Dis. **153**: 234-243.
49. CANTOR, P. C. 1976. Personality characteristics found among youthful female suicide attempters. J. Abnorm. Psychol. **85**(3): 324-319.
50. HENDERSON, A. S., J. HARTIGAN, J. DAVIDSON, et al. 1977. A typology of parasuicide. Br. J. Psychiatry **131**: 631-641.
51. CONTE, H. R. & R. PLUTCHIK. 1974. Personality and background characteristics of suicidal mental patients. J. Psychiatry Res. **10**: 181-188.
52. VINODA, K. S. 1966. Personality characteristics of attempted suicides. Br. J. Psychiatry **112**: 1143-1150.
53. MURTHY, V. N. 1969. Personality and the nature of suicidal attempts. Br. J. Psychiatry **115**: 791-795.
54. BIRTCHNELL, J. 1981. Some familial and clinical characteristics of female suicidal psychiatric patients. Br. J. Psychiatry **138**: 381-390.
55. PALLIS, D. J. & J. BIRTCHNELL. 1977. Serious of suicide attempt in relation to personality. Br. J. Psychiatry **130**: 253-259.
56. WEISSMAN, M. M., K. FOX & G. L. KLERMAN. 1973. Hostility and depression associated with suicide attempts. Am. J. Psychiatry **130**(4): 450-454.
57. PHILIP, A. 1970. Traits, attitudes and symptoms in a group of attempted suicides. Br. J. Psychiatry **116**: 475-482.
58. KELTIKANGAS-JARVINEN, L. 1978. Personality of violent offenders and suicidal individuals. Psychiatr. Fennica: 57-63.
59. TOPOL, P. & M. REZNIKOFF. 1982. Perceived peer and family relationships, hopelessness and locus of control as factors in adolescent suicide attempts. Suicide Life-threat. Behav. **12**(3): 141-150.
60. NELSON, V. L., E. C. NIELSEN & K. T. CHECKETTS. 1977. Interpersonal attitudes of suicidal individuals. Psychol. Rep. **40**: 983-989.

61. FARBEROW, N. L. & A. G. DEVRIES. 1967. An item differentiation analysis of MMPIs of suicidal neuropsychiatric hospital patients. Psychol. Rep. **20:** 607-617.
62. YUSIN, A., R. SINAI & K. NIHIRA. 1972. Adolescents in crises: evaluation of questionnaire. Am. J. Psychiatry **129:** 574-577.
63. RUSHING, W. A. 1969. Deviance, interpersonal relations and suicide. Hum. Relat. **22**(1): 61-76.
64. MEYHRYAR, A. H., H. HEKMAT & F. KHAJAVI. 1977. Some personality correlates of contemplated suicide. Psychol. Rep. **40:** 1291-1294.
65. FLOOD, R. & C. SEAGER. 1968. A retrospective examination of psychiatric case records of patients who subsequently committed suicide. Br. J. Psychiatry **114:** 443-452.
66. ROSS, M. W., J. R. CLAYER & R. L. CAMPBELL. 1983. Parental rearing patterns and suicidal thoughts. Acta Psychiatr. Scand. **67:** 429-433.
67. WETZEL, R. D. 1975. Self-concept and suicidal intent. Psychol. Rep. **36:** 279-282.
68. FARBEROW, N. L. & T. L. MCEVOY. 1966. Suicide among patients with diagnoses of anxiety reaction or depressive reaction in general medical and surgical hospitals. J. Abnorm. Psychol. **71:** 287-299.
69. SPALT, L. & J. B. WEISBAUCH. 1972. Suicide: an epidemiological study. Dis. Nerv. Syst. **33:** 23-29.
70. KAMANO, D. K. & C. S. CRAWFORD. 1966. Self-evaluations of suicidal mental health patients. J. Clin. Psychol. **22:** 278-279.
71. WILSON, L. T., G. N. BRAUCHT, R. W. MISKIMINS & K. L. BERRY. 1971. The severe suicide attempter and self-concept. J. Clin. Psychol. **27:** 307-309.
72. NEURINGER, C. 1973. Attitude toward self in suicidal individuals. Life-threat. Behav. **4:** 96-106.
73. NEURINGER, C. 1974. Self- and other-appraisals by suicidal, psychosomatic and normal hospitalized patients. J. Consult. Clin. Psychol. **42:** 306.
74. GOLDNEY, R. D. 1981. Attempted suicide in young women: correlates of lethality. Br. J. Psychiatry **139:** 382-390.
75. BRAATEN, L. J. & C. D. DARLING. 1962. Suicidal tendencies among college students. Psychiatr. Q. **36:** 665-692.
76. EASTWOOD, M. R., A. S. HENDERSON & I. M. MONTGOMERY. 1972. Personality and parasuicide: methodological problems. Med. J. Aust. **1:** 170-175.
77. GOLDNEY, R. D. 1981. Are young women who attempt suicide hysterical? Br. J. Psychiatry **138:** 141-146.
78. FARBEROW, N. L. 1950. Personality patterns of suicidal mental hospital patients. Gen. Psychol. Monogr. **42:** 3-79.
79. PALLIS, D. J. & J. BIRTCHNELL. 1976. Personality and psychiatric history in psychiatric patients. J. Clin. Psychol. **32:** 246-253.
80. LEONARD, C. V. 1977. The MMPI as a suicide predictor. J. Consult. Clin. Psychol. **45:** 367-377.
81. ROY, A. 1978. Self-mutilation. Br. J. Med. Psychol. **51:** 201-203.
82. IRFANI, S. 1978. Personality correlates of suicidal tendency among Iranian and Turkish students. J. Psychol. **99:** 151-153.
83. COLSON, C. E. 1972. Neuroticism, extraversion and repression-sensitization in suicidal college students. Br. J. Soc. Clin. Psychol. **11:** 88-89.
84. PALLIS, D. J. & J. S. JENKINS. 1977. Extraversion, neuroticism and intent in attempted suicides. Psychol. Rep. **41:** 19-22.
85. BEDROSIAN, R. C. & A. T. BECK. 1979. Cognitive aspects of suicidal behavior. Suicide Life-threat. Behav. **9**(2): 87-96.
86. BECK, A. T. 1963. Thinking and Depression. I. Idiosyncratic content and cognitive distortions. Arch. Gen. Psychiatry. **9:** 324.
87. MINKOFF, K., E. BERGMAN, A. T. BECK & R. BECK. 1973. Hopelessness, depression and attempted suicide. Am. J. Psychiatry **130**(4): 455-459.
88. BECK, R. W., J. B. MORRIS & A. T. BECK. 1974. Cross-validation of the suicidal intent scale. Psychol. Rep. **34:** 445-446.
89. MOTTO, J. 1977. Estimation of suicide risk by the use of clinical models. Life Threat. Behav. **74:** 237-245.

90. SCHOTTE, D. E. & G. A. CLUM. 1982. Suicide ideation in a college population: a test of a model. J. Consult. Clin. Psychol. 50(5): 690-696.
91. WETZEL, R. D., T. MARGULIES, R. DAVIS & E. KARAM. 1980. Hopelessness, depression and suicide intent. J. Clin. Psychiatry 41(5): 159-160.
92. WETZEL, R. D. 1976. Hopelessness, depression and suicide intent. Arch. Gen. Psychiatry 33: 1069-1073.
93. WENZ, F. V. 1977. Subjective powerlessness, sex, and suicide potential. Psychol. Rep. 40: 927-928.
94. BOOR, M. 1976. Relationship of internal-external control and United States suicide rates, 1966-73. J. Clin. Psychol. 32(4): 795-797.
95. PATSIOKAS, A. T., G. A. CLUM & R. L. LUSCOMB. 1979. Cognitive characteristics of suicide attempters. J. Consult. Clin. Psychol. 47(3): 478-484.
96. NEURINGER, C. 1964. Rigid thinking in suicidal individuals. J. Consult. Psychol. 28: 54-58.
97. LEVENSON, M. & C. NEURINGER. 1971. Intropunitiveness in suicidal adolescents. J. Proj. Tech. Personal Assess. 34: 409-411.
98. CLOPTON, J. R. & W. C. JONES. 1975. Use of the MMPI in the prediction of suicide. J. Clin. Psychol. 31: 52-54.
99. FOSTER, L. L. 1975. MMPI correlates of suiciding patients. Newsl. Res. Ment. Health Behav. Sci. 17: 9-10.
100. RAVENSBORG, M. R. & A. FOSS. 1969. Suicide and natural death in a state hospital population: a comparison of admission complaints, MMPI profiles and social competence factors. J. Consult. Clin. Psychol. 33: 466-471.
101. ROSEN, A., W. M. HALES & W. SIMON. 1954. Classification of "suicidal" patients. J. Consult. Clin. Psychol. 18: 359-362.
102. SENDBUEHLER, J. M., R. L. KINCEL, G. NEMETH & J. OERTEL. 1979. Dimension of seriousness in attempted suicide: significance of the Mf scale in suicidal MMPI profiles. Psychol. Rep. 44: 343-361.
103. SIMON, W. & H. GILBERSTADT. 1958. Analysis of the personality structure of 26 actual suicides. J. Nerv. Ment. Dis. 127: 555-557.
104. MARKS, P. A. & W. SEEMAN. 1963. The Actuarial Description of Abnormal Personalities. Williams & Wilkins. Baltimore, Md.
105. WATSON, C. G., W. G. KLETT, C. WALTERS & P. VASSAR. 1984. Suicide and the MMPI: a cross-validation of predictors. J. Clin. Psychol. 40(1): 115-119.
106. CLOPTON, J., R. POST & J. LARDE. 1983. Identification of suicide attempters by means of MMPI profiles. J. Clin. Psychol. 39(6): 868-871.
107. KRIEGER, G. 1974. The plasma level of cortisol as a predictor of suicide. Dis. Nerv. Syst. 35: 237-240.
108. BUNNEY, W. E., J. A. FAWCETT, J. M. DAVIS & S. GIFFORD. 1969. Further evaluation of urinary 17-hydroxycorticosteroids in suicidal patients. Arch. Gen. Psychiatry 21: 138-150.
109. GOTTFRIES, C. G., L. VON KNORRING & L. ORELAND. 1980. Platelet monoamine oxydase activity in mental disorders. II. Affective psychoses and suicidal behavior. Prog. Neuropsychopharmacol. 4: 185-192.
110. ZIPORYN, T. 1983. Depression, violent suicide tied to low metabolite level. JAMA 250: 3141-3142.
111. BANKI, C. M., M. VOJNIK, Z. PAPP, et al. 1985. Cerebrospinal fluid magnesium and calcium related to amine metabolites, diagnosis and suicide attempts. Biol. Psychiatry PS20: 163-171.
112. ASBERG, M., L. TRASKMAN & P. THOREN. 1976. 5 HIAA in the cerebrospinal fluid: a biochemical suicide prediction? Arch. Gen. Psychiatry 33: 1193-1197.
113. AGREN, H. 1980. Symptom patterns in unipolar and bipolar depression correlating with monoamine metabolites in the cerebrospinal fluid: suicide. Psychiatry Res. 3: 225-236.
114. VAN PRAAG, H. 1982. Depression, suicide and metabolism of serotonin in the brain. J. Affect. Disord. 4: 275-290.
115. BROWN, G. L., M. E. EBERT, P. F. GOYER, et al. 1982. Aggression, suicide and serotonin: relationships to CSF amine metabolites. Am. J. Psychiatry 139: 741-746.

116. TRASKMAN, L., M. ASBERG, L. BERTILSSON & L. SJOSTRAND. 1981. Monoamine metabolites in cerebrospinal fluid and suicidal behavior. Arch. Gen. Psychiatry **38:** 631-636.
117. LINKOWSKI, P., J. P. VAN WETTERE, M. KERKHOFE, et al. 1984. Violent suicidal behavior and the TRH-TSH test: a clinical outcome study. Neuropsychobiol. **12:** 19-22.
118. BROWN, G. L., F. K. GOODWIN, J. C. BALLENGER, et al. 1979. Aggression in humans correlates with CSF metabolites. Psychiatry Res. **1:** 131.
119. BANK, C. M., G. MOLNAR & M. VOJNIK. 1981. CSF amine metabolites, tryptophan and clinical parameters in depression: psychopathological symptoms. J. Affect. Discord **3:** 91.
120. ORELAND, L., A. WIBERG, M. ASBERG, et al. 1981. MAO activity and monoamine metabolites in CSF in depressed and suicidal patients and in healthy controls. Psychiatry Res. **4:** 21.
121. AGREN, H. 1983. Life at risk: markers of suicidality and depression. Psychiatry Dev. **1:** 87.
122. NINAN, P. T., D. P. VAN KAMMEN, M. SCHEINEN, et al. 1984. CSF 5 HIAA in suicidal schizophrenic pateints. Am. J. Psychiatry **141:** 566-569.
123. BROWN, G. L., F. K. GOODWIN & W. E. BUNNEY. 1982. Human aggression and suicide. In Serotonin in Biological Psychiatry. T. Ho et al., Eds.: 287-307. Raven Press. New York, N.Y.
124. ROY-BYRNE, P., R. M. POST, D. R. RUBINOW, et al. 1983. CSF 5 HIAA and personal and family history of suicide in affectively ill patients: a negative study. Psychiatry Res. **10:** 263-274.
125. ASBERG, M., L. BERTILSSON & B. MARTENSSON. 1984. CSF monoamine metabolites, depression and suicide. In Frontiers in Biochemical and Pharmacological Research in Depression. G. Usdin et al., Eds.: 87-97. Raven Press. New York, N.Y.
126. LIDBERG, L., J. R. TUCK, M. ASBERG, et al. 1985. Homicide, suicide and CSF 5 HIAA. Acta Psychiatr. Scand. **71:** 230-236.
127. VAN PRAAG, H. M. & S. DE HAAN. 1980. Depression vulnerability and 5HT prophylaxis. Psychiatry Res. **3:** 75-83.
128. SEDVALL, G., B. FRYO, B. GULBERG, et al. 1980. Relationships in healthy volunteers between concentrations of monoamine metabolites in CSF and family history of psychiatric morbidity. Br. J. Psychiatry **136:** 366-374.
129. ASBERG, M., L. BERTILSSON, E. RYDIN, et al. 1981. Monoamine metabolites in CSF in relation to depressive illness, suicidal behavior and personality. In Recent Advances in Neuropharmacology. B. Angrist et al., Eds.: 257-271. Pergamon Press. New York, N.Y.
130. BIOULAC, B., M. BENEZECH, B. RENAUD, et al. 1980. Serotoninergic dysfunction in the 47 XYY syndrome. Biol. Psychiatry **15(6):** 917-923.
131. SCHLUSINGER, F., S. KETY, D. ROSENTHAL, et al. 1979. A family study of suicide. In Origins, Prevention and Treatment of Affective Disorders. M. Schou & E. Stomgren, Eds. Academic Press. New York, N.Y.
132. DOUGLAS, J. D. 1967. The Meaning of Suicide. Princeton University Press. Princeton, N.J.
133. LINEHAN, M. M. 1981. A social-behavioral analysis of suicide and parasuicide. Depression: Behavioral and Directive Intervention Strategies. In J. Clarkin & H. Glazer, Eds.: 229-294. Garland Publishing. New York, N.Y.
134. DORPAT, T. L. & H. S. RIPLEY. 1960. The relationship between attempted suicide and committed suicide. Comp. Psychiatry **1:** 349-359.
135. KREITMAN, N., A. E. PHILIP, S. GREER & C. BAGLEY. 1969. Parasuicide. Br. J. Psychiatry **115:** 746-747.
136. BECK, A. T., J. H. DAVIS, C. J. FREDERICK, et al. 1973. Classification & nomenclatures. In Suicide Prevention in the 70's. H. Resnick & B. Hawthorne, Eds.: 7-12. U.S. Government Printing Office. Washington, D.C.
137. STENGEL, E. 1964. Suicide and Attempted Suicide. Penguin. Baltimore, Md.
138. KREITMAN, N. 1981. The epidemiology of suicide and parasuicide. Crisis **2:** 1-13.
139. ADAM, K. S. 1985. Attempted suicide. Psychiatry Clin. North Am. **8(2):** 183-203.

140. LIEBOWITZ, M. R. & D. F. KLEIN. Interrelationship of hysteroid dysphoria and borderline personality disorder. Psychiatry Clin. North Am. 4(1): 67-88.
141. LORANGER, A. W., V. L. SUSMAN & J. W. OLDHAM. 1984. Personality Disorders Examination (PDE). The New York Hospital-Cornell Medical Center. New York, N.Y.
142. STANGL, D., B. PFOHL & M. ZIMMERMAN. 1985. A Structured interview for DSM III personality disorders. Arch. Gen. Psychiatry 420: 591-596.
143. SPITZER, R. & J. B. WILLIAMS. 1983. Structured Clinical Interview for DSM III Personality Disorders (SCID II). Biometrics Research. New York State Psychiatric Institute. New York, N.Y.

Suicide in Schizophrenia

CELESTE A. JOHNS,[a] MICHAEL STANLEY,[b] AND BARBARA STANLEY[b,c]

[a]*Department of Psychiatry*
Hillside Hospital
Division of Long Island Jewish Medical Center
Glen Oaks, New York 11004

[b]*Department of Psychiatry*
Columbia University College of Physicians and Surgeons
and
New York State Psychiatric Institute
722 West 168th Street
New York, New York 10032

[c]*Department of Psychology*
John Jay College of Criminal Justice
444 West 56th Street
New York, New York 10019

Suicide represents a significant cause of death in patients with schizophrenia, and the rate of suicide in schizophrenia is many times higher than that of the general population. Estimates of the percentage of schizophrenic deaths that result from suicide vary from study to study, ranging from 1% to 13%;[1-5] most evidence suggests that the higher figure is correct. Several published studies have furthermore suggested that the suicide rate among schizophrenics has been increasing since the advent of modern psychiatric treatment in the 1950s.[3,6-9] The number of schizophrenic patients who attempt suicide is even larger than the number who complete it: more than 20% of patients hospitalized for schizophrenia attempt suicide at some time.[6,10]

The identification and treatment of suicidal schizophrenics is problematic, and has led to the clinical notion that suicide in schizophrenia is an impulsive act, unpredictable, and therefore impossible to forecast and prevent. Risk factors that would help establish a subgroup of schizophrenic patients who are suicide prone have not been clearly identified. However, a review of published data does suggest potential factors that predict toward suicide. Awareness of these factors may aid the clinician in managing the treatment of this group of patients, and suggests future avenues of investigation.

DEMOGRAPHICS

The first issue to be examined is the demographic characterization of schizophrenic patients who commit suicide. When the sex of these patients is examined, most studies find that 75% to 90% of schizophrenics who kill themselves are male.[5,11-13] In fact, there is such a preponderance of males in the group of schizophrenic suicides that some investigators have questioned whether female schizophrenics are at any increased risk of suicide over the general population.[5,14]

Schizophrenics who kill themselves tend to be young; suicide usually occurs before the age of 45.[8,9,15-17] The validity of this observation is bolstered by a study of older schizophrenic patients aged 57-77, in which the suicide rate was 3%.[2] This supports the observation that younger schizophrenic patients are more prone to suicide than are older patients, but demonstrates that older schizophrenic patients still remain at an increased risk of suicide when compared to the general population.

Absolute age at time of suicide may in fact be less meaningful than the number of years that elapse between the onset of schizophrenic illness and suicide. In examining this factor, it can be demonstrated that the majority of suicides occur relatively early in the course of illness: the first 10 years appear to be the years of highest risk for suicide.[3,12,13,18] One study of schizophrenic suicide attempters which divided patients into those with a late onset of psychosis (age 33-48) and those with an earlier age of onset supports this conclusion in attempters as well as completers. The temporal occurrence of suicide attempts in the older onset group of patients in relation to the actual age of onset corresponded closely with figures for the entire sample of schizophrenic patients. The authors conclude that it is the timing of the psychosis rather than age per se that determines suicidal acts.[10] It should be noted that, while suicides that occur within 10 years of onset of an illness are "early" suicides when considered in the context of a chronic lifelong illness such as schizophrenia, these suicides are not occurring acutely or at the first episode of psychosis. Those schizophrenic patients who commit suicide have typically experienced a severe, chronic relapsing form of illness with many exacerbations and hospitalizations by the time they commit suicide.[12] However, it must be noted that not all studies support this designation of the first 10 years as being those of highest risk: Tsuang found that mortality by suicide in the Iowa 500 schizophrenics was not clustered in the early years of follow-up, but continued evenly over the four decades in which the cohort was followed.[5,19]

Few data are available on the question of whether a differential rate of suicide in schizophrenic patients occurs by race. In one recent study, while only 57% of a nonsuicidal schizophrenic control group was white, whites accounted for 90% of the suicide group.[11] An earlier study, however, found no difference in the racial proportions of suicidal and control schizophrenic patients,[20] and no further conclusions can be drawn from the literature on this topic.

Similarly, few data exist concerning other demographic variables. Schizophrenics who commit suicide are typically single and unemployed,[9,12,21] but this is also characteristic of schizophrenic patients in general. Several studies do suggest that schizophrenic patients who suicide have a higher level of education than controls,[22,23] although other studies of this variable find no difference in the two groups of patients.[10]

DIAGNOSTIC SUBTYPES

Surprisingly, few published data address the issue of relative suicide risk in diagnostic subgroups of schizophrenics. While several uncontrolled clinical reports and studies have suggested that paranoid schizophrenics are at higher risk for suicide than are other diagnostic subgroups,[16,17,24] and one study specifically observed that hebephrenic patients have a lower suicide rate than paranoids do,[14] others find no difference in the percentage of suicides by subtype.[25] This paucity of data may be due in part to the nature of suicide research, in which a relatively small sample is studied, usually retrospectively, and subtyping, when sufficient data are available, would make samples impossibly small. At present, therefore, little is known concerning the relationship between subtype of schizophrenia and suicide liability.

CLINICAL PRESENTATION

The clinical course and symptom presentation of schizophrenic patients who commit suicide is an area of particular interest. It was stated earlier that schizophrenics who commit suicide tend to do so early in the course of their illness but not immediately after the onset of illness. Roy has demonstrated that schizophrenics who commit suicide are likely to have had a chronic episodic illness with many exacerbations and remissions,[12] and this has been demonstrated to hold true for patients who attempt suicide as well.[10] Given this, a logical question arises: Do patients who commit suicide do so during periods of psychotic decompensation, or during remission?

Perhaps contrary to expectations, a large proportion of patients show clinical improvement prior to their suicidal act, or do not appear to be acutely relapsed at the time of suicide.[9,11,26-28] In all of these studies, the majority of schizophrenic suicides occur in outpatients. Strikingly, most of these occur soon after discharge from a hospital—the majority within six months of discharge. Several studies suggest that the risk of suicide is highest immediately after hospital discharge, with as many as 50% of all schizophrenic suicides occurring within the first three months.[12,29] It must be remembered, however, that in this patient population which has multiple relapses and readmissions, being "recently discharged" may be a frequent, even continuous state.

Despite one investigator's description of agitation often accompanied by hallucinations or delusions preceding schizophrenic suicide attempts,[30] most well-controlled studies of completed suicide do not support a link between intense psychotic activity and suicide in all or even most cases. Roy found that command hallucinations occurred as frequently in his control patients as in those who committed suicide.[12] Shaffer found a borderline significant tendency for his suicide group to have a lesser incidence of hallucinations than his controls;[20] Warnes reported that over twice as many controls as suicides struggled with frightening hallucinations;[13] and Breier and Astrachan demonstrated that only 3 of 20 suicidal schizophrenics clearly had psychotic exacerbations prior to their suicides and none gave evidence of having experienced command hallucinations to kill themselves.[11] This should not be interpreted to mean that suicide in schizophrenics is rarely precipitated by psychotic symptoms. A subgroup of these suicides clearly occur in the context of delusions, agitation, or hallucinations; the literature shows, however, that this does not account for the majority of schizophrenic suicides.

Depression is one of the most frequently cited correlates of suicide in all populations, including schizophrenia. It represents, however, a particularly difficult area of study, as the definition of depression in schizophrenia is not clear. While many studies observe that suicidal schizophrenics are more likely to be depressed than are control schizophrenic patients,[8,20,22,24,26,27] few have used standardized measures of depression. The one study that used rigorously defined Research Diagnostic Criteria (RDC) for depression found that 53% of suicides but only 13% of controls met criteria for a major depressive episode.[12] Thus, although established criteria for depression have not been used uniformly, the consensus in the literature is that suicidal schizophrenic patients are far more likely to be depressed than their nonsuicidal counterparts.

Some investigators have suggested that depression may not be the most appropriate feeling to investigate in schizophrenia, suggesting such alternatives as emptiness, alienation, hopelessness, or negative attitudes. Hopelessness, or negative expectations about the future, has in particular been shown to correlate with suicidal intent in a group of schizophrenic patients,[31] and Beck has recently suggested that hopelessness can be quantified and utilized as a predictor of suicide.[32] Negative attitudes toward treatment, which might be construed as correlates of hopelessness, have also been reviewed by one investigator,[33] who found that suicidal schizophrenic patients had significantly more negative attitudes toward medication and psychiatric personnel than did nonsuicidal patients.

In the literature on suicide in all patient populations, it is stressed that both threats of suicide and prior attempts are strong predictors of suicide. A large proportion of schizophrenic patients who kill themselves have made prior attempts, and the presence of prior attempts is, statistically, an important if not the most important predictor of subsequent suicide.[20] However, twice as many schizophrenic patients attempt suicide as finally complete it,[12] thus limiting the predictive power of this variable. Threats of suicide are likewise of limited usefulness: a large proportion of schizophrenic patients make such threats and do not act on them, while a significant percentage make their first suicide attempt with no prior warning.[10,30]

PSYCHOSOCIAL FACTORS

Few studies have attempted to assess psychosocial characteristics of schizophrenics in order to relate them to suicidal behavior. Examples that may be fruitful areas of investigation include premorbid personality characteristics, life stressors, and negative symptoms such as impairment of social relations.

While the premorbid personality of schizophrenic suicides has not been systematically studied, Farberow and colleagues have demonstrated that schizophrenics who commit suicide have more education and higher military rank than do controls.[23] This led them to hypothesize that patients with better premorbid functioning are more prone to suicide. This is supported in part by the data of Noreik who, in a large sample of mixed diagnosis psychotic patients, found that patients with premorbid schizoid personality had a lower frequency of suicide attempts than those with other premorbid personality types,[14] although they did find that self-assertive premorbid personalities had similarly low suicide rates. The grouping of all patients for data analysis without abstracting the schizophrenic subgroup limits the applicability of these findings to schizophrenic suicides.

Social isolation is another variable that might be expected to correlate with suicide, but the retrospective nature of most published studies makes this a particularly difficult area of investigation. One report of a mixed-diagnosis group of psychiatric patients, the majority of whom were schizophrenic, did find that suicided patients were less likely than psychiatric controls to be involved in meaningful relationships.[21] The related but not identical issue of family support has been looked at by several investigators, who have noted an association between schizophrenic suicide and a lack of family support.[8,13] However, this is contradicted by the well-controlled studies of Roy[12] and

Shaffer,[20] both of whom found no significant difference in the percent of control and suicide patients who were living alone at the time of suicide.

The presence or absence of life stressors and their relationship to suicide have likewise been studied only minimally in the schizophrenic literature. Breier and Astrachan compared schizophrenic and nonschizophrenic patients who committed suicide, and found that the schizophrenic group consisted of significantly more subjects for whom no significant life event could be ascertained prior to suicide.[11] Of particular interest in view of the prior question of social isolation, however, is the finding that the most common significant life event for those schizophrenic suicide subjects in whom such as event could be identified was being told that they could no longer return to their family's home to live.

NEUROLEPTICS

Thus far, demographic and clinical variables that might differentiate suicidal from nonsuicidal schizophrenic patients have been reviewed. The role of treatment, particularly neuroleptics, in schizophrenic suicide has also been debated and studied. Do neuroleptics, by relieving psychotic symptoms, also decrease suicidality, or do they contribute to depressive episodes and thus promote suicide, or do they have no impact? Early studies suggested that neuroleptics and in particular, depot, long-acting neuroleptics gave rise to severe depressive moods and hence facilitated suicide,[34] but this has not been substantiated by later studies. A three-year follow-up study of patients on depot and oral medications found no significant difference in the incidence of depression or suicide between the two groups.[35] In a later study of a large group of schizophrenic suicides and schizophrenic controls, similar medication histories were found with the exceptions of significantly higher doses of prolixin enanthate but not prolixin decanoate in the suicidal patients and significantly greater prescription of concurrent antidepressants in the suicide group.[36] In both instances, causality is difficult to determine, as it can be argued that patients who are the most ill and the most depressed are both more likely to receive high-dose injectable neuroleptics and antidepressants, and are at a higher risk of suicide. Equal numbers of suicides and control patients were receiving neuroleptics in a study by Cohen and associates,[8] although a significant number of suicides reportedly occurred soon after abrupt medication discontinuation in these patients. Another investigation of this issue found that suicide completers took less neuroleptics than did controls.[13] Thus, while it has not been demonstrated that neuroleptics prevent suicide, it also appears that they do not precipitate such behavior. It must be noted, however, that there has been a recent case report of two patients who attempted suicide to relieve severe akathesia.[37] While this clearly needs further investigation, it does suggest a mechanism wherein neuroleptics might provoke suicidal behavior other than that of the induction of depression which was previously suggested.

CONCLUSION

In conclusion, suicide is prevalent in the schizophrenic population across all ages and diagnostic subtypes. A review of the literature leads to a profile of the schizophrenic patient who is most likely to commit suicide: this patient is young, male, and, although still within the first 10 years of the onset of illness, he has already experienced a severe chronic illness with multiple exacerbations and remissions. He is most likely, at the time of suicide, to have been recently discharged from a hospital, and to appear clinically depressed, hopeless, or negative toward his treatment. Rapid identification of such patients and prompt intervention with neuroleptics and antidepressants as clinically indicated would be appropriate treatment for these patients. Additional support and supervision should especially be given in periods of recompensation from psychotic episodes, when discharge is usually planned. At such times the patient is most likely to gain both insight into his illness and a recognition of the severity of his disability, which could lead to feelings of depression and suicide.

REFERENCES

1. BLEULER, M. 1978. The Schizophrenic Disorders: Long-term and Family Studies. Yale University Press. New Haven, Conn.
2. CIOMPI, L. 1976. Late suicide in former mental patients. Psychiatr. Clin. 9: 59-63.
3. LINDELIUS, R. & D. W. K. KAY. 1973. Some changes in the pattern of mortality in schizophrenia in Sweden. Acta Psychiatr. Scand. 49: 315-323.
4. MILES, C. 1977. Conditions predisposing to suicide. J. Nerv. Ment. Dis. 164: 231-246.
5. TSUANG, M. T. 1978. Suicide in schizophrenics, manics, depressives, and surgical controls. Arch. Gen. Psychiatry 35: 153-155.
6. ACHTE, K. A. 1961. Der verlauf der schizophrenien und der schizophreniformen psychosen. Acta Psychiatr. Scand. (Suppl.) 155: 1-273.
7. ARIETI, S. 1974. An Interpretation of Schizophrenia. 2nd edit.: 309. Basic Books. New York, N.Y.
8. COHEN, S., C. V. LEONARD, N. L. FARBEROW & E. S. SHNEIDMAN. 1964. Tranquilizers and suicide in schizophrenic patients. Arch. Gen. Psychiatry 11: 312-321.
9. YARDEN, P. E. 1974. Observations on suicide in chronic schizophrenics. Compr. Psychiatry 15(4): 325-333.
10. PLANANSKY, K. & R. JOHNSTON. 1971. The occurrence and characteristics of suicidal preoccupation and acts in schizophrenia. Acta Psychiatr. Scand. 47: 473-483.
11. BRIER, A. & B. M. ASTRACHAN. 1984. Characterization of schizophrenic patients who commit suicide. Am. J. Psychiatry 141(2): 206-209.
12. ROY, A. 1982. Suicide in chronic schizophrenia. Br. J. Psychiatry 141: 171-177.
13. WARNES, H. 1968. Suicide in schizophrenics. Dis. Nerv. Sys. (Suppl.) 29(5): 35-40.
14. NOREIK, K. 1975. Attempted suicide and suicide in functional psychoses. Acta Psychiatr. Scand. 52: 81-106.
15. BANEN, D. M. 1954. Suicide by psychotics. J. Nerv. Ment. Dis. 120: 349-357.
16. LEVY, S. & R. H. SOUTHCOMBE. 1953. Suicide in a state hospital for the mentally ill. J. Nerv. Ment. Dis. 117: 504-514.
17. VIRKKUNEN, M. 1974. Suicides in schizophrenia and paranoid psychoses. Acta Psychiatr. Scand. (Suppl.) 250: 1-305.
18. WILKINSON, D. G. 1982. The suicide rate in schizophrenia. Br. J. Psychiatry 140: 138-141.
19. TSUANG, M. T. & R. F. WOOLSON. 1978. Excess mortality in schizophrenia and affective disorders. Arch. Gen Psychiatry 35: 1181-1185.
20. SHAFFER, J. W., S. PERLIN, C. W. SCHMIDT & J. H. STEPHENS. 1974. The prediction of suicide in schizophrenia. J. Nerv. Ment. Dis. 159(5): 349-355.
21. WILSON, G. C. 1968. Suicide in psychiatric patients who have received hospital treatment. Am. J. Psychiatry 125(6): 752-757.
22. SLETTEN, I. W., M. L. BROWN, R. C. EVENSON & H. ALTMAN. 1972. Suicide in mental hospital patients. Dis. Nerv. Sys. 33: 328-334.
23. FARBEROW, N. L., E. S. SHNEIDMAN & C. NEURINGER. 1966. Case history and hospitalization factors in suicides of neuropsychiatric hospital patients. J. Nerv. Ment. Dis. 142: 32-44.

24. ACHTE, K., A. STENBACK & H. TERAVAINEN. 1966. On suicides committed during treatment in psychiatric hospitals. Acta Psychiatr. Scand. **42:** 272-284.
25. BOLIN, R. K., R. E. WRIGHT, M. N. WILKINSON & C. K. LINDNER. 1968. Survey of suicide among patients on home leave from a mental hospital. Psychiatr. Q. **42:** 81-89.
26. OTTO, U. 1967. Suicide attempts made by psychotic children and adolescents. Acta Paediatr. Scand. **56:** 349-356.
27. SEEMAN, M. V. 1979. Management of the schizophrenic patient. Can. Med. Assoc. J. **120:** 1097-1103.
28. SHNEIDMAN, E. S., N. L. FARBEROW & C. V. LEONARD. 1962. Suicide: evaluation of treatment of suicide risk among schizophrenic patients in psychiatric hospitals. Med. Bull. Vet. Admin. **8**(11): 1-20.
29. POKORNY, A. & H. KAPLAN. 1976. Suicide following psychiatric hospitalization. J. Nerv. Ment. Dis. **162:** 119-125.
30. PLANANSKY, K. & R. JOHNSTON. 1973. Clinical setting and motivation in suicidal attempts of schizophrenics. Acta Psychiatr. Scand. **49:** 680-690.
31. MINKOFF, K., E. BERGMAN, A. T. BECK & R. BECK. 1973. Hopelessness, depression, and attempted suicide. Am. J. Psychiatry **130**(4): 455-459.
32. BECK, A. T., R. A. STEER, M. KOVACS & B. GARRISON. 1985. Hopelessness and eventual suicide: a 10-year prospective study of patients hospitalized with suicidal ideation. Am. J. Psychiatry **142**(50): 559-563.
33. VIRKKUNEN, M. 1976. Attitude to psychiatric treatment before suicide in schizophrenia and paranoid psychoses. Br. J. Psychiatry **128:** 47-49.
34. DEALARCON, R. & M. W. CARNEY. 1969. Severe depressive mood changes following slow-release intramuscular fluphenazine injection. Br. J. Psychiatry **3:** 564-567.
35. NITURAD, A. & L. NICHOLSCHI-OPROIU. 1978. Suicidal risk in the treatment of outpatient schizophrenics with long-acting neuroleptics. Aggressologie **19:** 145-148.
36. HOGAN, T. P. & A. G. AWAD. 1983. Pharmacotherapy and suicide risk in schizophrenia. Can. J. Psychiatry **28:** 277-281.
37. DRAKE, R. E. & J. EHRLICH. 1985. Suicide attempts associated with akathisia. Am. J. Psychiatry **142**(4): 499-501.

Suicide and Bipolar Disorders[a]

KAY REDFIELD JAMISON

*UCLA Affective Disorders Clinic
Department of Psychiatry
UCLA School of Medicine
Los Angeles, California 90024*

The patients, therefore, often try to starve themselves, to hang themselves, to cut their arteries; they beg that they may be burned, buried alive, driven out into the woods and there allowed to die ... One of my patients struck his neck so often on the edge of a chisel fixed on the ground that all the soft parts were cut through to the vertebrae.
Kraepelin, *Manic-Depressive Insanity*

INTRODUCTION

Suicide represents the ultimate, final and most terrible consequence of manic-depressive illness. Those having the disease are at exceptionally high risk for committing suicide, constituting by far (with unipolar depressed patients) the single highest risk group for suicide. It is difficult to overemphasize that, in manic-depressive illness, suicide is a particularly real and dangerous possibility. Despite this, little is written about the unique pharmacological and psychological issues raised by this diagnostic group. The lack of research in this area is particularly surprising given the well-documented and extensive overlap between suicide, suicide attempts, and affective disorders.

The basic premises of this paper are several. First, suicide in untreated, inadequately treated, or treatment-resistant bipolar patients is not an uncommon outcome. Second, suicide in bipolar patients is usually, but by no means always, avoidable. Finally, although relatively little scientific literature deals specifically with this problem, there is enough known from the combination of recent biological studies, a formidable psychopharmacology literature, and an extensive clinical knowledge of manic-depressive illness to justify making specific suggestions for clinical management of suicidal bipolar patients.

RATES OF SUICIDE IN MANIC-DEPRESSIVE ILLNESS

General Issues

Determination of suicide rates under any conditions is a difficult task; the ascertainment of values for a population of individuals suffering from manic-depressive

[a] This paper is based on work presented in Goodwin, F. K. & K. R. Jamison. *Manic-Depressive Illness*. Oxford University Press. New York, N.Y. (In preparation.)

TABLE 1. Rates of Suicide in Manic-Depressive Illness

Author/Year	Patient & Study Characteristics	n	Findings
Bond & Braceland[2] 1937	Manic-depressive illness[a]	204	38% of deaths due to suicide
Slater[3] 1938	Manic-depressive illness[a]	138	15% of deaths due to suidcide
Langeluddecke[4] 1941	Manic-depressive illness[a]	341	15% of deaths due to suicide
Lundquist[5] 1945	Manic-depressive illness[a]	319	14% of deaths due to suicide
Ziskind et al[6] 1945	Manic-depressive illness[a]	109	60% of deaths due to suicide
Huston & Locher[7] 1948	Manic-depressive illness[a]	80	60% of deaths due to suicide
Huston & Locher[8] 1948	Manic-depressive illness[a]	93	36% of deaths due to suicide
Schulz[9] 1949	Manic-depressive illness[a]	2004	13% of deaths due to suicide
Fremming[10] 1951	Manic-depressive illness;[a] population survey	45	50% of deaths due to suicide
Stenstedt[11] 1952	Manic-depressive illness[a]	216	14% of deaths due to suicide
Watts[12] 1956	Manic-depressive illness[a]	368	19% of deaths due to suicide
Hastings[13] 1958	Manic-depressive illness[a]	238	35% of deaths due to suicide
Astrup et al.[14] 1959	Manic-depressive illness[a]	256	17% of deaths due to suicide
Robins et al.[15] 1959	Postmortem study of consecutive suides	134	46% of suicides were manic-depressives[a]

Study	Description	N	Findings
Seager[16] 1959	Manic-depressive illness[a]	206	54% of deaths due to suicide
Helgason[17] 1964	Manic-depressive illness;[a] population survey	103	51% of deaths due to suicide
Pitts & Winokur[18] 1964	Study of causes of death in first-degree relatives with affective disorders (index relatives depressed)[a]	56	16% of deaths due to suicide
Perris & d'Elia[19] 1966	Bipolar psychoses (F = 81, M = 57)	138	23% of all deaths in combined bipolar and unipolar samples due to suicide
Bratfos & Haug[20] 1968	Manic-depressive illness[a]	207	12% of deaths due to suicide
Barraclough[21] 1972	Postmortem study of consecutive suicides	100	64% of suicides had primary affective disorders
Taschev[22] 1974	Postmortem study of bipolar patients	122	27% of deaths due to suicide
James & Chapman[23] 1975	Bipolar patients & first-degree relatives with affective illness (Pts = 46, Rels = 52)	98	46% of deaths due to suicide
Winokur & Tsuang[24] 1975	30-40 year follow-up study of mortality in schizophrenics (Sch), manics (M), depressives (D), and surgical controls (S/C)	Sch = 170 M = 76 D = 182 S/C = 109	deaths due to suicide 10.1% 8.5–11.1% 9.3–10.6% 0.0%
Tsuang[25] 1978			
Dunner et al.[26] 1976	Bipolar manic-depressives. Follow-up 1–9 years postindex hospitalization	90	9% had committed suicide (BPI, 5.9%; BPII, 18.2%)
Helgason[27] 1979	Manic-depressive psychoses[a] in cohort of all Icelanders born 1895–1897 and alive in 1910		60% of probands who committed suicide had affective disorder (majority had manic-depressive psychosis)
Weeke[28] 1979	Manic-depressive patients[a] (M = 2840; F = 5296)	8136	Suicide risk in males: 11/1000 years, in females: 5/1000 years (see also FIGURE 2)

[a] Bipolar-unipolar distinction not made.

TABLE 2. Rates of Suicide Attempts in Manic-Depressive Illness

Author/Year	Patients & Study Characteristics	n	Findings
Kraepelin[29] 1921	Manic-depressive psychoses[a]	995	14.7% of females, 20.4% of males had made serious suicide attempts
Astrup et al.[14] 1959	Manic-depressive psychoses	96	Female bipolars far more likely to attempt suicide than bipolar or unipolar males, or unipolar females
Perris & d'Elia[19] 1966	Bipolar psychoses (F = 81, M = 57)	138	26% of bipolars had attempted suicide (37.0% of females, 10.5% of males)
Winokur et al.[30] 1969	Bipolar manic-depressive illness (F = 35, M = 26)	61	24.6% of bipolars had attempted suicide (40% of females, 4% of males, $p < 0.005$)
Woodruff et al.[31] 1971	Primary affective disorders (bipolar = 19, unipolar = 139)	158	32% of bipolars, 14% of unipolars had attempted suicide
Dunner et al.[26] 1976	Bipolar manic-depressive illness	90	38% of Bipolar Is and 56% of Bipolar IIs had attempted suicide
Johnson & Hunt[32] 1979	Bipolar patients and first-degree relatives (F = 19, M = 31)	50	20% of patients had made at least one attempt (26.3% of females, 16.1% of males). 90% of attempts serious enough to warrant hospitalization
Stallone et al.[33] 1980	Bipolar manic-depressive illness	125	38% of patients had attempted suicide (48% of females, 27% of males)

[a] Bipolar-unipolar distinction not made.

illness carries with it additional problems that are idiosyncratic to the disease. First and foremost, although completed suicides may be (relatively speaking) easily determined, suicidal ideation and behaviors form a tremendously complicated, and frequently unarticulated, spectrum from ideation through threats, attempted suicide, and completed suicide. The qualitative and predictive relationships of these various manifestations of suicidality have not been well studied, certainly not in bipolar patients. Just as mania and depression form a spectrum on many different continua, so too suicidal behaviors can vary in quality, quantity, duration, frequency, manifestation, and severity. When data on suicide rates are available, complicated and highly tentative interpretations are often necessary. For example, while such data generally reflect prelithium suicide rates, and thus probably yield a more realistic picture of the untreated natural course of the illness, they also reflect less sophisticated diagnostic and sampling techniques. Changes in suicide rates are also difficult to decipher. Diagnostic criteria vary across time, and new treatments are introduced—treatments for the illness itself and for the medical consequences of attempted suicide. Diagnostic criteria are also often unclear, and until recently, bipolar and unipolar distinctions seldom were made. Of particularly critical importance, follow-up periods across studies are enormously variable, thus creating severe difficulties in determining rates due to the highly variable periods at risk. Too, most studies concern hospitalized patients, skewing the data toward the more severely ill.

Rates of Suicide

Many early researchers noted the strikingly high rate of suicide in patients with manic-depressive illness, but Guze and Robins were the first to review and document systematically the extent of suicide risk in this population.[1] They reviewed 14 follow-up studies, 2 population surveys, and 1 family study. The findings of Guze and Robins were compelling: in no study was suicide found to be *less* than 12% of all deaths in manic-depressives; in 9 of the studies 12-19% of deaths were due to suicides; and in 8 studies the suicide rate ranged from 35-60%. They concluded that there was a "tendency for the ratio of suicides to all deaths to approach an asymptote at about 15% as the deaths approached 100%."[1]

Our review of 27 studies of suicide in manic-depressive patients[2-28] does not differ significantly from that of Guze and Robins. We found a range (9-60%) of manic-depressive deaths secondary to suicide; the modal figure was in the 10-30% range. A significant number of the studies (20%) concluded that at least 50% of their manic-depressive patients had died as a result of suicide. From a different perspective, Robins *et al.* found that 46% of those individuals who committed suicide also had manic-depressive illness;[15] Barraclough estimated that 64% of the suicides in his sample had a primary affective disorder;[21] and Helgason concluded that 60% of the suicides in his sample had an affective disorder.[27]

Rates of Attempted Suicide

Studies of attempted suicides in manic-depressive illness report that between 25% and 50% of bipolar patients attempt suicide at least once.[14,18,26,29-31] Johnson and Hunt, the only investigators to specify the severity of suicide attempts, classified 90% of them as serious enough to warrant hospitalization.[32] Combining data for both sexes resulted in an attempted suicide rate ranging from 20-56%. Women, however, were far more likely than men to attempt suicide, showing both a higher minimum and maximum rate, 15% and 48% respectively. The attempted suicide rate for men ranged from 4-27%.

Sex Differences in Rates of Attempted and Completed Suicide

Women demonstrate a consistently higher rate of attempted suicide, but sex differences diminish substantially in rates for completed suicide.[11,14,19,28-33] Almost all of the studies show a pronounced narrowing of the otherwise quite wide gap between the sexes in the overall population, where attempted suicide is three times more likely in women and completed suicide is three times more likely in men.

Effect of Lithium on Suicide Rate

One of the more interesting questions in preventive medicine today is the impact of lithium on suicide rates. There are no systematic data available at this time, although it can be hoped that a well-documented answer will be possible within the next 10 years. Until then, we must rely upon preliminary speculations and clinical observations. Barraclough hypothesized that because there was a high rate of suicide in affective disorders, and because lithium was very effective in the treatment of such disorders, lithium might well be expected to decrease the suicide rate.[21] He studied the records of 100 suicides in West Sussex and Portsmouth and found that 64 could be diagnosed as primary affective disorders (11% had been treated by a psychiatrist for mania); 16 others were excluded from consideration due to complications of alcoholism or a terminal physical illness. Of the 64 suicides with primary affective disorder, 44 had a history of a previous affective illness and 21 met Coppen's criteria for recurrent affective disorder, criteria that would tend to underestimate rather than overestimate the incidence of recurrent affective illness ("a clear history of affective disorder, and at least one affective illness per year for three years, or three affective illnesses in the previous two years, or two illnesses during the previous year. The affective illnesses could be manic or depressive or both").

On the basis of these figures, Barraclough estimated that had lithium been utilized, there would have been at least a 21% reduction in suicide. Although Barraclough probably underestimated the number of individuals in the sample who had recurrent affective illness, 44 out of 64 had histories of prior episodes, he also almost certainly overestimated the hypothetical lithium response rate and the compliance rate.

Kay and Petterson, in their follow-up of a group of bipolar patients (presumably at high risk for suicide), found no suicides.[38] They concluded that this was likely to be due to a relatively short follow-up period or the prophylactic effects of lithium. Yet another contributing factor may have been the highly specialized and competent medical care available at a clinic treating only affective disorders.

Weeke hypothesized that suicide was related to whether or not individuals were taking lithium at the time of their suicide.[28] He found that 22/222 (10%) of individuals who had committed suicide were on lithium at the time of their deaths; 18/222 (8%) had been on lithium at a previous time; and 182/222 (82%) had never been on lithium. He concluded that this,

> together with the information that 40% of the suicides during the observation period occurred within the first six months after first admission ... indicates that most suicides occur before lithium therapy has been considered. There are, however, no control figures for the use of lithium in the surviving manic-depressive patients at the same point in time after the first admission.[28]

It may be the case that lithium had been considered but rejected outright by a patient who had not yet been through enough episodes to accept the reality of the illness or, for some other reason, refused to take lithium. A related and important issue is the determination of the number of episodes necessary to warrant maintenance lithium. If suicides occur relatively early in the illness but lithium is not recommended unless a "sufficient" number of episodes elapse, the risk of suicide might be unnecessarily high. Clayton[39] points out that recent studies[40,41] indicate a lower suicide risk in bipolar patients than found in earlier investigations;[1] this might be attributable to a shorter follow-up period or to the effects of lithium. Relatedly, Prien et al., in their study of the efficacy of lithium, found that the only two suicides in their samples were the two patients on placebo rather than lithium.[42]

Additional data come from the clinical observations of Dr. Ronald Fieve (Columbia University and the Foundation for Depression and Manic-Depression in New York), Dr. Hagop Akiskal (University of Tennessee), and the Affective Disorders Clinic at the University of California at Los Angeles. Four suicides were reported in these combined clinical populations where over 9000 patients had or were receiving lithium treatment. The number is strikingly lower than would be expected from the overall suicide rate in this group of patients; it is all the more impressive as the most seriously ill are routinely referred to such specialty clinics. Clearly these figures represent only gross approximations; very little systematic follow-up on suicide has been done in these, or other, specialty clinics. The variety of highly specialized pharmacological and psychological treatments available at these clinics confounds any interpretations based on lithium as the sole reason for decreased suicide rates. However, it is impressive that within these clinics, treating a highly biased sample of particularly difficult bipolar patients (including, presumably, a disproportionately high rate of lithium noncompliers and nonresponders), there should be so few suicides in so many patients. The significantly low suicide rate in such a high-risk population is only suggestive, but extremely promising.

ASSOCIATED FEATURES

Diagnostic Considerations

One of the first steps in identifying individual bipolar patients at particularly high risk for committing suicide is to determine diagnostic subgroups with increased incidence. Dunner et al. classified 90 bipolar patients on the basis of whether they had experienced manic episodes (Bipolar I) or only hypomanic ones (Bipolar II).[26] They found that those patients with histories of hypomania but no mania had higher rates of both suicide and attempted suicide. Stallone *et al.*, using the same diagnostic system, classified 125 bipolar patients and replicated the finding that the rate of attempted suicide was higher in the Bipolar II than in the Bipolar I group.[33] The two groups did not differ significantly in rates of suicidal ideation, but overall, Bipolar Is were more often in the category of "nonsuicidal" than were the Bipolar IIs. Angst applied a similar designation of bipolar subtypes to 95 patients, and found that morbid risk of suicide in the first-degree relatives of his patients followed a similar pattern, i.e., the risk was higher in the Dm group (equivalent to Bipolar II) than in the MD group (Bipolar I); this rate, in turn, was higher than that for the Md group (predominance of manic symptomatology with little or no history of depression.[43] There were no patient suicides in the Dm ($n = 43$) or Md ($n = 16$) groups, but three of the 36 (8%) MD patients had killed themselves. This is at variance with the findings of Dunner *et al.*, but the sample sizes are small and problems inherent to retrospective diagnoses confound the results. Endicott *et al.*, in a recent study, found no significant difference between Bipolar I and Bipolar II patients in lifetime rates of suicide attempts.[44]

The separation of bipolar patients into subgroups—mixed, Bipolar I, Bipolar II, MD, Dm, and so on—may increase the ability of clinical researchers to predict suicide. It should be emphasized, however, that the diagnosis of bipolar manic-depressive illness itself remains the single best predictor of suicide.

Suicide and the Course of Illness

Little is known about suicide and the course of manic-depressive illness: for example, the point in the illness at which patients are most likely to kill themselves; the number of episodes likely to have occurred and/or the amount of time elapsing from the onset of the illness (or its first treatment) to suicide; the sequence of episode types carrying with them an increased suicide risk (e.g., depression following a manic or hypomanic episode; depression occurring independently of a manic episode; transitions between depressions and manias; and so on).

We are interested here in the occurrence of suicide in manic-depressive illness as a function of the amount of elapsed time from the onset of the illness to the suicide or suicide attempt.

Guze and Robins concluded that suicide was a particular risk early in the illness;[1] Tsuang and Woolson found that increased risk for suicide in patients with manias and depressions was largely limited to the first decade following first admissions;[45] and Weeke determined that 40% of suicides occurred within the first six months after first admission and more than 50% occurred within the first year.[28] These findings have obvious implications for the importance of early recognition, accurate diagnosis, and aggressive treatment.

Johnson and Hunt looked at the latency between the onset of illness and suicide attempts in bipolar patients.[32] Their study is one of the few to be carried out on bipolar patients specifically, and with details of timing specified. All of the suicide attempts were classified as serious, and 90% of them warranted hospitalization. The authors found that 30% of the suicide attempts occurred at the onset of the illness or during the first episode of depression, and that the median time latency was 5.5 years, indicating that the risk was greatest early in the course of illness. They also noted, after combining suicide attempts with other types of suicidal behaviors, more men (42%) than women (17%) manifested suicidal behaviors at the onset of illness.

Clinical State Preceding Suicide and Attempted Suicide

Communication of Suicidal Intent

It is known that patients who commit suicide generally communicate to others that they intend to do so. Dorpat and Ripley studied the records of 114 consecutive suicides and found that 83% had indicated suicidal intent in some manner, usually quite directly.[46] Robins et al., in their study of 134 consecutive suicides—approximately 50% of whom had manic-depressive illness— found that 68% of the manic-depressives had communicated their suicidal ideas, most frequently through a direct and specific statement of their intent to commit suicide.[15] They also observed that (1) men and women did not differ significantly in the frequency of suicidal communication; (2) expression of suicidal ideas was diverse, even from individual persons; (3) communications were repeated, and expressed to a number of different persons. The authors further noted that "in the vast majority of instances the relatives and friends did not regard these communications as efforts to manipulate the environment by playing on the emotions of the hearers."[15] Of the entire sample, 86% recently had expressed suicidal ideas for the first time, or had shown a recent intensification of these ideas. Suicidality most frequently was expressed to spouses and other relatives (60% and 51% respectively), and then to friends (35%) and physicians (18%).

Clinical State

Several clinical studies have looked at the relationship of the phase of the illness to suicide; others have examined changes in behavior, symptoms, and mental state in patients prior to committing suicide; a few have looked at clinicians' evaluations of suicide risk in patients who then went on to kill themselves. Robins et al., in their study of 134 suicides, found that no one had committed suicide in the manic phase; all were depressed at the time of death.[15] The presence or absence of mixed states was not specified; by their nature they are more difficult to elicit by history or postmortem questioning of family members and friends. Winokur et al. found no suicide attempts during mania, although suicidal ideation occurred during 7% of manic episodes.[30] They did find suicidal thoughts or attempts in 13% of depressive episodes following mania and a strikingly high rate of suicide threats and attempts in mixed states (43%). Suicidality during these mixed states was reported only in women. Kotin and Goodwin also have described the coexistence of suicidal behaviors and mixed states,[47] as of course did Kraepelin in his original clinical monograph.[29] Jameison described the mixed state as the most dangerous clinical state, or phase of illness, as far as suicide risk is concerned.[48] In his study of 100 suicides (50% with manic-depressive psychosis), he discussed as particularly lethal the combination of depressive symptoms, mental alertness, and tense, apprehensive, and restless behavior.

Clinical state and behavioral clues to suicide have been looked at by several authors. Insomnia and excessive concern about problems with sleep have been noted as correlates of increased suicidality,[49–52] as has the presence of pervasive hopelessness.[53,54] Severe depression, not surprisingly, also correlates with increased lethality.[28,48,51] Weeke, for example, found that at the time of death, 58% of patients were in a constant or worsening depressive state.[28] Interestingly, fully 30% of the patients were classified as "depressive state, recovering," a finding consistent with that of Jameison and Wall who found a sudden improvement in depression in many of their patients immediately prior to suicide.[49] Keith-Spiegel and Spiegel compared clinically rated affective states of 61 patients immediately preceding their suicides with 51 control patients of comparable age and diagnosis who had not committed suicide.[55] Those who killed themselves had histories of more severe depressions as well as more suicide attempts, threats, and suicidal ideation. Of interest to the discussion here, however, is that those who committed suicide were assessed just prior to death, by their clinicians, to be calmer and in better spirits than the control group. An "unwarranted" mood shift was observed in those who killed themselves. Weeke found that evaluation of suicide risk in patients who then went on to kill themselves resulted in 13% of the patients being assessed as "seriously suicidal," 58% assessed as "suicide possible, not likely," and 28% as "suicide quite unexpected."[28]

A final and rather consistent clinical observation in a significant number of patients who kill themselves is an increase in aggressiveness, violence, impulsivity, and irritability.[28,54,56] This perturbation is of particular importance to both a theoretical understanding of manic-depressive illness and its effective clinical management.

CLINICAL MANAGEMENT OF SUICIDE

Prevention of suicide in bipolar manic-depressive patients is, of course, inextricably bound to the prevention of further affective episodes. Thus, suicide prevention is most powerfully accomplished through the effective treatment of the illness itself. Early and accurate diagnosis is critical, as suicide is more likely to occur in the initial phases of the disease.[28,32,57,58] This early suicide risk period has significant implications for clinical management, ranging from the timing of medication maintenance therapy to possible intensification of clinical help (e.g., more frequent medication visits and psychotherapy) in the first months and years of the illness. The sophisticated and aggressive identification of bipolar patients, already at high risk for suicide, is important; so too is the identification of those bipolar patients at even higher risk because of personal or family history and perturbed clinical state.

Clinical Evaluation

Those aspects of history and diagnosis that are relevant to the prediction and clinical management of suicidal behaviors in patients with manic-depressive illness include the thorough assessment of personal and family history, the patient's present psychiatric status, interpersonal assets and liabilities, and treatment history.

Patients, and whenever possible their families, should be asked in detail about any history of *suicide, suicide attempts,* or *violence* in their *first-degree relatives.* Most clinicians acknowledge the importance of a *history of attempted suicide* in the determination of current or future suicide risk; the consistency of the research findings to this effect underscores the vital necessity for acquiring such a history, especially in bipolar patients.

Certain points in the *course of an illness,* and in the course of an individual episode, carry with them an increased risk for suicide.

A thorough history should include:

- Point in the overall course of the illness at which any past suicide attempts or severe suicidal ideation took place, especially:
  - latency from onset of illness;
  - latency from onset of diagnosis and treatment.
- Point in the sequence of episodes at which attempts or ideation took place, i.e., did patient attempt suicide in a depressive episode preceding, or following, a manic episode?
- Point in the individual episode at which patient appeared to be most vulnerable to suicidality. Was it:
  - in the transistion from manic to depressive, depressive to manic, manic or depressive to euthymic state?
  - relatively soon after the beginning of a depressive episode or well into it? (The duration of past episodes, treated and untreated, is important here.)
  - during the "recovery stage" of an episode? If so, did the patient perceive he was recovering or was it the perception of his physician, family, and friends?
- Point at which the patient, on the basis of past episodes (if any), might reasonably be expected to begin recovery, and to recover.
- Point in the menstrual cycle where the combination of that point and the affective episode might place patient in special jeopardy.
- Other points where patient might be at increased risk for suicide, e.g., postpartum, annual, seasonal, diurnal, or other patterns

It is difficult, but also extremely important, to elicit from the patient an accurate *history of violent feelings, thoughts, and behaviors.*

Dr. Marie Asberg (personal communication, 1982) has summarized what she sees as the primary suicide risk factors for bipolar patients:

1. Patient's opinion (does he think he may commit suicide?).
2. Previous suicide attempt, regardless of apparent intent and severity.
3. Low cerebrospinal fluid 5-hydroxyindoleacetic acid.
4. Apparent hostility (especially if expressed indirectly).
5. Lack of social support, and even more a lack of anyone (be it spouse, child, or pet) who is dependent on the patient.
6. Delusions and/or hallucinations.

To this list of high risk variables we would add:

1. Presence of mixed states, or history of same.
2. Family history of suicide.
3. Personal and/or family history of violence.

4. Short latency from onset of illness.
5. Poor lithium response or compliance.
6. Significant personal and interpersonal liabilities.

Clinical Management

Psychological Aspects

The psychological treatment of suicidal bipolar patients is often emotionally draining, time consuming, and usually of critical importance. The suicidal manic-depressive patient has many problems which may need the psychological support of psychotherapy or general counseling of an informational nature. Ongoing professional assessment of suicide potential is vital if the patient is to be treated as an outpatient. Often a suicidal depression will follow a manic episode, compounding the biological depression with many "precipitating" or "life" events—financial and employment chaos, marital problems, legal difficulties—which can intensify the postmanic depression. These often need adjunctive management. Other psychological problems arise from the illness itself, such as frustration and hopelessness due to lithium's delayed antidepressant effect, and devastation at having been insane or severely lacking in judgment. This can result in a syndrome analogous to a traumatic neurosis and is particularly common after the first manic episode.

Several general psychotherapeutic issues arise in treating suicidal bipolar patients.

Therapeutic style. Most clinicians agree that in-depth psychotherapy is contraindicated for most suicidal patients, especially in manic-depressives.[30,58] The therapist should be willing to take more initiative with severely depressed patients than would be appropriate in other psychotherapeutic situations. Directness with suicidal patients is imperative for several reasons: the gravity of the situation, the patient's paralysis of will, and the fact that most suicidal bipolar patients are hyperalert and hypersensitive, and uncannily able to sense fear, cautiousness, and mincing of words in their therapists. Directness on the part of the clinician can help allay unnecessary anxiety and unwarranted fantasies, decrease a rather pervasive sense of negative omnipotence, and establish a basis for trust which can extend to other aspects of clinical care.

Reassurance. The liberal and intelligent use of reassurance is an integral part of the effective psychological care of suicidal manic-depressive patients. The extension of hope is not an unreasonable thing when dealing with a treatable and spontaneously remitting illness. Winokur *et al.* suggest frequent reassurance to patients and families that (a) manic-depressive illness *is* an illness; (b) it is time limited; and (c) the clinician is familiar with this kind of problem.[30]

Medical Aspects

The sophisticated use of psychopharmacology in manic-depressive patients is the single best, although by no means complete, guarantee against suicide. We repeat, and again emphasize, the overlap between good medical management (acute and prophylactic) and effective suicide prevention. We present several very general points about psychopharmacology and electroconvulsive therapy.

Medication information and monitoring. The necessity for careful monitoring of medications and assistance from family members is apparent; to this we would add the importance of a limited prescription of lethal drugs.

Importance of symptomatic relief. Certain symptoms of manic-depressive illness are more disruptive, upsetting, and dangerous than others. Prominent among them are severe sleep disorders, delusions, aggressivity, and mixed states, and they should be vigorously treated with appropriate medication.

Use of electroconvulsive therapy. Electroconvulsive therapy (ECT) has been underutilized in the treatment of suicidal bipolar patients. There are various reasons for this: obstructive legal and bureaucratic pressures which make ECT a difficult and cumbersome procedure to use; litigation by patient advocacy groups, exacerbated by the fact that bipolar patients are often litigious when hypomanic; the availability of good, but not necessarily the best, alternative treatments, such as tricyclics and monoamine oxidase inhibitors; a "bad press" from outside the medical field and within the psychiatric field; and a lack of awareness of ECT's advantages in treating acutely suicidal patients. There are several advantages: a fast antidepressant response, an immediate lessening of suicidal risk, and time "bought" so that lithium can work—if not acutely, at least prophylactically.

Sophisticated use of lithium. Several common problems occur in the use of lithium that can increase the probability of relapse and associated risk of suicide: (1) lithium is not used in those patients whom it might benefit; (2) it is not used early enough; (3) insufficient attention is paid to noncompliance; (4) insufficient attention is paid to subclinical mood swings; (5) insufficient attention is paid to seasonal patterns; (6) too short a trial; (7) insufficient treatment of lithium side effects; and (8) nonoptimal lithium levels (too low or too high).

In summary, the prevention of suicide in bipolar manic-depressive illness is very possible, if challenging, but requires a sophisticated knowledge of the biology, pharmacology, and psychology of the disease.

REFERENCES

1. GUZE, S. B. & E. ROBINS. 1970. Suicide and primary affective disorders. Br. J. Psychiatry **117:** 437-438.
2. BOND, E. D. & F. J. BRACELAND. 1937. Prognosis in mental disease. Am. J. Psychiatry **94:** 263-274.
3. SLATER, E. 1938. Zure Erbpathologie des Manische-Depressiven Irreseins: die Eltern und Kindern von Manische-Depressiven. Gesamte Neurol. Psychiatr. **163:** 1-47.
4. LANGELUDDECKE, A. 1941. Uber Lebenserwartung und Ruckfallshaufigkeit bei Manisch-Depressiven. Z. Psych. Hyg. **14:** 1.
5. LUNDQUIST, G. 1945. Prognosis and course in manic-depressive psychoses. A follow-up study of 319 first admissions. Acta Psychiatr. Neurol. Suppl. No. 35: 1-96.
6. ZISKIND, E., E. SOMERFEID-ZISKIND & L. ZISKIND. 1945. Metrazol and electric convulsive therapy of the affective psychoses. Arch. Neurol. Psychiatry **53:** 212-217.

7. HUSTON, P. E. & L. M. LOCHER. 1948. Involutional psychosis. Arch. Neurol. Psychiatry **59:** 385-394.
8. HUSTON, P. E. & L. M. LOCHER.
9. SCHULTZ, B. 1949. Sterblichkeit Endogen Geisteskranker und Ihrer Eltern. Z. Menschl. Vererg. Konstitutions Lehre **29:** 338.
10. FREMMING, K. 1951. The expectation of mental infirmity in a sample of the Danish population. *In* Occasional Papers on Eugenics, No. 7. Cassel & Co. Ltd. London, England.
11. STENSTEDT, A. 1952. A study in manic-depressive psychosis: clinical, social and genetic investigations. Acta Psychiatr. Neurol. Scand. Suppl. No. 79.
12. WATTS, C. A. H. 1956. The incidence and prognosis of medical depression. Br. Med. J. **i:** 1392-1397.
13. HASTINGS, D. W. 1958. Follow-up results in psychiatric illness. Am. J. Psychiatry **114:** 1057-1066.
14. ASTRUP, C., A. FOSSUM & R. HOLMBOE. 1959. A follow-up study of 270 patients with acute affective psychoses. Acta Psychiatr. Neurol. Scand. Suppl. No. 135.
15. ROBINS, E., S. GASSNER, J. KAYES, R. H. WILKINSON & G. E. MURPHY. 1959. The communication of suicidal intent: a study of 134 consecutive cases of successful (completed) suicide. Am. J. Psychiatry **115:** 724-733.
16. SEAGER, C. P. 1959. Controlled trial of straight and modified electroplexy. J. Ment. Sci. **105:** 1022-1028.
17. HELGASON, T. 1979. Epidemiological investigations concerning affective disorder. *In* Origin, Prevention and Treatment of Affective Disorders. M. Schou & E. Strongren, Eds. Academic Press. London, England.
18. PITTS, F. & G. WINOKUR. 1964. Affective disorders. III. Diagnostic correlates and incidence of suicide. J. Nerv. Ment. Dis. **139:** 176-181.
19. PERRIS, C. & G. D'ELIA. 1966. X. Mortality, suicide and life cycles. Acta Psychiatr. Scand. Suppl. No. 194: 172-183.
20. BRATFOS, O. & J. O. HAUG. 1968. The course of manic-depressive psychosis: a follow-up investigation of 215 patients. Acta Psychiatr. Scand. **44:** 89-112.
21. BARRACLOUGH, B. 1972. Suicide prevention, recurrent affective disorder and lithium. Br. J. Psychiatry **121:** 391-392.
22. TASCHEVE, T. 1974. The course and prognosis of depression on the basis of 652 patients deceased. *In* Classification and Prediction of Outcome of Depression. J. Angst, Ed. Symposia Medica Hoechst. F. K. Schattauer Verlag. Stuttgart, FRG.
23. JAMES, N. M. & C. J. CHAPMAN. 1975. A genetic study of bipolar affective disorder. Br. J. Psychiatry **126:** 449-456.
24. WINOKUR, G. & M. TSUANG. 1975. The Iowa 500: suicide in mania, depression and schizophrenia. Am. J. Psychiatry **132:** 650-651.
25. TSUANG, M. T. 1978. Suicide in schizophrenics, manics, depressives, and surgical controls. Arch. Gen. Psychiatry **35:** 153-155.
26. DUNNER, D. L., F. S. GERSHON & F. K. GOODWIN. 1976. Hereditary factors in severity of affective illness. Biol. Psychiatry **11:** 31-42.
27. HELGASON, T. 1964. Epidemiology of mental disorders in Iceland: a psychiatric and demographic investigation of 5395 Icelanders. Acta Psychiatr. Scand. Suppl. No. 173.
28. WEEKE, A. 1979. Causes of death in manic-depressives. *In* Origin, Prevention and Treatment of Affective Disorders. M. Schou & E. Stromgren, Eds. Academic Press. London, England.
29. KRAEPELIN, E. 1921. Manic-Depressive Insanity and Paranoia. E. & S. Livingston, Ltd. London, England.
30. WINOKUR, G., P. CLAYTON & T. REICH. 1969. Manic-Depressive Illness: 108. Mosby. St. Louis, Mo.
31. WOODRUFF, R., S. GUZE & P. CLAYTON, P. 1971. Unipolar and bipolar primary affective disorder. Br. J. Psychiatry **119:** 33-38.
32. JOHNSON, G. F. & G. HUNT. 1979. Suicide behavior in bipolar manic-depressive patients and their families. Compr. Psychiatry **20:** 159-164.
33. STALLONE, F., D. L. DUNNER, J. AHEARN & R. R. FIEVE. 1980. Statistical predictions of suicides in depressives. Compr. Psychiatry **21:** 381-387.

34. ALSTROM, C. H. 1942. Mortality in mental hospitals with special regard to tuberculosis. Acta Psychiatr. Neurol. Scand. Suppl. No. 24.
35. DAHLGREN, K. G. 1945. On Suicide and Attempted Suicide. A Psychiatric and Statistical Investigation. Lund, Sweden.
36. RINGLE, E. 1953. Der Selbstmord. Wien. Dusseldorf, FRG.
37. ETTLINGER, R. 1964. Kan vi lita pa sjalvmordsstatistiken? Statistisk Tidskr. fs. 2: 119.
38. KAY, D. W. K. & U. PETTERSON. 1977. Mortality. Acta Psychiatr. Scand. Suppl. No.
39. CLAYTON, P. J. 1981. The epidemiology of bipolar affective disorder. Compr. Psychiatry 22: 31-43.
40. AKISKAL, H. S., A. H. BITAR, V. R. PUZANTIAN, et al. 1978. The nosological status of neurotic depression: a prospective three-to-four year follow-up evaluation in the light of the primary-secondary and unipolar-bipolar dichotomies. Arch. Gen. Psychiatry 35: 756-766.
41. PETTERSON, U. 1977. Manic-depressive illness: a clinical, social and genetic study. Acta Psychiatr. Scand. Suppl. No. 269.
42. PRIEN, R. F., C. M. CAFFEY & C. J. KLETT. 1973. Prophylactic efficacy of lithium carbonate in manic-depressive illness. Arch. Gen. Psychiatry 29: 420-425.
43. ANGST, J. 1981. Course of affective disorders. In Handbook of Biological Psychiatry. H. M. van Praag, et al., Eds.: 225-242. Marcel Dekker. New York, N.Y.
44. ENDICOTT, J., J. NEE, N. ANDREASEN, P. CLAYTON, M. KELLER & W. CORYELL. 1985. Bipolar II: combine or keep separate? J. Affect. Disord. 8: 17-28.
45. TSUANG, M. T. & R. F. WOOLSON. 1977. Mortality in patients with schizophrenia, mania, depression and surgical conditions. Br. J. Psychiatry 130: 162-166.
46. DORPAT, T. L. & H. S. RIPLEY. 1960. A study of suicide in the Seattle area. Compr. Psychiatry 1: 349-359.
47. KOTIN, J. & F. K. GOODWIN. 1972. Depression during mania: clinical observations and theoretical implications. Am. J. Psychiatry 129: 679-686.
48. JAMEISON, G. R. 1936. Suicide and mental disease: a clinical analysis of one hundred cases. Arch. Neurol. Psychiatry 36: 1-12.
49. JAMEISON, G. R. & J. H. WALL. 1933. Some psychiatric aspects of suicide. Psychiatr. Q. 7: 211-229.
50. SLATER, E. & M. ROTH. 1969. Clinical Psychiatry. 3rd edit. Bailliere, Tindall & Cassell. London, England.
51. BARRACLOUGH, B., J. BUNCH, B. NELSON & P. SAINSBURY. 1974. A hundred cases of suicide: clinical aspects. Br. J. Psychiatry 125: 355-373.
52. MOTTO, J. A. 1975. The recognition and management of the suicidal patient. In The nature and Treatment of Depression. F. F. Flach & S. C. Draghi, Eds. Wiley. New York, N.Y.
53. BECK, A. T., M. KOVAC & A. WEISMAN. 1975. Hopelessness and suicidal behavior. J. Am. Med. Assoc. 234: 1146-1149.
54. REICH, P. & M. J. KELLY. 1976. Suicide attempts by hospitalized medical and surgical patients. N. Engl. J. Med. 294: 298-301.
55. KEITH-SPEIGEL, P. & D. E. SPIEGEL. 1967. Affective states of patients immediately preceding suicide. J. Psychiatr. Res. 5: 89-93.
56. MYERS, D. H. & C. D. NEAL. 1978. Suicide in psychiatric patients. Br. J. Psychiatry 133: 38-44.
57. OTTOSSON, J. 1979. The suicidal patient—can the psychiatrist prevent his suicide? In Origin, Prevention and Treatment of Affective Disorders. M. Schou & E. Stromgren, Eds. Academic Press. London, England.
58. HANKOFF, L. D. 1982. Suicide and attempted suicide. In Handbook of Affective Disorders. E. S. Paykel, Ed. Guilford Press. New York, N.Y.

Suicide and Alcoholism

RICHARD J. FRANCES, JOHN FRANKLIN, AND
DANIEL K. FLAVIN

*Department of Psychiatry
New York Hospital-Cornell University Medical College
Westchester Division
21 Bloomingdale Road
White Plains, New York 10605*

Alcohol use and alcoholism are high risk factors for suicide. A fuller appreciation of causal relationships however will await understanding the interaction of intervening variables such as personality disorders, depression, other substance abuse, unemployment, recent loss, gender, age, and physical illness due to alcohol use. Methodologic problems in measuring these relationships include ambiguity of definition or means of measuring alcohol use, abuse, or dependency; reliably delineating natural history and depth of depressive mood; and accurately classifying overt and hidden self-destructive behavior. Alcohol use has been found to be associated with 50% of suicides and to increase the risk of suicidal behavior both for alcoholic and nonalcoholic populations. Between 5% and 27% of all deaths of alcoholics are caused by suicide.[1,2] The incidence of alcoholism among persons who commit suicide ranges from 6% to 30% in different studies with approximately 20% most frequently cited.[2,3] Lifetime risk for suicide is 1% in the general population, 15% for major affective illness, and 15% for alcoholism.[3-5] It is hard to evaluate how many of the 200,000 alcohol-related deaths per year are related to possible self-destructive behavior associated with motor vehicle accidents, serious medical illness such as cirrhosis of the liver, and being the victim of homicide. Menninger has said that alcoholism itself is a chronic form of suicide.[6] We will review the research literature on alcohol use, alcoholism, and suicide in relation to (1) depression, (2) toxic effects on mood, (3) interaction with other psychopathology, (4) social and interpersonal effects, and (5) common biologic markers. We will also discuss some of the diagnostic and management problems faced by clinicians in relation to alcohol use, alcoholism, and suicide.

ALCOHOL, ALCOHOLISM, DEPRESSION, AND SUICIDE

Alcoholics with depression have been found to have an increased risk for suicide. Recent attempts to better define criteria for the diagnosis of alcoholism and depression have aided in studying their relationship. The development of clearer criteria for defining alcohol abuse, alcoholism, major affective illness, etc., in the context of a multiaxial diagnostic system is an advance. Problems remain, however, in separating primary and secondary effects, as well as defining incidence. Depending on the instruments used, methods of measuring depression in alcoholics have produced estimates from 3% to 98%.[7-9] Hesselbrock found depression in the same alcoholics 62% of the time with the Minnesota Multiphasic Personality Inventory (MMPI), 54% with the Beck Depression Inventory, and 27% with the *Diagnostic and Statistical Manual*, third edition (DSM III).[10] Similarly, Weissman and Myers reported variable associations between alcohol and depression.[11] They believe these wide discrepancies result from various methods of assessing depression. O'Sullivan suggests that the percentage of depression is overrepresented in studied alcoholics because people who seek treatment are more likely to be depressed.[12]

Determining whether alcoholism or depression is primary or secondary is a difficult task in both groups. Making a diagnosis depends on the chronological sequence of drinking and depression, evaluation of discreet episodes, and careful family history, all of which may be hard to ascertain. Andreasen found that primary and secondary depression have the same symptoms, but in primary depression the symptoms are usually more severe.[13] Weissman *et al.* in a study of alcoholics with and without secondary depression found identical demographic characteristics, antisocial problems, and family history of affective disorder.[14]

Alcoholics are most likely clinically depressed at the time of suicide.[15] Distinguishing between first- and second-degree affective states may be of predictive significance. Martin found that second-degree depression carried a greater overall mortality as contrasted with primary depression.[16]

Assessment of the presence or absence of a depressive disorder has practical implications in the care of the suicidal alcoholic patient. Silver *et al.* found a positive relationship between the depth of depression and suicidal intent in alcoholics.[17] Schuckit suggests that female alcoholics with primary depression have a better overall prognosis.[18] Males who are depressed and alcoholic are at higher risk than females for suicide.

Khuri and Akiskal suggest that suicide is a late occurrence in chronic pure alcoholism whereas it appears earlier in affective illness.[19] Nakamura *et al.* describe a subset of alcoholics whose depression has as a central feature—the recognition of helplessness in the face of an addictive disease.[20] The longevity of drinking history is important. Cadoret and Winokur found that 62% of males who had secondary depression had alcoholic histories greater than 10 years.[21] Hamm's study indicated that clinical depressions are not common in young healthy male alcoholics not seeking treatment.[22] Early recognition and treatment of affective illness when it is present may help to prevent the secondary alcoholism that ultimately increases suicidal risk.

ALCOHOL AND MOOD

High levels of depressive symptomatology in previous studies may be secondary to the toxic effects of alcohol. Several experimental studies have demonstrated detrimental effects of alcohol on mood in alcoholics. McNamee's study showed that alcoholic subjects experienced an increase rather than a decrease in anxiety and depression during intoxication.[23] Tamerin and Mendelson found the anxiety reduction model to be generally inadequate to explain the motivation for alcohol use in alcoholics.[24] Prolonged drinking in an experimental situation produced progressive depression. Stopping alcohol was associated more with physical discomfort than psychic discomfort.

Mayfield, with an experimental injection of alcohol, found that alcoholics derived the least benefit from alcohol intoxication in terms of affective improvement, while depressed patients improved dramatically in mood.[25] This evidence suggests that alcohol in alcoholics may be more palliative than euphoric. Nonalcoholic drinkers may also experience depression while drinking.[26] Translation of these types of laboratory studies to natural environments with different cues and stimuli may be problematic.

The time during which the depression is studied is important in separating out toxic effects of alcohol and postwithdrawal depression. Schuckit sees most alcoholic depression related to short-lived toxic effects of alcohol.[26] Nakamura found that of 88 patients with alcoholism, 62 had depressive symptoms at the time of entry into the study.[20] At the end of four weeks, only 4 had residual symptoms. Hatsukami and Pickens found that the rates of depressive symptoms on subjects who were abstinent up to 1, 6, and 12 months after discharge were no higher than the general population.[27] In contrast, Pottenger, in a study of 61 outpatients, found that 57% were depressed and that the depression was found to persist over a one-year follow-up.[8] In a study of 72 alcoholics with 64 months of abstinence, 15% had serious depression which began after a mean of 35 months of sobriety.[28] It can be questioned whether this is related to a prior tendency for depression.

Alcohol may potentiate other methods of suicide such as pill overdose. It may interfere with the safe execution of an ambivalently conceived suicidal gesture such as wrist slashing. Schuckit suggests that the effect of alcohol and mood in suicidal alcoholics with depression is complicated by the often concomitant drug use.[26]

Mayfield and Montgomery found a bimodal distribution of two types of suicidal attempts in alcoholics.[29] One is an "abreaction attempt" which is an abrupt suicidal attempt while intoxicated. These attempts occur more in the context of interpersonal interaction of anger, aggression, and hyperactivity. Abreaction suicidal attempts usually are not necessarily repetitive in nature. These acts may be analogous to "crimes of passion" seen in homicidal cases, where intense affective stimuli may produce a dissociated state that results in violence. The second type is the depressive syndrome of chronic intoxication. These patients make their attempts after two weeks in which they experience increasingly depressive mood, motor retardation, and withdrawal. This type is the most lethal.

One integrative model for alcohol and suicide may include (1) external and internal cues that lead to drinking, (2) the expectation of relief of tension, (3) subsequent worsening of mood, (4) amnesia for the depression when sober, (5) guilt increase and low self-esteem with further drinking that finally results in suicide.

OTHER PSYCHOPATHOLOGY, ALCOHOL, AND SUICIDE

Alcoholics with dual psychiatric diagnoses are being recognized as a common problem. Sixty to seventy percent of alcoholics have an additional DSM III disorder.[10,30] Antisocial personality can be diagnosed in approximately 25% of alcoholics and 6% of suicides.[4,16,31] Nace et al. found that 12% of patients with alcoholism had a borderline personality disorder.[32] These patients were significantly younger and more likely to have a history of suicidal attempts and to be more sensitive to affective stimuli. Generalized anxiety disorder, panic attacks, attention deficit disorder, and post-traumatic stress syndrome also may produce intense dysphoric symptoms often ineffectively self-medicated with alcohol and ultimately may end in suicide. Further studies may clarify genetic relationships between these various personality disorders, suicide, and alcoholism.

Selzer found that psychopathology plays a specific role in accidents occurring in alcoholics.[33] When intoxicated they are more likely to express underlying illness. Alcoholics on the MMPI classically have impulsivity and low frustration tolerance. Interestingly, Tsuang et al. found a similar pattern of low frustration tolerance in accident victims.[34] He reviewed several studies which indicate that 50% of accidents and suicides are alcohol related by comparing coroner reports. Combs-Orme found that one-third of fatally injured adult pedestrians had positive blood alcohol levels.[35] Fifty percent of accident victims in Tabachnick's study had used alcohol before their accident, and 50% of these were people who were impulsive in nature.[36] It is hard to measure how many of the accident victims are hidden suicides and whether more of them are so when alcohol and alcoholism are also present.

Patients with recurrent hospitalizations for medical complications of alcohol abuse such as liver cirrhosis or gastrointestinal (GI) bleeding warrant psychiatric consultation for evaluation of hidden suicidal ideation. We have recently seen a number of alcoholic homosexuals who actively seek contacts with acquired immune deficiency syndrome (AIDS) or fantasize contracting AIDS as a passive suicidal act.

SOCIAL AND INTERPERSONAL EFFECTS OF CHRONIC ALCOHOLISM ON SUICIDAL BEHAVIOR

Suicide is often secondary to rejection or the perception of loss in alcoholics. In evaluating suicidal risk, a patient's social support system may be a crucial factor. Alcoholics face problem situations that in themselves have been known to be factors in nonalcoholic suicides. Murphy reported that a majority of suicidal alcoholics experienced serious job troubles, health problems, legal and money problems prior to their attempts.[37] Interpersonal loss in alcoholics may be the best predictor of suicidal risk. Murphy, in a study of 31 consecutive alcoholic suicides, showed that one-third had experienced interpersonal loss of a close relationship within six weeks.[37] Fawcett also found poor interpersonal relations a risk factor in suicide.[38] Berglund, in a prospective study of 88 alcoholics, found that alcoholics who later attempted suicide had a higher percentage of dysphoric symptoms, and were more brittle and sensitive to others.[2] Alcohol may decrease the ego's ability to ward off primitive superego pressure. Steer found intrapunitive self-attitudes as a factor in depression of alcoholics.[39] Bascue studied 69 surviving suicidal patients with alcoholism.[40] Past attempters continued to view themselves as a suicidal risk.

Communication of dependency needs is important in alcoholics. Alcoholics do not communicate suicidal thoughts readily. Beck found in outpatient alcoholics that hopelessness is a better indicator of suicidal ideation than is the level of depression or the number of past suicide attempts.[41] In a similar study of alcoholic and nonalcoholic suicidal attemptors, hopelessness was a key determinant of suicidal attempts in both groups.[3]

Careful evaluation of family dynamics may necessitate rapid stabilization of family support, with the clinician needing to make decisions to include or exclude family members or significant others. Alcoholics frequently alienate natural support systems protective against suicide. Alcoholics often have expectations of better acceptance from others when drinking and often see themselves as more sociable during these times. Alcoholism effects the whole family system; it is important to watch for depression and suicide in family members as an alcoholic patient improves, sometimes leading to symptomatic problems in another member of the system.

Support systems can include the family, Alcoholics Anonymous, schools, work place, and professional and community organizations. Alcoholics Anonymous is recognized as an important component of treatment for most alcoholics. Early identification and referral of suicidal members may play a preventative role. Similarly, early intervention programs for alcohol abuse in schools and the work place may help to identify high risk individuals. Bressler found that 40% of suicides in the medical community are alcohol related.[42] Physician assist programs may help to prevent the high rate of suicides in physicians.

A special note needs to be made of the relationship between alcohol use, other substance use, and suicide in the adolescent population. In a recent study of 20 children and adolescents who committed suicide, Shafir *et al.* found that fully 70% of the victims suffered from drug or alcohol abuse problems.[43] A similar association has been noted by other authors.[44] Effective assessment and intervention in this age group cannot be overemphasized.

Lester found that rates of suicide in the United States by states correlate positively with alcohol consumption rates.[45] Suicide rates in countries with low per capita consumption and high alcoholism such as Sweden could be compared with cultures such as Spain and Italy with higher per capita consumption, and lower alcoholism rates. It would be interesting to study the suicidal rates of cultures like the Amish, Chinese, and Islamic where traditionally there are low rates of alcoholism.

BIOLOGICAL MARKERS

Genetic transmission has been found to be important in both alcoholics and depression.[46,47] Biological markers in psychiatry tend to be relatively nonspecific at this time. For example, the dexamethasone suppression test (DST) is thought not to be helpful in recently intoxicated patients.[48] Platelet monoamine oxidase (MAO) levels are low in alcoholism, first-degree relatives of alcoholics, bipolar affective disorder, schizophrenia, and mountain climbers and therefore may be too broad to be of much use.[49,50]

Berglund found that peptic ulcer is predictive of late depressive alcoholic suicide in 21% of alcoholics vs. 7% in controls.[2] Ten percent of suicidal patients had a history of peptic ulcer disease. This may be indicative of a biological trait or a secondary personality factor. Knop and Fischer studied 1000 patients with a history of Billroth II resection.[51] Thirteen percent of these patients committed suicide, and alcoholism was found in 50% of these patients, with the most alcohol abuse developing after the surgery. The significance of these interesting findings is open to question.

Another major area of research has focused on neurotransmitters. There is evidence that low serotonin levels may be common in depression, suicide, and alcoholism. Asberg in a study of 68 depressed patients found low 5-hydroxyindoleacetic acid (5-HIAA) levels in the cerebrospinal fluid (CSF) in patients who attempted suicide.[52] The lowest levels of 5-HIAA were in suicides by the most violent means. Conversely, postmortem studies have shown no decrease in serotonin levels in brains of depressed suicides and alcoholics.[53] Goodwin has postulated the concept of a "serotonin deficit model as an etiology for alcoholism."[54] Branchy has associated depression with low ratios of tryptophan over amino acid levels.[55] In alcoholics there may be an association between suicidality and low tryptophan levels.

Animal models are being developed for alcoholism which may be used to study alcoholism in relation to neurotransmitters and to depression. Strains of rats and mice have been produced that either will or will not drink alcohol. Studying levels of transmitter in brains of these mice before and after drinking and in males and females may give information about what may lead to genetic transmission.[56] At the current time there is no accurate biological test to determine suicidal potential in alcoholic patients.

CLINICAL CONSIDERATIONS

The clinician working with patients with alcoholism is faced with difficult diagnostic, management, and ethical problems. Intoxicated suicidal emergency room patients often present with dramatic suicidal behavior that warrants immediate intervention to protect the person from self-harm, which may include involuntary commitment. Suicidal intent frequently clears during the sobering-up process. The immediate and long-term risks, however, are hard to predict. In the context of a society that values individual liberty, increasingly laws have restricted commitment of psychiatric patients. Emergency management requires containment, and the committability of the alcoholic patient requires consideration of prior suicidal attempts, frequency of alcohol intoxication, degree of depression and other psychiatric illness, and evaluation of the patient's insight into the situation. Psychiatrists need to consider alcoholism and the likelihood of a quick return to drinking as one of the risk factors in making this decision. It is also true that in the long run, patients with alcoholism will not be able to be helped unless they become motivated for treatment and repeated hospitalization or attempts on the part of clinicians may sometimes become part of an enabling process that can include the family and health care provider. At some point, patients may face a choice between accepting help or going further downhill and the therapist may not be able to prevent further deterioration. Close cooperation between police, hospital emergency rooms, and hospitals is needed to assure immediate protection of intoxicated, depressed and suicidal patients until a more complete evaluation is possible.

Management of these patients with alcoholism and additional psychiatric diagnosis requires astute diagnostic evaluation, good general psychiatric care, and knowledge and skill of application of treatment options for both the alcoholism and additional psychiatric disorders. Alcoholics at high suicidal risk are not straightforward cases. Psychiatry must play a prominent role in the management of these patients. Treatment plans must be tailored to best suit individual needs. Many alcohol treatment facilities have inadequate psychiatric support to identify and treat patients at suicide risk. A treatment approach that emphasizes confrontation and community support may have negative effects on the severely depressed suicidal alcoholic. Alcoholics Anonymous self-help groups have been an essential component in the treatment of alcoholics. Unfortunately, some AA group members may advise against taking medication or seeking psychiatric care though it is indicated.

The psychiatrist should play a prominent role in diagnosis, triage, and treatment of these patients in a variety of treatment settings. So far the study of the right combination of treatments tailored to each patient with alcoholism needs new and useful outcome research. A recent survey of psychiatrists found that 2/3 do supportive individual work, 1/3 do insight-oriented therapy, 85% utilize AA, 50% use antabuse, and 45% frequently recommend group therapy.[57] At our present state of technology, the therapist must decide which approach or combination of approaches is best for each patient.

Clinical Case 1

A 39-year-old, homosexual man without formal psychiatric history was admitted to the Alcoholism Treatment Service with a 10-year history of alcohol dependence characterized by increased tolerance, mild withdrawal symptoms upon the cessation of use, blackouts, significant daily consumption, and psychosocial sequelae. For three years prior to admission he noted periods of free-floating anxiety as well as lability of mood not diagnostic of bipolar illness. Prominent were features of social withdrawal, lethargy, guilty ruminations, and suicidal ideation. A strong positive history of alcoholism was noted. His suicidal ideation was chronic, and after several defined failed attempts on his own life, he deliberately sought out sexual partners with acquired immune deficiency syndrome. He stated that he wished to die but found it difficult to take his own life; subsequently he engaged in multiple high risk sexual contacts exposing himself and possibly others to the illness. He saw alcohol as a means to reduce the chronic anxiety and to distance himself from his actions. Clinically the diagnosis was alcohol dependence continuous in an individual with a mixed character disorder with histrionic and narcissistic features. His Axis III diagnosis was pre-AIDS syndrome.

During the initial weeks of his sobriety, his anxiety worsened coupled with depressed mood when a immunological investigation revealed the diagnosis of AIDS. Nevertheless, he continued to reach out for help and actively participate in the rehabilitation program. Psychological testing suggested a chronic predilection toward anxiety and depressed mood, coupled with sexual identity conflicts. He was discharged six weeks after admission with an improved sense of self and appropriate follow-up recommendations.

This case illustrates that suicidal behavior can take many, often bizarre forms. For this man, his actions took on the dramatic quality of a love suicidal fantasy, upon which he acted with his multiple partners. His chronic use of alcohol facilitated use of another individual as executioner, reminiscent of the pattern Asch spoke of when he described the projection of murderous wishes in seeking out another as an executioner.[58] Murderous wishes were also evident in our patient given his awareness that he could transmit the disease to others through multiple sexual contacts and that he proceeded to continue this pattern of relationships. Chronic use of alcohol may certainly facilitate impulsive behavior in a variety of forms, in this case related to sexual contacts with AIDS victims.

For this patient, the combination of his depressed mood, social isolation, and long-term alcohol use contributed to conflicts surrounding his homosexuality and the struggle for acceptance of this aspect of his life by both the patient and his family. During the course of treatment he was better able to confront the defensive denial associated with his alcoholism, homosexuality, and the diagnosis of the pre-AIDS syndrome, and he began working through acceptance of each of these issues with improved self-esteem. It was unclear as to how much the awareness of his illness led to appeasement of self-punitive superego demands. By the end of his hospitalization, bargaining and a wish to live became more apparent with intense sadness at the awareness of having begun an irreversible process.

Clinical Case 2

A 64-year-old married retired man was admitted to the alcoholism treatment service with a 10-year history of alcohol dependence characterized by increased tolerance, withdrawal symptoms upon cessation of use, binging, and threatened job loss. A 6-month period of sobriety ended 6 months prior to admission, after he was forced to retire. One-and-a-half months before coming into the hospital he attempted suicide during an alcoholic binge by ingesting an overdose of his bronchodilator, requiring extended medical management in an intensive care unit. He had acknowledged a similar overdose attempt 20 years earlier, though he related no formal psychiatric contacts previously. Chronic marital discord was noted as was a positive family history of alcoholism and psychiatric illness. Themes of early childhood loss marked his developmental history. Sporadic attempts at outpatient management of his alcohol abuse were unsuccessful, prompting referral to our facility.

Initially he appeared to be a tearful, circumstantial, anxious, and depressed man with subjective complaints of decreased energy and libido as well as social withdrawal. He acknowledged passive suicidal ideation. Psychological testing revealed a predilection toward depressive mood and somatization without cognitive deficit. Throughout his stay he participated in individual and group psychotherapy and lectures; he was an active participant in the vocational services part of the program. Family involvement was sporadic and marked by a sense of hopelessness and counterproductive behavior encouraging the patient to disregard carefully made disposition plans. He was discharged seven weeks after admission, intending to follow through on our follow-up recommendations. He was without subjective complaints of depressed mood or suicidal ideation.

It is interesting that in this case the patient was able to maintain two-and-a-half years of sobriety when threatened with job termination, only to return to alcohol use shortly after he was forced to retire. Though forced loss may occur at any time, it is especially a cogent issue for geriatric populations and may serve as a risk factor as well as for alcohol abuse. Here it appears that his depressed mood was secondary both to situational factors and chronic alcohol use. Facilitation of impulsive behavior was most dramatically displayed by his serious suicide attempt while intoxicated, underscoring the potential interrelationship of alcoholism, suicidal gestures, and psychiatric illness.

The importance of family systems in the treatment of alcoholics cannot be overemphasized; here a sense of hopelessness on the part of the family may have contributed to a death wish toward the patient, here overtly displayed by intransigence and active attempts at undermining treatment. It is difficult to say with accuracy to what degree this may have contributed to his suicidal attempt. Efforts to contain the family psychopathology were the focus of family therapy.

CONCLUSION

In summary, alcohol, alcoholism, sadness, depression, suicide, and accidents are correlated and share common intervening variables; however, more work is needed to clearly establish causal relationships. Methodological problems have included clearly defining each category, sample selection, and accounting for demographic variables. Both alcoholism and suicide may be forms of escape from interpersonal problems and depression. Clinicians should be aware of alcoholism as a significant risk factor for suicide.

REFERENCES

1. RUSHING, W. A. 1968. Individual behavior and suicide. *In* Suicide. J. P. Gibbs, Ed.: Suicide. 96-121. Harper and Row. New York, N.Y.
2. BERGLUND, M. 1984. Suicide in alcoholism: a prospective study of 88 suicides. I. The multidimensional diagnosis at first admission. Arch. Gen. Psychiatry **41:** 888-891.
3. BECK, A. T., A. WEISSMAN & M. KOVACS. 1976. Alcoholism, hopelessness and suicidal behavior. J. Studies Alcohol **37:** 66-76.
4. MILES, C. P. 1977. Conditions predisposing to suicide: a review. J. Nerv. Ment. Dis. **164:** 231-243.
5. GUZE, S. B. & E. ROBINS. 1970. Suicide and primary affective disorders. Br. J. Psychiatry **117:** 437-483.
6. MENNINGER, K. A. 1938. Man against Himself. Harcourt Brace. New York, N.Y.
7. PETTY, F. & H. A. NASRALLAH. 1981. Secondary depression in alcoholism: implications for future research. Compr. Psychiatry. **22:** 587-595.
8. POTTENGER, M., J. MCKERNON, L. E. PATRIE, M. M. WEISSMAN, H. L. RUBEN & P. NEWBERRY. 1978. The frequency and persistence of depressive symptoms in the alcohol abuser. J. Nerv. Ment. Dis. **166:** 562-569.
9. KEELER, M. H., I. TAYLOR & W. C. MILLER. 1979. Are all recently detoxified alcoholics depressed. Am. J. Psychiatry. **136:** 586-588.
10. HESSELBROCK, M. N., V. M. HESSELBROCK, H. TENNEN, R. E. MEYER & K. L. WORKMAN. 1983. Methodological considerations in the assessment of depression in alcoholics. J. Consult. Clin. Psychol. **53:** 399-405.
11. WEISSMAN, M. M. & J. K. MYERS. 1980. Clinical depression in alcoholism. Am. J. Psychiatry **137:** 372-373.
12. O'SULLIVAN, K. O. 1984. Depression and its treatment in alcoholics. Can. J. Psychiatry **29:** 379-384.
13. ANDREASEN, N. C. & G. WINOKUR. 1979. Secondary depression: familial, clinical, and research perspectives. Am. J. Psychiatry **136:** 62-66.
14. WEISSMAN, M. M., M. POTTENGER, H. KLEBER, H. L. RUBEN, D. WILLIAMS & W. D. THOMPSON. 1977. Symptom patterns in primary and secondary depression. Arch. Gen. Psychiatry **34:** 854-862.
15. FOWLER, R. C., B. I. LISKOW, V. L. TANNA. 1980. Alcoholism, depression, and life events. J. Affect. Disord. **2:** 127-135.
16. MARTIN, R. L., R. CLONINGER, S. B. GUZE & P. J. CLAYTON. 1985. Mortality in a follow-up of 500 psychiatric outpatients. Arch. Gen. Psychiatry **42:** 47-54.
17. SILVER, M. A., M. BOHNERT, A. T. BECK & D. MARCUS. 1971. Relation of depression to attempted suicide and seriousness of intent. Arch. Gen. Psychiatry **25:** 573-576.
18. SCHUCKIT, M. A. & G. WINOKUR. 1972. A short term follow-up on women alcoholics. Dis. Nerv. Sys. **33:** 672-678.

19. KHURI, R. & H. S. AKISKAL. 1983. Suicide prevention: the necessity of treating contributory psychiatric disorders. Psychiatr. Clin. North Am. 6: 193-207.
20. NAKAMURA, M. M., J. E. OVERALL, L. E. HOLLISTER & E. RADCLIFFE. 1983. Factors affecting outcome of depressive symptom alcoholics. Alcohol. Clin. Exp. Res. 7: 188-193.
21. CADORET, R. & G. WINOKUR. 1972. Depression in alcoholism. Ann. N.Y. Acad. Sci. 233: 34-39.
22. HAMM, J., L. F. MAJOR & G. BROWN. 1979. The quantitive measurement of depression and anxiety in male alcoholics. Am. J. Psychiatry 136: 580-582.
23. MCNAMEE, H. B., N. K. MELLO & J. H. MENDELSON. 1968. Experimental analysis of drinking patterns of alcoholics: concurrent psychiatric observations. Am. J. Psychiatry 124: 1063-1069.
24. TAMERIN, J. S. & J. H. MENDELSON. 1969. The psychodynamics of chronic inebriation: observations of alcoholics during the process of drinking in an experimental group setting. Am. J. Psychiatry 125: 886-899.
25. MAYFIELD, D. & D. ALLEN. 1967. Alcohol and affect: a psychopharmacological study. Am. J. Psychiatry. 11: 1346-1351.
26. SCHUCKIT, M. 1983. Alcoholic patients with secondary depression. Am. J. Psychiatry 140: 711-714.
27. HATSUKAMI, D. & R. W. PICKENS. 1982. Post treatment depression in an alcohol and drug abuse population. Am. J. Psychiatry 139: 1563-1566.
28. BEHAR, D., G. WINOKUR & C. J. BERG. 1984. Depression in the abstinent alcoholic. Clin. Res. Rep. 141: 1105-1106.
29. MAYFIELD, D. G. & D. MONTGOMERY. 1972. Alcoholism, alcohol intoxication, and suicide attempts. Arch. Gen. Psychiatry 27: 349-353.
30. POWELL, B. J., E. C. PENICK, E. OTMMER, S. F. BINGHAM & A. S. RICE. 1982. Prevalence of additional psychiatric syndromes among male alcoholics. J. Clin. Psychiatry 43: 404-407.
31. CADORET, R., E. TROUGHTON & R. WIDMER. 1984. Clinical differences between antisocial and primary alcoholics. Compr. Psychiatry 25: 1-8.
32. NACE, E. P., J. J. SAXON & N. SHORE. 1983. A comparison of borderline and non-borderline alcoholic patients. Arch. Gen. Psychiatry 40: 54-56.
33. SELZER, M. L., C. E. PAYNE, F. H. WESTERVELT, et al. 1967. Automobile accidents as an expression of psychopathology in an alcoholic population. Q. J. Stud. Alcohol. 28: 505-516.
34. TSUANG, M. T., M. BOOR & J. A. FLEMING. 1985. Psychiatric aspects of traffic accidents. Am. J. Psychiatry 142: 538-546.
35. COMBS-ORME, T., J. R. TAYLOR, E. B. SCOTT & S. J. HOLMES. 1983. Violent deaths among alcoholics: a descriptive study. J. Stud. Alcohol. 44: 938-949.
36. TABACHNICK, N., R. E. LITMAN, M. OSMAN, W. L. JONES, J. COHN, A. KASPER & J. MOFFAT. 1966. Comparative psychiatric study of accidental and suicidal death. 14: 60-68.
37. MURPHY, G. E., J. W. ARMSTRONG, S. L. HERMELE, J. R. FISCHER & W. W. CLENDININ. 1979. Suicide and alcoholism. 36: 65-69.
38. FAWCETT, J., M. LEFF & W. E. BUNNEY. 1969. Suicide. Arch. Gen. Psychiatry 21: 129-137.
39. STEER, R. A., M. G. MCELROY & A. T. BECK. 1982. Structure of depression in alcoholic men: a partial replication. Psychol. Rep. 50: 723-728.
40. BASCUE, I. O. & L. EPSTEIN. 1980. Suicide attitudes and experiences of hospitalized alcoholics. Psychol. Rep. 47: 1233-1234.
41. BECK, A. T., R. A. STEER & M. G. MCELROY. 1982. Relationships of hopelessness, depression and previous suicide attempts to suicidal ideation in alcoholics. J. Stud. Alcohol. 43: 1042-1045.
42. BRESSLER, B. 1976. Suicide and drug abuse in the medical community. Suicide Life-threat. Behav. 3: 169-178.
43. SHAFIR, M., S. CARRIGAN, J. R. WHITTINGHILL & Z. A. DERRICK. 1985. Psychological autopsy of completed suicide in children and adolescents. Am. J. Psychiatry 142: 1061-1067.
44. RYDELIUS, P. A. 1984. Deaths among child and adolescent psychiatric patients. Acta Psychiatr. Scand. 70: 119-126.

45. LESTER, D. 1980. Alcohol and suicide and homicide. J. Stud. Alcohol. 141: 1220-1223.
46. MERIKANGAS, K. R., J. F. LECKMAN, B. A. PRUSOFF, D. L. PAULS & M. M. WEISSMAN. 1985. Familial transmission of depression and alcoholism. Arch. Gen. Psychiatry. 42: 367-372.
47. GOODWIN, D. W., F. SCHULSINGER, J. KNOP, S. MEDNICK & S. B. GUZE. 1977. Alcoholism and depression in adopted-out daughters. Arch. Gen. Psychiatry. 34: 751-755.
48. RAVI, S. D., W. DORUS, Y. NAMPARK, M. C. COLLINS, R. W. REID & G. F. BORGE. 1984. The DST test and depressive symptoms in early and late withdrawal from alcohol. Am. J. Psychiatry 141: 1445-1448.
49. BELMAKER, R. H., H. S. BRACHA & R. B. EBSTEIN. 1980. Platelet monoamine oxidase in affective illness and alcoholism. Schizophrenia Bull. 6: 130-133.
50. ALEXOPOULOS, G. S., K. W. LIEBERMAN, R. C. YOUNG, et al. 1984. Platelet MAO activity and age at onset of depression in elderly depressed women. Am. J. Psychiatry 141: 1276-1278.
51. KNOP, J. & A. FISCHER. 1981. Duodenal ulcer: suicide, psychopathology and alcoholism. Psychiatr. Scand. 63: 346-355.
52. ASBERG, M., L. TRASKMAN & P. THOREN. 1976. 5-HIAA in the cerebrospinal fluid. A biochemical suicide predictor. Arch. Gen. Psychiatry 33: 1193-1197.
53. COCHRAN, E., E. ROBINS & S. GROTE. 1976. Regional serotonin levels in brain: suicides vs. controls. Biol. Psychiatry 11: 283-294.
54. GOODWIN, W. D. 1985. Alcoholism and genetics. Arch. Gen. Psychiatry 42: 171-174.
55. BRANCHEY, L., M. BRANCHEY, S. SHAW & C. S. LIEBER. 1984. Depression, suicide, and aggression in alcoholics and their relationship to plasma amino acids. Psychiatry Res. 12: 219-226.
56. Report of the 1983 Research Planning Panel: National Institute on Alcohol Abuse and Alcoholism. U.S. Government Printing Office. Washington, D.C.
57. MILLER, S. I. & R. J. FRANCES. 1986. Psychiatrists and the treatment of addictions, perceptions and practices. Am. J. Alcohol Drug Abuse. 12(3): 187-199.
58. ASCH, S. S. 1980. Suicide and the hidden executioner. Int. Rev. Psychoanal. 7: 51-60.

Generalizable Treatment Strategies for Suicidal Behavior

SUSAN J. BLUMENTHAL[a] AND DAVID J. KUPFER[b]

[a]*Suicide Research Unit*
Center for Studies in Affective Disorders
National Institute of Mental Health
Parklawn Building, Room 10C27
5600 Fishers Lane
Rockville, Maryland 20857

[b]*Department of Psychiatry*
University of Pittsburgh School of Medicine
Western Psychiatric Institute and Clinic
3811 O'Hara Street
Pittsburgh, Pennsylvania 15213

INTRODUCTION

The parts of this volume on the psychobiology of suicidal behavior have focused on suicidal behavior, its description, and various risk factors, as well as possible neurochemical and genetic correlates of suicide. This paper summarizes the section on suicidal behavior associated with major psychiatric syndromes and emphasizes the need for improved methodology for more precise clinical reporting of suicide attempts and completions; and argues that improved data will aid in developing more information about risk factors. Such efforts will help maximize our ability to detect high-risk individuals and devise better treatment strategies for suicidal behavior.

One of the problems in reaching any level of consensus on appropriate interventions for suicidal behavior has been a certain degree of neglect to the classification of suicidal behaviors and the ways in which intervention and management should differ for each behavior group. As suggested by Beck and colleagues,[1,2] individuals who are suicidal can be divided into those with suicidal ideation, suicide attempters, and those who complete suicide. Although these groups do not represent a necessary continuum, it has clearly been shown that there is overlap between these two groups and that one risk factor for completed suicide is a previous suicide attempt. Approximately one-third of attempters will ultimately end their life by suicide.[3] Attempters should be further separated into a group who did not intend for the gesture to be lethal and a group of "accidental survivors" (attempters with highest lethality). In all cases, factors of intent, method, and degree of lethality need to be included when suicidal behavior is reported.

Before commenting on generalizable treatment strategies for suicidal behavior, it is useful to reemphasize several of the risk factors that have been discussed in this volume. As shown in TABLE 1, the most important risk factors for completed suicide do not point to a homogeneous population at risk, nor does a listing of these factors

TABLE 1. People at Highest Risk for Suicide

- White males
- Aged 24-35 or over 50
- Recently widowed, separated, or divorced
- History of suicide attempts
- History of psychiatric disorder, in particular depression, alcoholism, or schizophrenia
- Low CSF 5-HIAA or serotonergic deficiency
- Family history of suicidal behavior and/or affective disorders

imply that we can simply add up the various risk factors to determine a risk and lethality score for each individual. Previous research designed to accomplish this task has been largely unrewarding.[2,4,5]

A matrix or multiaxial approach may be the most appropriate model for considering the major risk factors for clinical investigation.[6] Several alternative strategies can be used to integrate current research data into this model. One model for suicide completion, akin to the "final common pathway" suggested for the pathogenesis of other psychiatric illnesses such as depression, would enable even one factor to contribute almost totally to a completed suicide, i.e., loss of job leads to suicide or suffering from depression results in suicide. However, we believe that an overlapping model with several domains, which can be visualized as a series of interlocking Venn diagrams, is a more compelling alternative (FIGURE 1). With this latter model, the task of research would be to develop weights for each of the major component factors. For example, in this model, loss of job might be the final precipitating humiliating experience that triggers a depressive episode in an individual with inadequate social supports and with a family history of affective disorder. The interaction of these risk factor domains increases the individual's vulnerability (risk) for suicide. Or, for example, what distinguishes the 15% of people who suffer from an affective disorder and end their lives by suicide while the other 85% do not? We would hypothesize, using this matrix model, that the subgroup of affective disorder patients who commit suicide have a greater overlap of risk factors such as increased hopelessness, a higher level of impulsivity, decreased social supports, recent humiliating life experience, and an increased family history of affective disorder or suicidal behavior.

Regardless of which model one considers, strategies that attempt to understand and intervene with suicidal behavior should include five different components.[6] The first two factors involve *subgrouping the various risk factors according to psychiatric diagnosis and personality style.* It has been suggested that behaviors relating to suicide, such as aggression, impulsivity, and hopelessness, are important in and of themselves in characterizing suicide[7,8] since they may represent "personality traits" that cut across diagnostic groupings. A third factor is concerned with *psychosocial risk factors such as social supports, life events, and chronic medical illness.* Early loss, increased negative life events, and decreased social supports increase risk for suicide.[9-17] A fourth area is the *identification of both genetic and family factors.* It has already been suggested that the genetics of suicide may be independent of the genetics and family history of a specific psychiatric disorder such as affective disorder.[18,19] The fifth factor in the matrix relates to the *neurochemical and biochemical factors,* currently under active investigation, that may identify either an abnormality or a vulnerability state.[20-45] Each of these five components and their individual "weights" must be addressed as they relate to the other four before we can approach treatment strategies. Individual differences might also be explained by the contribution of the various weights of each risk factor. Naturally, we should assume that different constellations of risk factors will be present for suicide attempters than for suicide completers. While a certain level of overlap is likely to be present, this paper will pay particular attention to those risk factors relating to suicide completers.

PSYCHIATRIC DIAGNOSIS AND PERSONALITY FACTORS

With respect to the issue of specific psychiatric diagnoses in association with increased risk for suicide, the studies presented at this conference relating to depressive disorders, bipolar affective disorders, personality disorders, schizophrenia, and substance abuse[8,46-49] have not been able to easily identify common factors for suicide risk across diagnostic categories. This may, in part, be due to the lack of standardized diagnostic criteria and systematized data collection procedures across studies. This dearth of consistently collected data reinforces the need for collaborative research efforts on the relationship of different psychiatric diagnoses to suicide in order to address this issue systematically and to identify criteria that influence suicidal behavior within each diagnosis [i.e., some *Diagnostic and Statistical Manual,* third edition (DSM III) disorders include suicidal behavior or ideation in their criteria such as major depressive episode and histrionic and borderline personality disorder]. Existing evidence implicates depressive disorders as bearing a major relationship to the overall suicide rate at any age.[10,11,46,50-56] In addition, impulsive, aggressive behaviors such as conduct disorders in youth and antisocial personality disorder and borderline personality disorder in adults have been associated with suicide.[35,36,57-60] This point is discussed further in the treatment section.

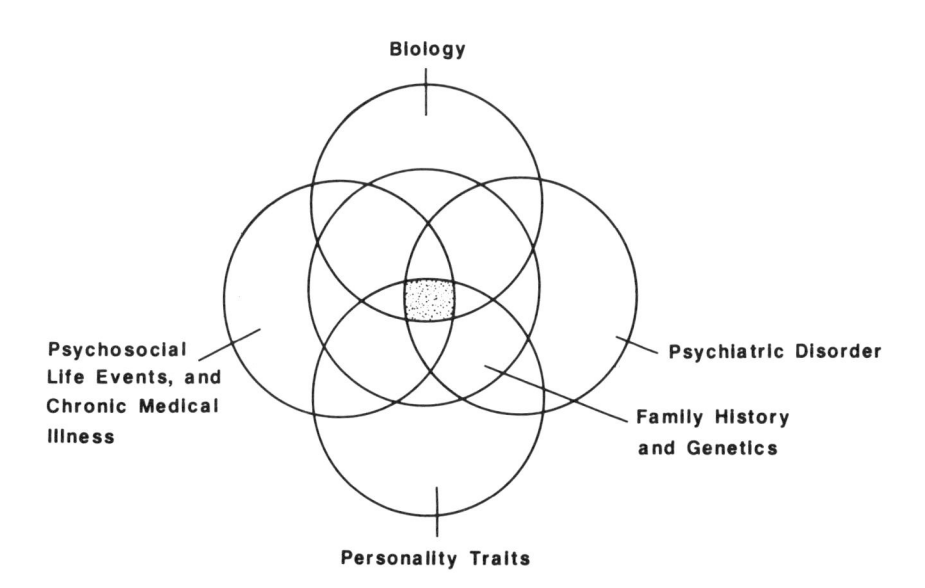

FIGURE 1. Overlap model (five domains).

With respect to diagnosis, it should be pointed out that DSM III Axis I diagnoses are not sufficient to complete the diagnostic task. Axis II diagnoses are particularly important when examining comorbidity issues relevant to suicidal behavior. However, suicide research and reporting methodology should include more than Axis I and II disorders; it must document personality style and traits (i.e., aggressivity, impulsivity, hopelessness) as well. Finally, we also need to understand that Axis III is important in assessing the patient since concurrent medical diseases have been identified as a risk factor for suicide at any age.[11,50,54,55] Terminal illnesses across the life cycle and multiple medical problems in the elderly are especially important to note. Unfortunately, while the reviews in this volume on psychiatric diagnosis[46-49] address specific Axis I diagnoses, they do not deal explicitly with concurrent psychiatric diagnoses (comorbidity) including substance abuse and personality disorders. For instance, Beck found in his study of 472 attempters that 18 of the 25 patients who eventually killed themselves had a history of alcoholism.[7,61] Similarly, in a psychological autopsy study of adolescent suicide, 70% of the victims had a history of drug or alcohol abuse.[60] How these comorbidity issues of Axis I, II, and III interrelate are important for increasing the clinician's ability to identify persons at highest risk for suicide.

Most studies that examine the relationship of psychiatric diagnosis to suicide have been performed in adult populations. If we sum the findings from the major large studies of suicide in the adult literature,[11,50,54,55,62] we find that over 90% of the people who end their lives by suicide are suffering from a psychiatric disorder; less than 10% of people who kill themselves have no documentable psychiatric illness. Of the 90% with a psychiatric disorder, 60-80% suffer from a major affective illness. However, since three of the four investigations that have reached this conclusion were retrospective studies, their methodology may limit the generalizability of the findings. However, Robins reexamined the initial sample of his elegant study, applied Research Diagnostic Criteria (RDC) to the diagnoses made in the 1950s investigation, and concluded that the initial diagnoses of major affective disorder remained unchanged.[54,55] As best we can tell from available data, 15% of people with an affective disorder will end their life by suicide;[56] 15% of people with schizophrenia will do the same.[49,63,64] Affective disorders followed by alcoholism are the major psychiatric diagnoses associated with suicide.[50,54,55,62] Therefore, the early detection and treatment of depression and alcoholism, in particular, represent major prevention strategies for completed suicide.[10] Not only is appropriate psychopharmacologic treatment critical when necessary, but psychotherapeutic intervention aimed at decreasing hopelessness and altering the cognitive distortions that may accompany depression is essential to effective treatment. So, too, are strengthening social supports and promoting better interpersonal relationships for these individuals.

In youth suicide, the diagnostic picture is less clear. Only a few studies on completed suicide have been conducted in this age group.[57-60] A study by Shafii *et al.* suggests that 70% of youngsters who end their lives by suicide have associated substance abuse, 70% have a history of antisocial behaviors, 65% have "inhibited" personality traits, and 50% have made a previous suicide attempt.[60] Suicidal behavior of parents, relatives, and friends, along with a parental history of emotional problems and abuse, were also significant variables. A study by Shaffer suggests several personality traits of youngsters who end their lives by suicide, including those who tend to be withdrawn, perfectionistic, impulsive, or aloof.[57] Preliminary data from an ongoing large psychological autopsy study of adolescents[59] suggest that at least a third of the young people in the study who ended their lives by suicide had an associated conduct disorder and that one-quarter of the sample population were suffering from a depressive disorder. Approximately 50% of these young people had a family history of suicidal behavior. Suicide attempts in this age group have likewise been linked to depressive symptoms.[52]

The comorbidity of antisocial and depressive symptoms appears to be a particularly lethal combination in youth.[51,59] It is likely that this combination of aggressivity, impulsivity, and depressive symptomatology represents a major contribution to risk for suicide across the life cycle.[10]

Antisocial and borderline personality disorders have been described as being particularly associated with suicidal behavior in adults.[8] This is true for adolescent suicide as well, where conduct disorders and borderline personality disorder are highly associated with suicide.[57–60,65] Secondly, personality traits and their severity (i.e., degree of impulsivity or degree of hopelessness) may not only be correlates of suicide but may also be related to a biological abnormality (i.e., serotonergic deficiency). Moreover, in the presence of certain environmental stressors or triggers, specific personality traits may make some individuals more vulnerable to suicide. However, in order to separate out these behavioral dimensions related to a specific psychiatric diagnosis from those core personality/behavioral components, attention must be devoted to the reliability and validity of clinical and self-ratings which measure behavioral dimensions independent of diagnosis. How well can aggressive behavior be separated from impulsive behavior? How well can hopelessness be delineated from the symptom constellation in a depression? Does change on a hopelessness scale toward hopefulness relate to risk reduction, or is it a general property of reduced symptom severity? Finally, behavioral dimensions need to be measured over time to ascertain the effectiveness of a given treatment strategy. Most studies of suicidality and personality have measured personality at the time or near time of the suicide attempt so that the subjects in these studies are troubled, agitated, or depressed at the time of the assessment, decreasing the validity of personality measurement. In summary, attention must be given to more accurate detection and documentation of DSM III Axis I, II, and III diagnosis as well as personality traits. In this way, the important issues of comorbidity as increasing suicidal risk may be adequately addressed.

PSYCHOSOCIAL FACTORS, LIFE EVENTS, AND CHRONIC MEDICAL ILLNESS

The advent of more sophisticated diagnostic instruments has improved the reliability of psychiatric diagnoses and has provided more precise documentation of family history of suicidal behavior and psychiatric disorders. However, as we are increasing our knowledge about diagnosis, family history, and biological factors associated with suicidal behavior, it is critical to continue to consider the important role of the psychosocial environment and specific life events in refining our understanding of suicidal behavior. Recent bereavement, separation or divorce, early loss, decreased social supports, loss of job, and significant humiliation are all potentially important factors that can affect the "lethality" of a suicide attempt.[9,10] In a similar manner, the presence of a chronic medical illness can have a devastating impact on a person's ability to deal with stress. In particular, diseases with chronic debilitating courses are frequent "stimuli" to suicidal behavior.[9–11,13,15,50,54,55,58,66] Individuals suffering from psychiatric illnesses may be more vulnerable to environmental stressors or to a loss in social support systems. Conversely, recent losses, a humiliating life event, or recent exposure to suicide may precipitate psychiatric vulnerability. In these ways, psychosocial factors may be particularly important as one of the contributing weights in the matrix model that explain individual differences across high-risk groups.

FAMILY HISTORY/GENETICS

A family history of suicide is a significant risk factor for suicide. Explanations for this association include identification with and imitation of a family member who has committed suicide, transmission of genetic factors for suicide, and transmission of genetic factors for psychiatric disorders such as affective disorders.[10,19,67-70]

A number of clinical studies report a higher incidence of suicidal behavior among relatives of persons with suicidal behavior. Further, a study of psychiatric inpatients revealed that (1) half of the persons with a family history of suicide had attempted suicide themselves, and (2) more than half of all patients with a family history of suicide had a primary diagnosis of affective disorder.[17,71] A study of the Amish, a religious group with a 100-year history of nonviolence, no alcohol or drug abuse, a high degree of social cohesion, no divorce or family dissolution, and a philosophy of suicide as the ultimate sin, has demonstrated an unexpected finding: suicides do occur among this group. Twenty-six suicides have occurred among the Amish of southeastern Pennsylvania between 1880 and 1980. Twenty-four of the 26 individuals who committed suicide were diagnosed with a major affective disorder, and the suicides occurred in four primary pedigrees. This research suggests possible genetic factors in both the transmission of affective disorders and suicide.[72] Another study of suicides in the general population found that six of 100 suicide completers also had a parent who committed suicide. This rate was 88 times higher than predicted.[73]

Investigations have suggested a high concordance rate for suicide in identical twins.[19,74,75] While 10 sets of identical twin pairs who have both committed suicide have been reported in the literature, there has been no report in which both fraternal twins have committed suicide.[76] In another study, a greater incidence of suicide was found in the relatives of psychiatric patients who committed suicide than in the relatives of the control group in this study.[69] In the well-known Copenhagen adoption study, a greater incidence of suicide was found in the biological relatives of adoptees who committed suicide than in their adoptive relatives (as compared to adoptee controls).[18,68] Of 57 adoptees who committed suicide, there were 269 biological relatives, of whom 12 committed suicide (4.5%) and no adopting relatives who committed suicide. By comparison, only 2 of the 269 biological relatives of 57 matched control adoptees (0.7%) and none of 150 adopting relatives committed suicide. In another adoption study of suicide in persons with known depressive illness and matched controls, these same investigators again found a greater incidence of suicide among the biological relatives of the probands (3.7%). Of 407 biological relatives of probands, 15 (0.5%) committed suicide; only 1 of 187 adopting relatives committed suicide.

These studies suggest that we may be able to separate out the contribution of a family history of suicide and a family history of affective disorder to isolate high-risk groups for both research and clinical purposes. Issues of family history and genetic factors are complicated not only by concordance for psychiatric diagnoses in families but also by the environment in terms of identification and imitation of suicidal behavior by family members over long periods of time.

BIOLOGICAL FACTORS

Recent biochemical investigations of suicidal behavior have shown that suicide victims and violent suicide attempters have alterations in the function of a brain neurotransmitter, serotonin. Furthermore, reduced central serotonergic activity is associated with suicidal behavior, not only when there is a diagnosis of unipolar depressive disorder, but also an association with a range of other psychiatric disorders. This research has found a common biochemical association between aggression, impulsivity, and reduced serotonergic function. Some studies suggest that the findings of decreased serotonin and violent suicide attempts may increase the risk of completed suicide 10-fold at one-year follow-up.[30] Arsonists, for example, show a very high incidence of violent suicide attempts.[23,38] But even with the promising 5-hydroxyindoleactic acid (5-HIAA) data, we must urge caution. While low 5-HIAA levels are associated with violent suicide attempts and completions, low 5-HIAA levels are also found in patients with diverse psychiatric illnesses and in groups of normal controls.[36] An increased incidence of depressive illness has been found in the relatives of both patients[45] and normals[42] with decreased cerebrospinal fluid (CSF) 5-HIAA. These neurochemical levels appear to be consistent over time.[29] While the serotonergic data represent the most compelling current evidence for a biological correlate of suicidal behavior, other biologic factors (neuroendocrine, neurophysiological) are actively being investigated. It is expected that information derived from such studies will strengthen the data base on biology as playing a key role in assessing relative weights in the matrix model (e.g., links with personality factors).

TREATMENT STRATEGIES

As mentioned in the Introduction, we felt that a more pointed discussion of treatment strategies for suicidal behavior is possible if an integration of the key risk factors is first made explicit. Therefore, we have presented a matrix approach which involves five components: psychiatric diagnosis; personality factors; psychosocial factors, life events and chronic medical illness; family history/genetics; and biological factors. These components taken together with varying individual weights point to the expectation that we may be able to identify and tag high-risk individuals. Our treatment strategies might, therefore, reflect selective types of intervention depending on the specific and additive contributions of the five risk factor domains. As shown in TABLE 2, a variety of treatment strategies and interventions to prevent suicide have been attempted for suicidal ideation and behavior over the last several decades. In understanding these interventions, we have to realize that some have been geared to dealing with suicide ideators or attempters while others have been targeted to those at high risk for completed suicide. This is especially true of such aggressive outreach programs as the suicide prevention centers that were started in the 1960s. Careful evaluation of these centers and programs has, at best, yielded equivocal results, in part due to the methodological problems plaguing these studies.[77–81]

On the other hand, strategies geared to the treatment of specific psychiatric syndromes may be more likely to prevent suicidal behavior. Examples of this approach would be the use of lithium carbonate early in the course of bipolar affective disorder to prevent future manic episodes or the continued use of neuroleptics in the treatment of schizophrenia. It has been demonstrated that suicide risk is probably high in the early years of illness for both bipolar disorder and schizophrenia.[48,49] Therefore, aggressive treatment during this period might indeed reduce the risk of completed suicide.

The first overall treatment strategy in the matrix model approach would be to treat the associated psychiatric condition, but at the same time "red flag" the high-risk patient and especially pay particular attention to environmental stresses and

TABLE 2. Treatment of High-Risk Groups

- Identification of high-risk groups
- Treatment
  - Crisis intervention
  - Early detection and treatment of psychiatric disorder
    Psychotherapy (behavioral, cognitive, interpersonal psychodynamic, family)
    Pharmacotherapy
  - Environmental interventions

psychosocial supports. Psychotherapeutic and psychosocial treatment modalities used in conjunction with pharmacotherapy may increase the compliance rate in the treatment of these high-risk individuals who are most prone to commit suicide. In addition, psychotherapeutic treatment may improve interpersonal relationships and reduce the cognitive distortions that frequently occur with depression and suicidal thinking. Since suicidal patients are difficult to sustain in treatment and are noncompliant, the use of clinic facilities, clinic support, or network systems to ensure that such individuals continue in treatment is an important strategy. In addition, such programs provide a type of social support where patients, families, and clinicians form a treatment alliance which provides education, treatment, and family support over long periods of time. For example, studies of affective disorder clinic facilities in New York, Tennessee, and California confirm this phenomenon.[48] These surveys suggest that the rates of suicide in these patient groups are lower than would be expected and that such system approaches have a "protective role."

While most attention has been given to treatment of the specific illness associated with suicidal behavior, more recently a number of approaches have attempted to ameliorate the conditions that theoretically would predispose an individual to suicidal behavior[82] (for example, the reduction of suicidal ideation by behavioral treatments). This would be the second treatment strategy in the matrix model approach. An evaluation of such studies suggests that the number of suicide attempts has not been affected appreciably by these treatments but that these strategies may alter suicidal plans and improve social adjustment.[83] In the future, designing modalities to treat specific suicidal behaviors, apart from psychiatric syndromes, may represent an important approach. For example, several studies have used behavioral/cognitive techniques, which have demonstrated a reduction of hopelessness.[7,84] In a similar way, it would be useful to design treatment modalities that might specifically address how to reduce aggressive, impulsive behavior, and other high-risk personality traits. Such an approach using behavioral treatments might be efficacious, since efforts to treat antisocial behavior in groups of prisoners have shown success.[82]

A third area for action is the promise of new psychopharmacologic modalities. Several studies suggest that the correction of "serotonergic deficiencies" (that is, using specific drugs with serotonergic reuptake blockade properties)[21] may more specifically affect suicidal behavior. In addition, there may be a suicidal subgroup of depressed patients in whom these medications may be most beneficial. However, it is still unclear whether the depressive phenomena are indeed related to serotonergic metabolites or whether serotonergic abnormalities are possibly related to specific personality characteristics such as aggressivity and impulsivity. A sufficient data base is not currently available to conclude one way or the other with respect to these psychopharmacologic interventions, but research offers promise for pharmacologic treatment strategies for some suicidal individuals.

A fourth area that needs to be addressed is the identification of individuals with a family history of suicidal behavior. Direct educational efforts may be helpful in addressing this high-risk group and could represent a strategy for prevention of completed suicide.

A fifth type of intervention is education. Evidence is also available to indicate that more education about suicide is needed, especially of primary care physicians, regarding recognition of the signs and symptoms of depression and suicidal behavior and the selection of appropriate treatment strategies and interventions for the suicidal patient. We know that as many as 80% of people who end their lives with suicide have seen a physician within several months prior to completion.[50,55,62] Many have used medication given to them by their physicians to end their lives. These findings underscore the importance of increasing physician awareness and knowledge about suicide and changing their behavior regarding assessment and intervention. Specialized training courses should be provided as part of medical school education, the psychiatric residency, and other mental health specialists' and health care professionals' educational experiences as well as in postgraduate education settings, critical care and emergency medicine residencies, and continuing education programs, to ensure that clinicians dealing with suicidal patients have the greatest amount of expertise currently available for detecting and treating suicidal individuals. In addition, education of the media about psychiatric disorders, suicidal behavior, and where to go for treatment will help to increase public awareness about these problems and motivate high-risk individuals to seek treatment.

A final area that requires special attention is suicide among young people. Suicide is the third leading cause of death in this age group. The rate of suicide for young people has tripled over the past 30 years.[10] Between 1970 and 1980, 49,496 of the nation's youth 15-24 years of age committed suicide. The suicide rate for this age group increased 40% (from 8.8 deaths per 100,000 population in 1970 to 12.3 per 100,000 in 1980), while the rate for the remainder of the population remained stable. Young adults (20-24 years of age) had approximately twice the number and rate of suicides as teenagers 15-19 years old. This increase in youth suicide is due primarily to an increasing rate of suicide among young men: rates for males increased by 50% (from 13.5 to 20.2) compared with a 2% increase in females (4.2 to 4.3), so that by 1980 for this age group the ratio of suicides committed by males to those committed by females was almost 5 to 1.[85] Treatment interventions for this age group need to pay specific attention to those risk factors in the early years that may be different from risk factors for suicide in older individuals. As shown in TABLE 3, such factors in young people more clearly include antisocial behavior, family history of suicidal behavior, and being the victim of child abuse as well as depressive symptoms in the younger years. In addition, particular attention to family treatment, increasing social support, and enhancing self-esteem in this age group is needed. Our difficulty in recognizing and treating suicidal behavior in teenagers today is analogous to the difficulty we had in diagnosing and treating affective disorders some 5 to 10 years

TABLE 3. Adolescent Suicide—Risk Factors

- History of previous suicide attempt
- Family history of suicidal behavior and/or affective disorders
- Associated with substance abuse
- Associated with conduct disorders (and impulsive disorders, i.e., eating disorders)
- Associated with affective disorders
- Precipitating humiliating life event

ago. Just as we have significantly improved our current ability to diagnose and treat affective disorders in adolescents, we are hopeful that comparable advances will be made in the early detection and treatment of suicidal behavior in young people.

A recommendation for clinical investigators working in the area of suicide is to realize that the majority of scientific articles dealing with suicidal behavior appearing in peer-reviewed journals do not contain certain data considered essential to the accumulation of standardized clinical and research information about suicide attempts and completions. A consensus process is necessary to develop guidelines that would be helpful in interpreting clinical research reports on psychiatric, psychosocial, biological and genetic factors as well as treatment studies related to suicidal behavior. This relatively small step would stimulate increased communication among investigators and clinicians across different disciplines.

Finally, with respect to clinical interventions and the design of future research studies, there are issues that cut across the different domains of the matrix model. We need to realize that antidepressants may be useful for specific aspects of suicidal behavior across psychiatric syndromes (i.e., increased aggressivity and impulsivity associated with decreased serotonin). We need to establish randomized clinical trials in all age groups for suicidal behavior comparing psychotherapeutic interventions (cognitive behavioral/psychodynamic) with psychopharmacologic therapy and their combination. Interventions aimed at strengthening and increasing social supports are also needed. Ideal assessment and treatment studies would provide a comprehensive approach aimed at psychiatric diagnosis, personality traits, specific correlates of suicidal behavior, social supports, family and genetic history, and the possibility of obtaining sufficient plasma, urine, and in certain cases cerebrospinal fluid to ascertain whether there are neurochemical or genetic abnormalities in particular individuals. While we have not yet identified a neurochemical or genetic suicide "test" or "marker" (i.e., DNA probe), the hope exists that within the relatively near future such breakthroughs will be made. In addition, treatment should include interventions aimed at mobilizing and strengthening social supports in the patient's environment.

It is only with the use of the five-component matrix assessing psychiatric, personality, psychosocial, genetic, and biological information that we will be able to achieve a much greater precision and success in the early detection and treatment of suicidal individuals. Recognition of this approach with its components provides the rationale for treating the psychiatric syndrome, the personality disorder and traits, and suicidal behavior concurrently. Furthermore, it emphasizes the need for environmental interventions, the identification of high-risk genetic loading for affective disorders and suicidal behavior, and reinforces the search for possible biological abnormalities in vulnerable individuals. Given the increased focus on suicidal behavior, its public health consequences, and the tragic loss of human life that it represents, it is expected that advances in our understanding of this major public health problem should be forthcoming.

REFERENCES

1. BECK, A. T., J. H. DAVIS, C. J. FREDERICK, S. PERLIN, A. D. POKORNY, R. E. SCHULMAN, R. H. SEIDEN & B. J. WITTLIN. 1973. Classification and nomenclature. *In* Suicide Prevention in the Seventies. H. L. P. Resnik & B. C. Hawthorne, Eds. National Institute of Mental Health. Rockville, Md.

2. BECK, A. T., H. L. P. RESNIK & D. J. LETTIERI. 1974. The Prediction of Suicide. Charles Press. Bowie, Md.
3. AVERY, D. & G. WINOKUR. 1978. Suicide, attempted suicide, and relapse rates in depression. Arch. Gen. Psychiatry 35: 749-753.
4. MOTTO, J. A. 1977. Estimation of suicide risk by the use of clinical models. Suicide Life Threat. Behav. 7: 236-245.
5. WEISSMAN, A. & W. WORDEN. 1972. Risk rescue rating in suicide assessment. Arch. Gen. Psychiatry 26: 553-560.
6. BLUMENTHAL, S. J. & D. J. KUPFER. Models and criteria for the description of suicidal behavior. (Submitted for publication).
7. BECK, A. T. Hopelessness as a predictor of suicide. Ann. N.Y. Acad. Sci. (This volume.)
8. FRANCES, A., M. FYER & J. CLARKIN. Personality and suicide. Ann. N.Y. Acad. Sci. (This volume.)
9. HIRSCHFELD, R. & S. BLUMENTHAL. Personality, life events and other psychosocial factors in adolescent depression and suicide: a review. *In* Suicide among Adolescents and Young Adults. G. Klerman, Ed. American Psychiatric Press. Washington, D.C. (In press.)
10. BLUMENTHAL, S. J. 1984. An overview of suicide risk factor research. Presented at the Annual Meeting of the American Psychiatric Association, Los Angeles, May 1984.
11. DORPAT, T. L. & H. S. RIPLEY. 1960. A study of suicide in the Seattle area. Compr. Psychiatry 1: 349-359.
12. SLATER, J. & R. A. DEPUE. 1981. The contribution of environmental events and social supports to serious suicide attempts in primary depressive disorder. J. Abnorm. Psychol. 90: 275-285.
13. PAYKEL, E. S., B. A. PRUSOFF & J. K. MYERS. 1975. Suicide attempts and recent life events: a controlled comparison. Arch. Gen. Psychiatry 32: 327-333.
14. HAGNELL, O. & B. RORSMAN. 1980. Suicide in the Lundby study: a controlled prospective investigation of stressful life events. Neuropsychobiology 6: 319-332.
15. BORG, E. S. & M. STAHL. 1982. A prospective study of suicides and controls among psychiatric patients. Acta Psychiatr. Scand. 65: 221-232.
16. DORPAT, T. L., J. K. JACKSON & H. S. RIPLEY. 1965. Broken home and attempted suicide and completed suicide. Arch. Gen. Psychiatry 12: 213-216.
17. ROY, A. 1984. Suicide in recurrent affective disorder patients. Can. J. Psychiatry 29: 319-322.
18. KETY, S. Personal Communication.
19. ROY, A. Genetics of Suicide. Ann. N.Y. Acad. Sci. (This volume.)
20. ÅSBERG, M., P. NORDSTRÖM & L. TRÄSKMAN-BENDZ. Cerebrospinal fluid studies in suicide: an overview. Ann. N.Y. Acad. Sci. (This volume.)
21. STANLEY, M., J. J. MANN & L. S. COHEN. Serotonin and serotonergic receptors in suicide. Ann. N.Y. Acad. Sci. (This volume.)
22. MANN, J. J., P. A. MCBRIDE & M. STANLEY. Postmortem monoamine receptor and enzyme studies in suicide. Ann. N.Y. Acad. Sci. (This volume.)
23. ROY, A., M. VIRKKUNEN, S. GUTHRIE & M. LINNOILA. Indices of serotonin and glucose metabolism in violent offenders, arsonists, and alcoholics. Ann. N.Y. Acad. Sci. (This volume.)
24. VAN PRAAG, H., R. PLUTCHIK & H. CONTE. The serotonin hypothesis of (auto) aggression. Ann. N.Y. Acad. Sci. (This volume.)
25. BROWN, G. L. & F. K. GOODWIN. Cerebrospinal fluid correlates of suicide attempts and aggression. Ann. N.Y. Acad. Sci. (This volume.)
26. MELTZER, H. Y. & R. C. ARORA. Platelet markers of suicidality. Ann. N.Y. Acad. Sci. (This volume.)
27. AGREN, H. 1983. Life at risk: markers of suicidality and depression. Psychiatr. Dev. 1: 87-103.
28. AGREN, H. 1980. Symptom patterns in unipolar and bipolar depression correlating with monoamine metabolites in the cerebrospinal fluid: suicide. Psychiatry Res. 3: 225-236.
29. ASBERG, M., L. BERTILSSON, E. RYDIN, D. SCHALLING, P. THOREN & L. TRASKMAN-BENDZ. 1981. Monoamine metabolites in CSF in relation to depressive illness, suicidal behavior and personality. *In* Recent Advances in Neuropsychopharmacology. B. Angrist,

G. D. Burrows, M. Lader, O. Lingjaerde, G. Sedvall & D. Wheatley, Eds.: 257-271. Pergamon Press. New York, N.Y.
30. ASBERG, M., L. TRASKMAN & P. THOREN. 1976. 5-HIAA in the cerebrospinal fluid: a biochemical suicide prediction. Arch. Gen. Psychiatry 33: 1193-1197.
31. ASBERG, M., L. BERTILSSON & B. MARTENSSON. 1984. CSF monoamine metabolites, depression and suicide. In Frontiers in Biochemical and Pharmacological Research in Depression. E. Usdin, M. Asberg, L. Bertilsson & F. Sjoqvist, Eds.: 87-97. Raven Press. New York, N.Y.
32. BANKI, C. M., G. MOLNAR & M. VOJNIK. 1981. Cerebrospinal fluid amine metabolites, tryptophan and clinical parameters in depression. II. Psychopathological symptoms. J. Affect. Disord. 3: 91-99.
33. BANKI, C. M., M. VOJNIK, Z. PAPP, Z. B. KATLIN & M. ARATO. 1985. Cerebrospinal fluid magnesium and calcium related to amine metabolites, diagnosis and suicide attempts. Biol. Psychiatry 20: 163-171.
34. BROWN, G. L., M. H. EBERT, P. F. GOYER, D. C. JIMERSON, W. J. KLEIN, W. E. BUNNEY & F. K. GOODWIN. 1982. Aggression, suicide and serotonin: relationships to CSF amine metabolites. Am. J. Psychiatry 139: 741-746.
35. BROWN, G. L., F. K. GOODWIN, J. C. BALLENGER, P. F. GOYER & L. F. MAJOR. 1979. Aggression in humans correlates with cerebrospinal fluid amine metabolites. Psychiatry Res. 1: 131-139.
36. BROWN, G. L., F. K. GOODWIN & W. E. BUNNEY. 1982. Human aggression and suicide: their relationship to neuropsychiatric diagnosis and serotonin metabolism. In Serotonin in Biological Psychiatry. B. T. Ho, J. C. Schooler & E. Usdin, Eds.: 287-307. Raven Press. New York, N.Y.
37. LIDBERG, L., J. R. TUCK, M. ASBERG, G. P. SCALIA-TOMBA & L. BERTILSSON. 1985. Homicide, suicide and CSF 5-HIAA. Acta Psychiatr. Scand. 71: 230-236.
38. LINNOILA, M., M. VIRKKUNEN, M. SCHEININ, A. NUUTILA, R. RIMON & F. K. GOODWIN. 1983. Low cerebrospinal fluid 5-hydroxyindoleacetic acid concentration differentiates impulsive from nonimpulsive violent behavior. Life Sci. 33: 2609-2614.
39. NINAN, P. T., D. P. VAN KAMMEN, M. SCHEININ, M. LINNOILA, W. E. BUNNEY, JR. & F. K. GOODWIN. 1984. CSF 5-hydroxyindoleacetic acid levels in suicidal schizophrenic patients. Am. J. Psychiatry 141: 566-569.
40. ORELAND, L., A. WIBERG, M. ASBERG, L. TRASKMAN, L. SJOSTRAND, P. THOREN, L. BERTILSSON & G. TYBRING. 1981. Platelet MAO activity and monoamine metabolites in cerebrospinal fluid in depressed and suicidal patients and in healthy controls. Psychiatry Res. 4: 21-29.
41. ROY-BYRNE, P., R. M. POST, D. R. RUBINOW, M. LINNOILA, R. SAVARD & D. DAVIS. 1983. CSF 5HIAA and personal and family history of suicide in affectively ill patients: a negative study. Psychiatry Res. 10: 263-274.
42. SEDVALL, G., B. FYRO, B. GULLBERG, H. NYBACK, F. A. WIESEL & B. WODE-HELGODT. 1980. Relationships in healthy volunteers between concentrations of monoamine metabolites in cerebrospinal fluid and family history of psychiatric morbidity. Br. J. Psychiatry 136: 366-374.
43. TRASKMAN, L., M. ASBERG, L. BERTILSSON & L. SJOSTRAND. 1981. Monoamine metabolites in cerebrospinal fluid and suicidal behavior. Arch. Gen. Psychiatry 38: 631-636.
44. VAN PRAAG, H. 1982. Depression, suicide and metabolism of serotonin in the brain. J. Affect. Disord. 4: 275-290.
45. VAN PRAAG, H. M. & S. DE HAAN. 1980. Depression vulnerability and 5HT prophylaxis. Psychiatry Res. 3: 75-83.
46. FAWCETT, J. 1985. Depressive disorders and suicide. Paper presented at the Conference on Psychobiology of Suicidal Behavior. New York, N.Y., Sept. 18-20. (This volume.)
47. FRANCES, R. J., J. FRANKLIN & D. K. FLAVIN. Suicide and Alcoholism. Ann. N.Y. Acad. Sci. (This volume.)
48. JAMISON, K. R. Suicide and bipolar disorders. Ann. N. Y. Acad. Sci. (This volume.)
49. JOHNS, C. A., M. STANLEY & B. STANLEY. Suicide in schizophrenia. Ann. N.Y. Acad. Sci. (This volume.)
50. BARRACLOUGH, B., J. BUNCH, B. NELSON & P. SAINSBURY. 1974. A hundred cases of suicide: clinical aspects. Br. J. Psychiatry 125: 355-373.

51. CHILES, J. A., L. M. MILLER & G. B. COX. 1980. Depression in an adolescent delinquent population. Arch. Gen. Psychiatry 37: 1179-1184.
52. CRUMLEY, F. 1982. Adolescent suicide attempts and melancholia. Tex-Med. 78: 62-65.
53. CRUMLEY, F. E. 1982. The adolescent suicide attempt: a cardinal symptom of serious psychiatric disorder. Am. J. Psychother. 36: 158-165.
54. ROBINS, E. 1981. The Final Months. Oxford University Press. New York, N.Y.
55. ROBINS, E., G. E. MURPHY, R. H. WILKINSON, S. GASSNER & J. KAYES. 1959. Some clinical considerations in the prevention of suicide based on a study of 134 successful suicides. Am. J. Public Health 49: 889-899.
56. GUZE, S. B. & E. ROBINS. 1970. Suicide and primary affective disorder. Br. J. Psychiatry 117: 437-438.
57. SHAFFER, D. 1974. Suicide in childhood and early adolescence. J. Child Psychol. Psychiatry 15: 275-291.
58. SHAFFER, D. & P. FISHER. 1981. The epidemiology of suicide in children and adolescents. J. Am. Acad. Child Psychiatry 20: 545-565.
59. SHAFFER, D., M. GOULD & P. TRAUBMAN. 1985. Paper presented at the Conference on the Psychobiology of Suicidal Behavior, New York, N.Y., Sept. 18-20.
60. SHAFII, M., S. CARRIGAN, J. R. WHITTINGHILL & A. DERRICK. 1985. Psychological autopsy of completed suicide in children and adolescents. Am. J. Psychiatry 142: 1061-1064.
61. BECK, A. T., R. A. STEER, M. KOVACS & B. GARRISON. 1985. Hopelessness and eventual suicide: a 10-year prospective study of patients hospitalized with suicidal ideation. Am. J. Psychiatry 142: 559-563.
62. HAGNELL, O., J. LANKE & B. RORSMAN. 1981. Suicide rates in the Lundby study: mental illness as a risk factor for suicide. Neuropsychobiology 7: 248-253.
63. MILES, D. 1977. Conditions predisposing to suicide: a review. J. Nerv. Ment. Dis. 164: 231-246.
64. POKORNY, A. D. 1964. Suicide rates in various psychiatric disorders. J. Nerv. Ment. Dis. 139: 499-506.
65. CRUMLEY, F. 1981. Adolescent suicide attempts and borderline personality disorder: clinical features. Southwest. Med. J. 74: 546-549.
66. LUSCOMB, R. L., G. A. CLUM & A. T. PATSIOKAS. 1980. Mediating factors in the relationship between life stress and suicide attempting. J. Nerv. Ment. Dis. 168: 644-650.
67. ROY, A. 1983. Family history of suicide. Arch. Gen. Psychiatry 40: 971-974.
68. SCHULSINGER, F., S. S. KETY, D. ROSENTHAL & P. H. WENDER. 1979. A family study of suicide. In Origins, Prevention and Treatment of Affective Disorders. M. Schou & E. Stromgren, Eds.: 277-287. Academic Press, Inc. New York, N.Y.
69. TSUANG, M. 1983. Risk of suicide in the relatives of schizophrenics, manics, depressives and controls. J. Clin. Psychiatry 44: 396-400.
70. TSUANG, M. 1977. Genetic factors in suicide. Dis. Nerv. System 38: 498-501.
71. ROY, A. 1982. Risk factors for suicide in psychiatric patients. Arch. Gen. Psychiatry 39: 1089-1095.
72. EGELAND, J. A. & J. N. SUSSEX. 1985. Suicide and family loading for affective disorders. JAMA 254: 915-918.
73. FARBEROW, N. & M. SIMON. 1969. Suicide in Los Angeles and Vienna: an intercultural study of two cities. Public Health Rep. 84: 389-403.
74. HABERLANDT, W. 1967. Aportacion a la genetica del suicidio. Folio Clin. Int. 17: 319-322.
75. HABERLANDT, W. 1965. Der suizid als genetisches problem (zwillings-and familier analyse). Anthrop. Anz. 29: 65-89.
76. ZAW, K. 1981. A suicidal family. Br. J. Psychiatry 189: 68-69.
77. JENNINGS, C., B. M. BARRACLOUGH & J. R. MOSS. 1978. Have the Samaritans lowered the suicide rate? A controlled study. Psychol. Med. 8: 413-422.
78. MILLER, H. L., D. W. COOMBS, J. D. LEEPER & S. N. BARTON. 1984. An analysis of the effects of suicide prevention facilities on suicide rates in the United States. Am. J. Public Health 74: 340-343.
79. LESTER, D. 1974. Effects of suicide prevention centers on suicide rates in the United States. Health Serv. Rep. 89: 37-39.
80. LESTER, D. 1972. The myth of suicide prevention. Compr. Psychiatry 13: 555-560.

81. BRIDGE, T. P., S. G. PLOTKIN, W. W. K. ZUNG 7 B. J. SOLDO. 1977. Suicide prevention centers. J. Nerv. Ment Dis. **164:** 18-24.
82. GIBBONS, J. S., J. BUTLER, P. URWIN & J. L. GIBBONS. 1978. Evaluation of a social work service for self-poisoning patients. Br. J. Psychiatry **133:** 111-118.
83. LIBERMAN, R. P. & T. ECKMAN. 1981. Behavior therapy vs. insight-oriented therapy for repeated suicide attempters. Arch. Gen. Psychiatry **38:** 1126-1130.
84. KOVACS, M., J. RUSH, A. BECK & S. HOLLON. 1981. Depressed outpatients treated with cognitive therapy or pharmacotherapy. A one year follow-up. Arch. Gen. Psychiatry **38:** 33-39.
85. CENTERS FOR DISEASE CONTROL. 1985. Suicide Surveillance, 1970-1980. Department of Health and Human Services. U.S. Public Health Service. Atlanta, Ga.

Suicide Prevention

Current Efficacy and Future Promise

CYNTHIA R. PFEFFER

*Child Psychiatry Inpatient Unit
New York Hospital-Cornell Medical Center
Westchester Division
21 Bloomingdale Road
White Plains, New York 10605*

It is almost the centennial year of the publication of Emil Durkheim's great sociological book *Le Suicide* (1897) and almost 75 years since the historic 1910 Vienna Psychoanalytic Society meeting devoted to discussing the problems of suicide. Yet, facts indicating that there has been a threefold increase in rates of suicide for 15- to 24-year-olds in the past 20 years,[1] an increase in suicide rates as one ages, and higher suicide rates for cohorts of people born in more recent years[2,3] offer a worrisome reminder that the prevention of suicide has not been satisfactorily accomplished. Nevertheless, the present volume clearly highlights scientific achievements used to study suicidal behavior. Our current body of information points out multidimensional features of suicidal behaviors and suggests that prevention must have a multidisciplinary orientation that includes psychobiological, psychosocial, philosophical, and sociocultural components. All these components have value in understanding the etiology, treatment, and natural course of suicidal behavior and prevention of suicidal acts.

Achievements in suicide prevention have occurred in a number of areas. Most notable are insights from epidemiological investigations that suicide prevention must be aimed toward large numbers of people as well as focused on unique features of particular individuals. Public health models of disease prevention that attempt to increase resistance to illness, to discover cases of illness in its early stages, and to provide services to large numbers of vulnerable individuals are being applied to suicide prevention. These techniques, however, should not exclude more traditional clinical approaches in which individually planned treatment is offered by a physician or a mental health professional to a patient.

CLARIFICATION OF TERMINOLOGY

A number of principles for suicide prevention have been delineated. While many of these premises are based on a disease model reflecting that cause of an illness is based on interactions between host, agent, and environment, the complex nature of psychological processes must be recognized For example, the relationship between cause of psychological illness and effect of interventions is often difficult to demonstrate. Also, it is essential to clarify terminology regarding suicide prevention.

Concepts of Prevention

Brown pointed out two important concepts for suicide prevention.[4] First, suicide mortality refers to the rate of suicide. Second, suicide morbidity is the combined rates of suicide and attempted suicide. He suggested that these concepts are associated with two levels of prevention that employ different approaches. The primary level focuses on reduction of morbidity by improving knowledge and treatment of psychiatric illness. The second level focuses on reduction of mortality by reducing the lethality of suicide acts and improving acute treatment of the effects of the suicide methods.

Definition of Suicide

Shneidman, feeling uneasy about the adequacy of current definitions of suicide, offered a definition that focuses on how "acts of suicide should be understood and how they should be regarded, especially by the academic and professional communities [page 3]."[5] His definition emphasizes the psychological, contextual, and needful state of an individual who, by means of suicide, wishes to end an intolerably painful state. Shneidman proposed the following definition: "Currently in the western world, suicide is the conscious act of self-induced annihilation, best understood as a multidimensional malaise in a needful individual who defines an issue for which the suicide is perceived as the best solution [page 203]."[5]

Based on this definition, Schneidman suggested a number of practical prevention measures that included reducing pain, fulfilling an individual's frustrated needs, providing a viable answer and indicating alternatives, giving transfusions of hope, playing for time to decrease ambivalent thinking, increasing the processes for self-awareness, listening for the need to involve others, blocking the suicidal action, and invoking previous positive patterns of successful coping. The purposes of these complex suicide prevention operations are to reduce the person's degree of perturbation or state of unrest or distress, and the lethality of thinking. A number of basic and practical principles for suicide prevention, which are compatible with these concepts, will be highlighted in the remaining sections of this paper.

LETHALITY OF SUICIDAL METHODS

Brown believes that "the most likely causes of the decline of suicide mortality [in Britain] are extraneous and fortuitous developments that aid in reducing the number of deaths 'secondary prevention' by reducing the lethality of some commonly used modes of suicide [page 1124]."[4] He pointed out that these "secondary prevention" approaches involved "reduction in toxicity in domestic gas supplies, reduced lethality of prescription sedatives, and improved treatment for self-poisoning [page 1123]."[4] He noted that individuals infrequently substitute one type of suicide method when a more available form of socioculturally accepted method is reduced. This observation has impelled others to support the contention that making it harder to carry out socioculturally accepted methods of suicide may lower suicide mortality.[6]

Interventions of limiting the number and type of sedatives and antidepressant tablets prescribed at a given time,[7] fencing in observation platforms of high buildings and bridges,[8] reducing toxic gas in automobile exhausts,[9] and removing guns from homes[6,10] have been advocated. For example, Boor determined that "virtually all the increases in the suicide rates [in the United States] for each of the four sex-ethnic groups between 1962 and 1975 can be attributed to increases in the rates of suicide by firearms [page 73]."[6] His finding that "suicide rates are affected by the availability of preferred, socioculturally accepted methods of suicide suggests that some suicides in the United States could be prevented by decreasing the availability of firearms to suicidal individuals [page 74]."[6]

Several practical clinical principles follow from this suggestion. Therapists working with suicidal individuals should ascertain the methods being considered to carry out suicidal intent. Warning family members to remove potentially lethal agents such as pills, guns, and knives is indicated. Improvement in the medical management of the lethal effects of suicide methods is necessary.[11-13] Furthermore, strict gun control legislation may decrease the United States suicide rates.[14]

EFFICACY OF SUICIDE PREVENTION CENTERS

The Samaritans, incorporated in the United Kingdom in 1953, is an international organization of lay individuals involved in providing crisis intervention. Its mandates include primary prevention of suicide and alleviation of other emotional problems. Suicide prevention centers with similar mandates have developed throughout the World during the 1960s and 1970s. Research about the efficacy of these suicide prevention centers varies and suggests that there is no evidence that suicide prevention centers influence suicide rates.[4] However, such investigations have been hampered by methodological problems especially because of the numerous confounding variables in research on suicide.[4,15] Nevertheless, a recent comparison of suicide rates in United States counties with and without suicide prevention centers suggested an association between presence of a center and reduction in suicide rates of young white females,[15] the most frequent group of individuals who call such centers. This finding provides a basis for additional research and "suggests that future research can now attempt to analyze the factors that are responsible for this reduction and extend the principles to other populations which, while not reached by prevention centers, are at greater risk for suicide [page 343]."[15]

PREDICTION OF SUICIDE RISK

Prediction of suicide in individuals who are at risk has been a hoped for method of suicide prevention. However, Murphy pointed out a number of difficulties in prediction that depend on evidence from empirical studies. He advocated the need to define terms: "If, by prediction, we mean the identification of persons who at some time in the future will commit suicide, the problem is largely a statistical one and its difficulties are immense. But if, by prediction, we mean the identification of persons who are at immediate or near term risk of suicide, the focus is clinical, and the problems are different [page 331]."[16]

One approach for prediction is to classify populations at risk by demographic attributes or psychiatric illness. Such classifications, however, are too general for suicide prediction because they include many individuals who will never become suicidal. Another approach depends upon prospective studies of at-risk populations and the identification of risk factors from data when suicide outcome is known.[17,18] The clinical value of such risk predictors has been negligible because of the problem of statistically predicting infrequent events. Even if these suicide risk predictors had high sensitivity and specificity, they would produce too many false positives. The application of suicide intervention techniques to the false positive individuals would be both unfeasible and unwarranted especially because they require extensive time, effort, cost, and may even produce untoward treatment side effects.

Murphy emphasized that "when base rates are low, predictions inevitably suffer grievously [page 343]."[16] He pointed out another reason why "the prediction of suicide at a definite or indefinite future time is not likely to meet reasonable standards of accuracy.... All evidence points to the conclusion that suicidal intent is not constant within an individual person. It waxes, wanes, and disappears, and it may surface abruptly. This fact suggests that the suicidal urge is state-dependent [page 343]."[16] These propositions emphasize the contextual quality of suicide.

Pokorny suggested that the clinician's work in suicide prediction, in contrast to statistical predictions, involves a different approach that consists of a sequence of small decisions. "For example, in suicide prediction, the first decision might be based on some alerting note or sign, and the decision would be to investigate further ... in each case, the decision is not what to do for all times, but rather what to do next, for the near future [page 257]."[18] Such a clinical method is based on a process of multiple assessments of the person who is in a suicidal crisis.

There is evidence that clinicians can make short-term reliable and rational predictive assessments about suicidal behavior.[19] Furthermore, reliability may be enhanced by the use of semistructured or standard interview formats, clinical instruments to highlight suicidal risk,[20] and experience in working with suicidal individuals. Biological parameters may add a promising dimension to the scope of immediate suicide risk assessment. Thus, clinical suicide prediction is work based on a "different time frame, dealing in minutes, hours, or days [page 257]."[18] It is work "done at close quarters [page 344]."[16]

TREATMENT ISSUES

It has been shown that suicide rarely occurs in the absence of psychiatric disorder[21-24] and that suicidal individuals often make contact with clinical agencies prior to their suicidal behavior.[25] In fact, only 3% to 5% of individuals threatening suicide are certain that they want to die[26] and the majority are ambivalent about their death intent. Thus, there are a large number of suicidal individuals for whom suicide prevention, when effectively carried out, can be life-saving. Therefore, effective recognition of the suicidal individual as well as treatment aimed at reducing the components of suicide risk and the underlying psychiatric disorder is a key factor in suicide prevention. Treatment may include psychotherapy, medication, hospitalization, and/or social changes.

Clinicians must be knowledgable about the most current approaches to risk assessment and appropriate intervention strategies. Unfortunately, several studies have suggested that many mental health professionals and physicians do not have adequate training in recognizing suicide signs.[18,22,25,27,28] In fact, many suicide victims who have consulted a professional before committing suicide have either been misdiagnosed or ineffectively treated.[29-32] To insure that this does not occur, prevention efforts must include an educational component that regularly updates clinicians about suicidal phenomena, diagnostic approaches that include interviewing and biological techniques, and modalities of treatment.

Suicide can be prevented especially if warning signs are recognized and immediate intervention is offered.[16,25,30] The high rate of suicide among individuals with affective disorders and chronic alcoholism as well as among those with schizophrenia, personality disorders, neurosis, and chronic brain syndromes has been definitively documented.[21,22,24,33] One study has shown that aggressive treatment of primary affective disorders in an outpatient population reduced suicide in this population.[30] Similarly, Enzell noted that depressed patients who participated in a periodic health checkup, in contrast to those who did not participate in the program, did not commit suicide.[34] Furthermore, estimates of a relatively sizable lifetime risk of suicide in different psychiatric disorders (15% of primary depressives, 15% of chronic alcoholics, 10% of schizophrenics, 10% of neurotic depressives, 6% of sociopaths, and 5% of personality disorders and mixed neuroses)[23] points out the long-term need for follow-up, repeated biological and psychosocial interventions, and careful monitoring of warning signs of individuals with psychiatric disorders. In general, the prevention of suicide morbidity requires that the treatment of suicidal individuals be a long-term process using specific interventions for psychiatric disorder, approaches that minimize dropping out of clinical care, and the establishment of networks of people who are skilled in recognizing a suicidal individual.

SOCIAL STIMULATION OF SUICIDAL BEHAVIOR

A relationship between imitation and suicide morbidity has been demonstrated in a number of ways and is now an important new focus for prevention efforts. A startling phenomenon that highlighted this occurred in the eighteenth century with the publication of Goethe's book, *The Sorrows of Young Werther*, about a young man who committed suicide by shooting himself. This book was believed to have stimulated an epidemic of imitative suicides in young adults.

Philips studied the effects of sensational newspaper reports on suicide and concluded that there is a significant association between the increase in suicides and the extent of publicity.[35] Ashton and Donnon studied a 1978 epidemic of self-burning in England and Wales.[36] Within a year, there were 82 suicides by burning compared to the usual incidents of 23 per year between 1963 and 1978. The apparent trigger for this epidemic was a young woman's suicide motivated by political reasons. Among the 82 imitative suicides, the victims were predominantly young single men or older married women. A large number of these victims had documented psychiatric histories.

Furthermore, none of the suicides appeared to be politically motivated. Ashton and Donnon concluded that imitative suicides occurred in vulnerable individuals and were mediated by news coverage.[36] Furthermore, they suggested that "in the short-term, suicides are related to reporting and that, in the long-term, methods of suicide are related to public knowledge; it is clear that some form of code of practice for the reporting of suicides is required [page 739]."[36]

Identification with an individual who has committed suicide has been observed among psychiatric inpatients,[37] and evidence for the occurrence of clusters of self-destructive behavior among adolescents in residential treatment has been offered.[38] The role of clustering phenomena in increasing the adolescent suicide rate in the United States has been a major issue confronting prevention efforts. Adolescent suicides in Westchester County, New York, and Plano, Texas, have raised questions about whether adolescent suicides cluster within a defined time period and if they are interrelated. A recent study of teenage suicide attempts in a suburban community in 1982 and 1983, found that in 1982, teenage suicide attempts preceded a widely publicized cluster of adolescent suicide in that community in 1983.[39] In addition, geographic clustering of suicide attempts by neighborhood occurred and enrollment in the same school in which a teenager committed suicide was positively correlated with suicide attempts of other teenagers. Specific social linkages between the adolescents who attempted and those who committed suicide were demonstrated in that study.

These studies point out the need to decrease factors associated with cluster effects and imitative suicidal behaviors. Further research is required to determine which adolescents are particularly vulnerable to these phenomena as well as to delineate practical intervention and prevention procedures.

PUBLIC EDUCATION AND THE NEED TO RESPOND

A critical aspect of prevention involves educating the general public about recognition of high-risk individuals and, most importantly, utilization of intervention services. It seems likely that a uniform approach to public education is less effective than specifically planned programs that address the unique characteristics of a given community or population at risk. Recently, school suicide prevention programs have been developed to educate parents, school staff, and students about teenage suicidal behavior. However, the efficacy of these programs to prevent suicide has not been evaluated.

Another important new issue for prevention involves planning approaches to enhance adaptive skills and self-preservative behaviors. Such approaches need to address psychological, social, and developmental factors. For example, Pokorny believed that it is necessary to "instill some ethical or moral barriers to the act of suicide, making such behavior less 'available' to the patient. It is questionable whether this could be done in adulthood, after suicidal behavior or preoccupation has already appeared. It may work only if taught or instilled during childhood [page 249]."[18]

In keeping with Pokorny's ideas, Khantzian and Mack noted that "the complex functions relating to self-preservation, self-protection and survival are relatively neglected in contemporary psychoanalytic literature despite the special urgency of these matters for many of our patients [page 209]."[40] These psychoanalysts proposed that there is a complex set of functions involved in "self-care" and that failure in the operation of these functions may contribute to self-destructive behavior. They suggested that "people are often not so much compelled or driven in their behavior as they are impaired or deficient in self-care functions that are otherwise present in the mature ego [page 210]."[40] The types of self-care functions that they proposed include (1) sufficient positive self-esteem to feel oneself to be worth protecting; (2) the capacity to anticipate dangerous situations; (3) the ability to control impulses; (4) pleasure in mastering inevitable situations of risk; (5) knowledge about the outside world and oneself for survival; (6) the ability to be self-assertive or aggressive enough to protect oneself; and (7) the ability to choose relationships with others who will enhance one's protection or at least not jeopardize one's existence. Such functions are developmentally determined and are based on factors associated with personal experiences, psychological maturation, and constitutional background.

Implications for suicide prevention related to these theoretical ideas include a focus on the fundamental structure of family and social life.[41] For example, it is necessary to teach adequate parenting skills and to intervene in a variety of psychosocial and biological ways against such parental problems as affective disorders,[42,43] sexual and violent abuse, and alcoholism that hamper a parent's ability to raise children and to promote the child's development of self-care skills. Furthermore, it is necessary to be aware of methods for early detection of psychiatric disorder such as depression or tendencies toward dyscontrol in offspring of affected parents.[44] Finally, research must be directed to learning about the responses of survivors of a suicide in a family and the prevention of suicide morbidity among such family members.[45,46]

Extensive social change that affects intrafamilial relationships and social roles has been found to be associated with adolescent suicide. This phenomenon has been dramatically evident in the post-World War II society of Micronesia, where there has been an eightfold increase in male adolescent suicide between 1960 and 1980.[47] This observation highlights the necessity to ameliorate the adverse effects of social dissolution prompted by family breakups, mobility, social role changes, and loss of extrafamilial support groups. On a more global scale, suicide prevention should promote awareness of the threat of a nuclear holocaust and provide an impetus for arms control, diplomacy, and better world cohesion that can serve to thwart the possibility of human self-annihilation.

Finally, suicide prevention must promote an immediate response from everyone to the voices of those individuals who are particularly distressed. Currently, adolescents are a large group who are calling out for help in a variety of ways. An excerpt from the following poem, "A Time of Hurt and Confusion," written by an anonymous 16-year-old high school student, is a voice that depicts pain and despair but also hope and a wish to have others respond:

> In the hand with which I've been writing
> I have held two weapons.
> One a knife
> A knife that I have used to cut myself. . . .
> The second weapon—a pen. . . .
> That can hurt only the illness
> That won't leave me.
> The pen that can forever rid me of hurt
> Just as a knife.
> I only hope the pen will be successful
>   in this hateful war.
> Don't be too late!
> Tell someone of this conflict
> Before it's too late.
> The knife has won too many battles.[48]

CONCLUSION

Our present knowledge of suicidal behavior points out that it is a preventable phenomenon. Many principles of suicide prevention are known and are being practiced. Future efforts require that research be devoted to evaluating prevention approaches especially for specific high-risk groups, to educating professionals and the public about this problem, and to continuing exploration of biological and psychosocial interactions that characterize persons at risk for suicide morbidity. It has become increasingly evident that suicide prevention must shift away from the isolated work of individual clinicians and toward an approach that involves networks of scientists, clinicians, the general public, and at-risk individuals in working together to recognize and treat the components of suicidal risk as well as to develop protective mechanisms against suicidal tendencies.

Our suicide prevention efforts, although difficult to discern, must be vigorous, skilled, and sanguine. Murphy emphasized that if suicide prevention is successful, "the patient will live. A suicide will have been prevented. Yet to quantify this effect is impossible. It is important to realize that the absence of a suicide generates no data. Thus, we can never prove what has been accomplished. Yet we can hardly doubt that it occurs" [page 347]."[49] Thus, the most important conclusion that can be drawn is that suicide prevention must involve the cooperative efforts of everyone.

REFERENCES

1. 1984. Monthly Vital Statistics Report. National Center for Health Statistics.
2. HELLON, C. P. & M. I. SOLOMON 1980. Suicide and age in Alberta, Canada, 1951 to 1977: the changing profile. Arch. Gen. Psychiatry 37: 505-510.
3. SOLOMON, M. I. & C. P. HELLON. 1980. Suicide and age in Alberta, Canada, 1951 to 1977: a cohort analysis. Arch. Gen. Psychiatry 37: 511-513.
4. BROWN, J. H. 1979. Suicide in Britain: more attempts, fewer deaths, lessons for public policy. Arch. Gen. Psychiatry 36: 1119-1124.
5. SHNEIDMAN, E. 1985. Definitions of Suicide. John Wiley and Sons. New York, N.Y.
6. BOOR, M. 1981. Methods of suicide and implications for suicide prevention. J. Clin. Psychol. 37: 70-75.
7. O'BRIEN, J. P. 1977. Increase in suicide attempts by drug ingestion: the Boston experience 1964-1974. Arch. Gen. Psychiatry 34: 1165-1169.
8. PRASAD, A. & G. G. LLOYD. 1983. Attempted suicide by jumping. Acta Psychiatr. Scand. 68: 394-396.
9. HAYS, P. & R. A. BORNSTEIN. 1984. Failed suicide attempt by emission gas poisoning. Am. J. Psychiatry 141: 592-593.1.
10. BOYD, J. H. 1983. The increasing rate of suicide by firearms. N. Engl. J. Med. 308: 872-874.
11. CONN, L. M., B. F. RUDNICK & J. R. LION. 1984. Psychiatric care for patients with self-inflicted gunshot wounds. Am. J. Psychiatry 141: 261-263.
12. PETERSON, L. G., M. PETERSON, G. J. O'SHANIEK & A. SWANN. 1985. Self-inflicted gunshot wounds: lethality of method versus intent. Am. J. Psychiatry 142: 228-231.
13. SAWYER, W. T., J. L. CANDILL & M. J. ELLISON. 1984. A case of severe acute desimpramine overdose. Am. J. Psychiatry 141: 122-123.
14. LESTER, D. & M. MURRELL. 1980. The influence of gun control laws in suicidal behavior. Am. J. Psychiatry 137: 121-122.
15. MILLER, H. L., D. W. COOMBS, J. D. LEEPER & S. N. BARTON. 1984. An analysis of the

effects of suicide prevention facilities on suicide rates in the United States. Am. J. Public Health **74:** 340-343.
16. MURPHY, G. E. 1983. On suicide prediction and prevention. Arch. Gen. Psychiatry **40:** 343-344.
17. MOTTO, J. A. 1984. Suicide in male adolescents. *In* Suicide in the Young. H. S. Sudak, A. B. Ford & N. B. Rushforth, Eds. John Wright PSG, Inc. Boston, Mass.
18. POKORNY, A. D. 1983. Prediction of suicide in psychiatric patients: report of a prospective study. Arch. Gen. Psychiatry **40:** 249-257.
19. KAPLAN, R. D., D. B. KOTTLER & A. J. FRANCES. 1982. Reliability and rationality in the prediction of suicide. Hosp. Commun. Psychiatry **33:** 212-215.
20. MOTTO, J. A., D. C. HEILBRON & R. P. JUSTER. 1985. Development of a clinical instrument to estimate suicidal risk. Am. J. Psychiatry **142:** 680-686.
21. BARRACLOUGH, B., J. BUNCH, B. NELSON & P. SAINSBURY. 1974. A hundred cases of suicide: clinical aspects. Br. J. Psychiatry **125:** 355-373.
22. DORPAT, T. L. & H. S. RIPLEY. 1960. A study of suicide in the Seattle area. Compr. Psychiatry **1:** 349-359.
23. GUZE, S. B. & E. ROBINS. 1970. Suicide and primary affective disorder. Psychiatry **117:** 437-448.
24. ROBINS, E., G. E. MURPHY, R. H. WILKINSON, JR., S. GASSNER & J. KAYES. 1959. Some clinical considerations in the prevention of suicide based on a study of 134 successful suicides. Am. J. Public Health **49:** 888-899.
25. MORGAN, H. G. 1981. Management of suicidal behavior. Br. J. Psychiatry **138:** 259-260.
26. LITMAN, R. E. & N. L. FARBEROW. 1961. Emergency evaluation of self-destructive behavior. *In* The Cry for Help. N. Farberow & E. Shneidman, Eds. McGraw-Hill. New York, N.Y.
27. BURDICK, B. M., C. B. HOLMES & R. F. WALN. 1983. Recognition of suicide signs by physicians in different areas of specialization. J. Med. Educ. **58:** 716-721.
28. HOLMES, C. B. & M. E. HOWARD. 1980. Recognition of suicide lethality factors by physicians, mental health professionals, ministers, and college students. J. Consult. Clin. Psychol. **48:** 383-387.
29. KHURI, R. & H. S. AKISKAL. 1983. Suicide prevention: the necessity of treating contributory psychiatric disorders. Psychiatr. Clin. North Am. **6:** 193-207.
30. MARTIN, R. L., R. CLONINGER, S. B. GUZE & P. J. CLAYTON. 1985. Mortality in a followup of 500 psychiatric outpatients: cause-specific modality. Arch. Gen. Psychiatry **42:** 58-66.
31. MURPHY, G. E. 1975. The physician's responsibility for suicide: errors of ommission. Ann. Intern. Med. **82:** 305-309.
32. ROY, A. 1982. Risk factors for suicide in psychiatric patients. Arch. Gen. Psychiatry **39:** 1089-1095.
33. KRAFT, D. P. & H. M. BABIGIAN. 1976. Suicide by persons with and without psychiatric contacts. Arch. Gen. Psychiatry **33:** 209-215.
34. ENZELL, K. 1984. Mortality among persons with depressive symptoms and among responders and non-responders in a health check-up. Acta Psychiatr. Scand. **69:** 89-102.
35. PHILLIPS, D. P. 1974. The influence of suggestion on suicide: substantive and theoretical implications of the Werther effect. Am. Socio. Rev. **39:** 340-354.
36. ASHTON, J. R. & S. DONNON. 1981. Suicide by burning as an epidemic phenomenon: an analysis of 82 deaths and inquests in England and Wales in 1978-1979. Psychol. Med. **11:** 735-739.
37. SACKS, M. & S. ETH. 1981. Psychological identification as a cause of suicide on an inpatient unit. Hosp. Commun. Psychiatry **32:** 36-40.
38. WALSH, B. W. & P. ROSEN. 1985. Self-mutilation and contagion: an empirical test. Am. J. Psychiatry **130:** 468-471.
39. DAVIDSON, L. 1985. Parasuicide changes during a teen suicide cluster. *In* New Research Program and Abstracts: 115. American Psychiatric Association. Dallas, Tex.
40. KHANTZIAN, E. J. & J. E. MACK. 1983. Self-preservation and the care of the self. Psychoanal. Study Child **38:** 209-232.
41. YESAVAGE, J. A. & L. WIDROW. 1985. Early parental discipline and adult self-destructive acts. J. Nerv. Ment. Dis. **173:** 74-77.

42. DAVENPORT, Y. B., C. ZAHN-WAXLER, M. L. ADLAND & A. MAYFIELD. 1984. Early child-rearing practices in families with a manic-depressive parent. Am. J. Psychiatry 141: 230-235.
43. ZAHN-WAXLER, C., D. H. MCKNEW, E. M. CUMMINGS, Y. B. DAVENPORT & M. RADKE-YARROW. 1984. Problem behaviors and peer interactions of young children with a manic-depressive parent. Am. J. Psychiatry 141: 230-235.
44. WEISSMAN, M. M., P. WICKRAMARATNE, K. R. MERIKANGAS, J. F. LACKMAN, B. A. PRUSOFF, K. A. CARUSO, K. K. KIDD & G. GAMMON. 1984. Onset of major depression in early adulthood: increased familial loading and specificity. Arch. Gen. Psychiatry 41: 1136-1143.
45. MURPHY, G. & R. D. WETZEL. 1982. Family history of suicidal behavior among suicide attempters. J. Nerv. Ment. Dis. 170: 86-90.
46. RUDESTAM, K. E. & D. IMBROLL. 1983. Societal reactions to a child's death by suicide. J. Consult. Clin. Psychol. 51: 461-462.
47. RUBINSTEIN, D. H. 1983. Epidemic suicide among Microesian adolescents. Soc. Sci. Med. 17: 657-665.
48. 1984. A time of hurt and confusion. Suicide Life-Threat. Behav. 14: 284.
49. MURPHY, G. E. 1984. The prediction of suicide: why is it so difficult? Am. J. Psychother. 38: 341-349.

Suicide, Aggression, and Depression

A Theoretical Framework for Future Research

FREDERICK K. GOODWIN

*Office of Scientific Director
Intramural Research Program
National Institute of Mental Health
Building 10, Room 4N-224
Bethesda, Maryland 20892*

I have been asked to provide some overview comments focusing on future directions for research on suicide. First, we need to ask ourselves these questions: (1) What has been firmly established by widely replicated studies? (2) What are the emerging areas of consensus? (3) What are the remaining areas of complete ignorance? The field of suicide research has, until recently, lagged behind the mainstream of advances in clinical psychiatry—advances that have been so dramatic in the past two decades. The papers presented in this volume are a healthy indication that the methods and concepts fruitful to research in psychopharmacology and in the major mental disorders (particularly, the affective disorders) can also invigorate suicide research.

In the past, the study of suicide has evolved in a peculiar way—that is, in two separate intellectual traditions, each maintaining an isolation from the other. On the one hand has been the *psychosocial* focus of the suicide prevention movement, and, on the other hand, the *clinical* focus on suicide as an integral part of major psychiatric illness. The suicide prevention focus has primarily derived its experience from working with people who *threaten or attempt suicide,* while the clinical-medical focus comes primarily from dealing with *completed or nearly completed suicide* as part of psychiatric illness, most often major depression. Although the domains of attempters and completers do overlap somewhat, by and large they represent distinctly different populations.[1] Unfortunately, this distinction has too often been glossed over; a problem to which others in this volume have pointed, as well. In my view, this important distinction should orient future research on suicide.

The presentations here serve to reemphasize what is already clear from the literature: the single most important risk factor for *actual* suicide is the presence of a major mental disorder, particularly major depression or manic-depressive illness, and, less frequently, personality disorders, alcoholism, schizophrenia and organic disorders.[2] It strikes me that one could conceptualize the affective disorders as conveying the "core" vulnerability to suicide, while the other disorders contribute additional risk factors such as impulsivity psychosis, and reduced cognitive function.

Another fundamental reality repeatedly emphasized here is that of genetic vulnerability. TABLE 1 illustrates the data from the Schulsinger *et al.* study,[3] which employed the adoption strategy, one of the better ways to tease apart "nature" from "nurture." What is most interesting about these results is that the association between suicide in a subject and a family history of suicide in the biological parents (but not the rearing parents) was independent of the presence of a psychiatric diagnosis. That is to say, in some of the suicide cases in which there was an indicated genetic predisposition, no major psychiatric illness had been diagnosed in the relatives who suicided, suggesting there are some genetic factors that can contribute to suicide independent of a major psychiatric disorder. Suicide is much more likely to occur when a genetic vulnerability both to suicide *and* to affective illness is present, as recently shown by Egeland *et al.*[4]

Another recurrent focus in this symposium is that the biological factors associated with suicide may interact with biological changes associated with a particular psychiatric illness. Thus, although central serotonin systems have been most consistently associated with suicide across a variety of diagnoses, there are, in the major depressive disorders, some indications that dopaminergic function may also be involved. However, those studies that have focused on aggression/impulsivity independent of psychiatric diagnoses consistently implicate serotonergic systems; furthermore, this relationship is most consistent with a wide range of animal literature.

Another lesson from this symposium should be that the role of psychosocial variables in suicide cannot usefully be considered in isolation from the clinical context of suicide. In spite of substantial effort sustained over many years, the role of psychosocial factors per se as risk factors for *actual* suicides is yet to be demonstrated

TABLE 1. Suicides among Relatives of 57 Adopted Suicide Victims[a]

	Nonpsychiatric		Psychiatric	
	Biological	Adoptive	Biological	Adoptive
Index (269, 148)	6	0	6	0
Controls (269, 150)	1	0	1	0

[a] Data from Reference 3.

in a way that separates them from the risks conveyed by psychiatric illness and biological predisposition. It is interesting to note that psychosocial research on the relationship between child abuse and later adult aggressive behavior tends to assume that the association reflects psychological transmission. But what of the obvious possibilities that the relationship reflects a genetic pattern of an aggressive, abusing parent producing a child prone to violence or an unusually aggressive child (genetically predisposed) provoking aggressive behavior in parents? Of course, it is not easy to tease apart psychosocial and biological contributions but theoretical constructs should be broad enough to include both explanations, as well as the interactions between them.

Another important issue critically reviewed in this symposium was that of methodology. With regard to diagnostic precision, we must accept that diagnostic methods and concepts continue to evolve; this evolution can be a problem when one tries to integrate recent findings with previous literature. Of course, we must use standardized diagnostic methodologies, although there is a certain risk of "overstandardizing" too early. This methodological problem might happen, for example, when multiple investigators in various settings collaborate in an attempt to obtain a large homogeneous sample. Another methodological problem is sample selection typically determined and limited by the kinds of patients who come to a particular treatment setting. The next generation of clinical-biological studies in psychiatry should undertake sample selection using standardized epidemiological techniques. A relevant example of the need for epidemiological techniques derives from the reports of suicide "clusters." It is not at all clear that these reports will stand up to rigorous epidemiological replications. For example, the initial reports of "clusters" of leukemia were not substantiated by subsequent, controlled epidemiological study.

Another critical conceptual issue highlighted in this volume is the distinction between "trait" and "state." Even when one can demonstrate a trait variable, it is difficult to assess the degree to which it may be influenced by overlying state effects. To deal with this problem, I suggest that we focus on intensive, longitudinal studies with small numbers of patients carefully selected as being in a high-risk group. Only in this way can we accomplish the multiple simultaneous measures that will permit a teasing apart of trait and state variables. Then one can tackle the larger populations, with sharpened hypothoses and instruments more likely to yield results in which one can have confidence. This longitudinal approach should be at two levels: (1) the entire life course of an illness (which admittedly is not likely to be funded with the current short-term oriented research grant policy); and (2) short-term longitudinal studies *within* an episode of illness. Biologically, one has no reason to assume that the initial phase of an illness episode is the same as later (compensated?) phases. For example, with rapidly cycling manic-depressive patients, there are biological changes that accumulate with an increasing number of episodes. These changes imply that each episode functions as a stress, with the development of a "sensitization" reaction. With relation to suicide, Dr. Jamison asked when in the course of a particular illness is the risk for suicide greatest? This question should be studied.

Dr. Åsberg reviewed the common sources of variance in biological studies in psychiatry. I think it is fair to say that none of us who work in these areas has consistently been able to control for all of these variables in the same study at the same time. Incidentally, one of the most interesting sources of variance is season.[5] FIGURE 1 illustrates the seasonal peak in suicides, derived from a review of numerous studies. This information should allow us to factor out some of the variance in the literature and to focus high-risk studies at the appropriate time, i.e., early spring.

I would like to discuss briefly some newer approaches to enlarging our understanding of suicide. Important as the linkage between suicide and major diagnosis is, it would, nevertheless, be helpful if more studies could focus on suicidal behavior as the independent variable, relating it to a whole range of clinical, biological, and psychological assessments. And there are many clinical questions to be answered. For example, psychometric and psychophysiological correlates of aggression/impulsivity would be of particular interest. Sensation seeking, the evoked response, reaction time, field dependence, to name a few of the traditional measures, should all be explored.

It is very important to stick to a commonsense hypothesis. There are far too many instances where an investigator becomes inundated by massive amounts of data obtained without benefit of a coherent hypothesis. The data are then turned over to a computer and a statistician, associations are produced, and then *post hoc* conceptual formulations are derived; this turns the process upside down. It is foolhardy to crunch large numbers of observations through powerful discriminate function analyses so as to produce "significant" associations and then to expect, *de novo*, to extract biological or clinical meaning. Any associations so generated should be considered meaningless until replicated in a fresh sample. Unfortunately, the literature too often stops with the interesting initial association and we never see the replications. More commonsense "eyeballing" of the data would allow us to make better use of powerful statistics.

Another issue is that of special populations that might advance our suicide research.

Especially important, in my view, would be a focus on first-degree relatives of those who have committed suicide in the *absence* of a psychiatric diagnosis and/or the absence of a family history of psychiatric illness. Or consider the normal subjects who fall in the "suicide" range in an associated biological [e.g., 5-hydroxyindoleacetic acid (5-HIAA)] or personality (e.g., impulsive) measure. For example, are the low 5-HIAA normal controls more likely to have a trait of impulsivity?

One especially important population is the one with bipolar manic-depressive illness—the subgroup at the highest risk for suicide. The data described here suggest that for the bipolar patients, the serotonin-suicide association may not pertain. If true, this suggests one of two possibilities: (1) The illness itself is so dominant as a risk factor for suicide that it "overrides" the serotonin-impulsivity contribution seen in

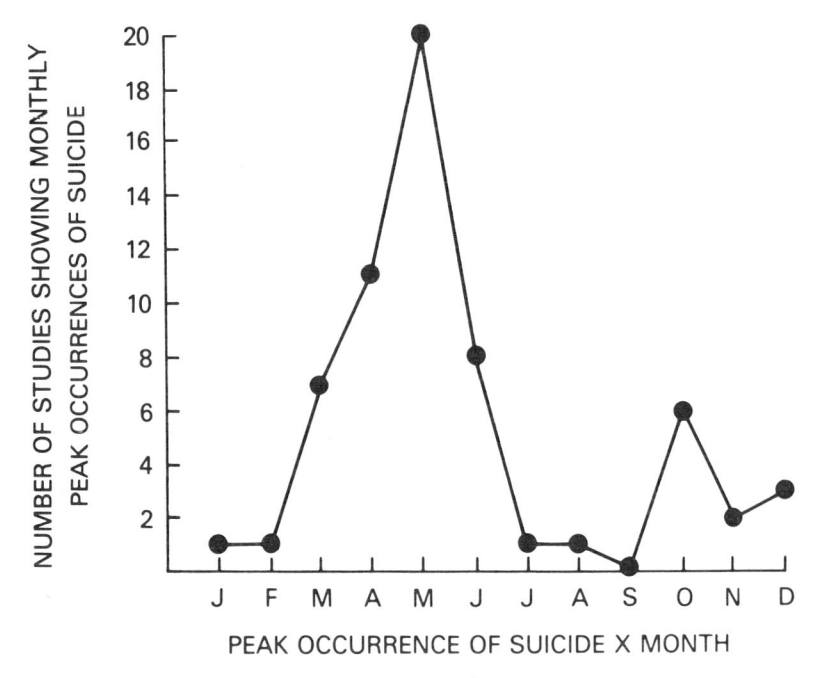

FIGURE 1. Monthly peak occurrences of suicide: a review of studies.

other diagnostic groups. (2) Serotonin alterations are imbedded in the pathophysiology of bipolar illness itself, thus washing out serotonin-suicide correlations. There is some evidence suggesting that bipolar illness may involve serotonin disturbances more than other subgroups of depressed patients. It is, therefore, possible that it is a lowered serotonin function in bipolar illness that contributes to the high suicide rate among these patients.

This volume has also reminded us that we need to look at the epidemiology of treatment. These are not only scientific issues, but urgent public health questions. To what extent does vigorous treatment of major depressive illness prevent suicide? What has been the impact of successful lithium prophylaxis for bipolar disorder on the suicide rate? Dr. Jamison presented some intriguing data from three major lithium clinics indicating a substantial reduction in suicide in this population (lithium is also known to enhance and stabilize central serotonin systems); controlled studies are needed.

The horizons of biological research are expanding rapidly as a result of new technology. Once we have carefully defined the appropriate questions and the appropriate populations, we will, no doubt, find these techniques of great potential benefit. For example, brain-imaging strategies should allow us to evaluate whether the disturbed areas of brain identified from postmortem examination might be reflected in these *in vivo* measures. Not only can we now study regional metabolic activity, but also we can now look at specific receptor types including serotonin receptors. Related to these research questions is a robust literature on animal models of depression and of aggressive behavior and even of self-destructive behavior. Animal models are convenient because they allow us to ask a question that has always fascinated me: Not only is there the more often asked question of what is the impact of a neurobiological substrate on psychosocial change, but, further, what is the impact of psychosocial change on a neurobiological substrate?

It has been encouraging to note here the beginnings of an apparent rapprochement between psychosocial approaches to suicide and the clinical-biological tradition.

REFERENCES

1. CLAYTON, P. J. 1985. Suicide. Psychiatr. Clin. North Am. **8:** 203-214.
2. POKORNY, A. D. 1964. Suicide rates in various psychiatric disorders. J. Nerv. Ment. Dis. **139:** 499-506.
3. SCHULSINGER, F., S. S. KETY, D. ROSENTHAL & P. H. WENDER. 1979. A family study of suicide. *In* Origin, Prevention and Treatment of Affective Disorders. M. Schou & E. Stromgren, Eds.: 277-287. Academic Press. London, England.
4. EGELAND, J. A. & J. N. SUSSEX. 1985. Suicide and family loading for affective disorders. JAMA **254:** 915-918.
5. GOODWIN, F. K. & K. R. JAMISON. Manic-Depressive Illness. Oxford University Press. New York, N.Y. (In preparation.)

Index of Contributors

Adam, K. S., 63-76
Agren, H., 189-196
Arató, M., 221-230, 263-270
Arora, R. C., 271-280
Åsberg, M., 168-174, 243-255

Banki, C. M., 221-230, 263-270
Beck, A. T., 90-96
Berrettini, W. H., 197-201
Bissette, G., 263-270
Black, D. W., 106-113
Blumenthal, S. J., 327-340
Breier, A., 189-196
Brown, G. L., 175-188
Brown, R. P., 175-188, 256-262

Candy, J. M., 128-142
Clarkin, J., 281-293
Cohen, J., 34-41
Cohen, L. S., 122-127
Colison, J., 189-196
Conte, H., 150-167
Cross, A. J., 128-142
Cross, C. K., 77-89, 231-242

Depue, R. A., 47-62
Doran, A., 189-196

Ferrier, I. N., 128-142
Flavin, D. K., 316-326
Frances, A., 281-293
Frances, R. J., 316-326
Franklin, J., 316-326
Fyer, M., 281-293

Gershon, E. S., 197-201
Gillin, J. C., 143-149
Goodwin, F. K., 175-188, 351-355
Guthrie, S., 202-220

Hirschfeld, R. M. A., 77-89

Jamison, K. R., 301-315
Janowsky, D. S., 143-149
Johns, C. A., 294-300

Katz, M. M., 231-242
Kaufman, C. A., 143-149

Kelsoe, J. R., Jr., 143-149
Kennedy, S., 256-262
Kilts, C. D., 221-230
Kleinman, J. E., 143-149
Kocsis, J. H., 231-242, 256-262
Koslow, S., 231-242
Kulbok, P. A., 1-15
Kupfer, D. J., 327-340

Linehan, M. M., 16-33
Linnoila, M., 202-220

Maas, J. W., 231-242
Mann, J. J., ix, 114-121, 122-127, 256-262
Mason, B., 256-262
McBride, P. A., 114-121
McKeith, I. G., 128-142
Meltzer, H. Y., 271-280

Narrow, W., 197-201
Nemeroff, C. B., 263-270
Nordström, P., 243-255
Nurnberger, J. I., Jr., 197-201

Perry, E. K., 128-142
Perry, R. H., 128-142
Pfeffer, C. R., 341-350
Pickar, D., 189-196
Plutchik, R., 150-167

Risch, S. C., 143-149
Robins, L. N., 1-15
Roy, A., 97-105, 189-196, 202-220

Schalling, D., 168-174
Secunda, S. K., 231-242
Simmons-Alling, S., 197-201
Spoont, M. R., 47-62
Stanley, B., 42-46, 294-300
Stanley, M., ix, 114-121, 122-127, 294-300

Träskman-Bendz, L., 168-174, 243-255

Van Praag, H. M., 150-167
Virkkunen, M., 202-220

Winokur, G., 106-113
Wolkowitz, O., 189-196